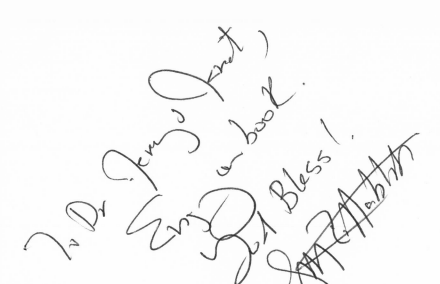

To Dr. Jerry's Great)
Enjoy the book.
God Bless !

THE BETTER LIFE INSTITUTE™
FAMILY HEALTH PLAN

THE BETTER LIFE INSTITUTE™
FAMILY HEALTH PLAN

Steven M. Zifferblatt, Ph.D.
Patricia M. Zifferblatt
AND
Norm Chandler Fox

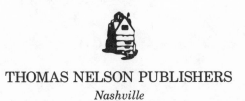

THOMAS NELSON PUBLISHERS

Nashville

Copyright © 1991 by Steven M. Zifferblatt, Patricia M. Zifferblatt, and Norm Chandler Fox.

Published in Nashville, Tennessee, by Thomas Nelson, Inc., and distributed in Canada by Lawson Falle, Ltd., Cambridge, Ontario.

Scripture quotations are from the NEW KING JAMES VERSION of the Bible, Copyright © 1983, 1982, 1980, 1979, by Thomas Nelson Publishers.

Library of Congress Cataloging-in-Publication Data

Zifferblatt, Steven M.
    The Better Life Institute family health plan / Steven M.
Zifferblatt, Patricia M. Zifferblatt, and Norm Chandler Fox.
      p. cm.
    ISBN 0-8407-7651-9
    1. Health. I. Zifferblatt, Patricia M. II. Fox, Norm Chandler.
III. Title.
RA776.Z54 1991
613—dc20
                                      91–3456
                                      CIP

Printed in the United States of America
1 2 3 4 5 6 7 — 95 94 93 92 91 90

This book is dedicated to Rich and Jay who shared their dream with us so that we can share our dream with others.

PAT AND STEVE ZIFFERBLATT

*   *   *

For my partner in life, Loreen Arbus, who is my inspiration, my muse, and the most intelligent and trusting, the dearest human being I'll ever know.

NORM CHANDLER FOX

Acknowledgments

■ ■

No project is ever complete until all the i's are dotted and all the t's are crossed. This means saying thank you to those people who have had a significant impact on our lives. Thank you to:

Bill Nicholson, who in his special way creates new lives and destinies for others—especially us. He's a friend, confidant, and teacher.

Helen DeVos for her unfailing love and support.

The late Nathan Pritikin and his wife, Ilene. They paved the way.

To the man called "Z," who asked us to "look into my eyes" and helped us to see our true selves.

To Bruce Barbour for being a "cool dude."

To Steve Van Andel, Dan DeVos, Claire Zevalkink, Bob Kerkstra, Ken McDonald, Bob Blanchard, Pat Sullivan, and Kim Bruyn. We call them the "ramrod team."

To Kim Ter Haar who pushed her way through three very difficult weeks while suffering from "morning sickness" twenty-four hours a day.

To the Better Life Institute staff, who are wonderful: Marilyn, Barb, Molly, and Lynn.

Steven wishes especially to thank:

Dr. Jack Farquhar for his many years of mentoring. He was and still is a true guiding light in my life.

Dr. Robert I. Levy and Dr. Basil Rifkind, who lead us through the muddy scientific waters of cholesterol and heart disease during difficult times.

The late B. F. Skinner, whose mentoring helped forge my value for practicality and objectivity.

My son, Jonathon. His love and support made the difficult times manageable.

Patricia wishes especially to thank:

My entire Italian family. They know who they are!

Theodore R. Walters, my first teacher.

My children, who are my life: Michelle, Ted, Mary, Thomas, Damian, Julia, Amy, Ange, and Marti.

My daughters-in-law and my sons-in-law. I love them. They are my children.

My most wonderful grandchildren, who bring me joy in my graying years.

To: J. T., who taught me about unconditional love and doesn't even know that he did!

We thank one another. Without our love, friendship, and mutual support, these pages and the Better Life Institute could never be.

And we thank God for His love and His belief in us. He is our Guiding Light.

STEVEN AND PATRICIA

Forewords *John Farquhar*

■ ■ ■ ■ ■ ■ ■ ■ ■ ■ ■ ■ ■ ■ ■ ■ ■ ■ ■ ■

The United States is in the middle of a health revolution that has led millions of Americans to change dietary and exercise habits, to stop smoking, to reduce alcohol abuse, and to become aware of the need to avoid stress. We have much to be proud of. For example, cigarette smoking has fallen by more than 30 percent, and now only 27 percent of adult Americans smoke. We lead the world in this retreat from smoking. We can also be pleased that we have made fairly important changes in diet that have lowered the average American's cholesterol levels. Consequently, both heart attacks and strokes are much less common than they were twenty years ago.

However, we have to admit that most of these beneficial changes have occurred in older adults, especially in those who have been motivated to change because of a special level of personal risk or through exposure to a friend or family member who developed lung cancer, a heart attack, or a stroke because of smoking, high blood cholesterol, or high blood pressure.

But what have we been missing? Why haven't more of us at all ages changed our unhealthy habits? One reason, I think, is that almost all the books on health have addressed adults as single beings, without spouses or children. But this book by the Zifferblatts fills the void. It adds the missing ingredient by focusing on families, covering all ages and taking advantage of the potential strengths of a family unit in creating the right environment for change, in providing loving support for change, and by taking the longer view that families can have.

Such an approach is badly needed. We, as a country, have failed our children and adolescents in matters of health. While many adults have made improvements in personal health habits, sadly this is not the case for many of our young people. For example, obesity has steadily increased among our children, due to inadequate exercise (often a function of watching television) and to our avalanche of fatty snack and fast foods. Various forms of substance abuse remain as formidable problems among the young. Even if school-based health programs were to become universal, the addition of a "family health program" would be an important ingredient.

This book will open windows of opportunity for families and help them work on risk factors together as a unit. You will find the practicality of the book a delight and a blessing. Often we hear *what* we should do, such as "get more exercise" or "eat less than 30 percent of your calories from fat." But we are not told *how* to do all this. The Zifferblatts, however, give the how, including ways to maintain changes over the long haul.

Humans live most productively in families. Often, modern society tears down that natural unit. This book upholds the family—*your* family—and it will help you keep it together on the road to good health.

John Farquhar, M.D.
Professor of Medicine, Stanford University School of Medicine

Philip Sunshine

■ ■ ■ ■ ■ ■ ■ ■ ■ ■ ■ ■ ■ ■ ■ ■ ■ ■ ■

While numerous books have been written about nutrition, exercise, and various approaches to improving the quality of life, Patricia and Steven Zifferblatt have taken a unique approach to these issues. They address all of these topics, but emphasize a family approach to maintaining a proper diet, participating in exercise programs, and cultivating a healthy lifestyle.

Many of the goals outlined in this book are lofty indeed. However, families can achieve a great deal with relative ease if they are sufficiently motivated to do so. I firmly believe that any improvement in the health of children must take place in a family setting, with each member participating as best as he or she is able. It is a sad state of affairs, that only 12 percent of twelve-year-old children actually participate in regular athletic activities.

Parents must, therefore, act not only as teachers, but as role models for their children. By exposing their children to "healthy" eating habits at an early age, and by making eating a "wonderful family activity," the child will learn these habits in a positive way.

The authors also stress the importance of including grandparents in family activities, including meals, exercise, and "the family circle." In this era when extended families do not typically spend much time together, it will take more effort to include them in as many family activities as possible. I have often been impressed by how well grandparents and grandchildren relate to each other. They share a warmth and fondness that bonds them together.

The authors lucidly describe various degenerative diseases and how diet and exercise can actually reverse some of these processes. These are important concepts for parents to know because steps taken now can affect not only their lives, but the lives of their children.

Lastly, the authors have used excellent illustrative techniques to enhance their presentation. They empathize with the difficulties in changing lifestyles, eating patterns, and exercise habits. They even stress "the 60 percent solution"—one must not abandon a project just because one does not achieve perfection. They also note that new habits should become a regular activity so that these are as natural as "brushing your teeth or taking a shower."

This is a book that you will read and re-read and encounter new ideas with which to relate at each exposure.

Philip Sunshine, M.D.
Professor and Vice-Chairman, Department of Pediatrics, USC School of Medicine
Head, Department of Pediatrics, Children's Hospital of Los Angeles

Contents

■ ■ ■ ■ ■ ■ ■ ■ ■ ■ ■ ■ ■ ■ ■ ■ ■

Why Are We Writing This Book?

Preface

■ ■ ■ ■ ■ ■ ■ ■ ■ ■ ■ ■ ■ ■ ■ ■ ■ ■ ■

Our Children, Our Families, Our Future

While many people are rightfully unhappy over the declining level of education in our nation today, many are also confused and alarmed by the incredibly high proportion of kids whose poor health habits are already affecting their longevity as well as their lifestyles. According to a recent survey by the President's Council for Physical Fitness, about one in four children under the age of sixteen is considered to be at risk for heart disease because of overweight, high cholesterol, or lack of regular exercise. And the American Institute for Cancer Research estimates that one of four children born today will die prematurely of cancer. The health facts of their parents are even worse. Sixty million American adults have high blood pressure, fifty million have high blood cholesterol, ten million deal with adult onset diabetes, 100 million are overweight, and countless millions are headed toward a deadly date with cancer. And many have two or more of these conditions simultaneously.

As we see succeeding generations of Americans becoming greater health risks, we are taking it upon ourselves to do something to turn things around. Wanting to start somewhere, we are writing this book. We will focus on all kinds of families—the "Ozzie and Harriet" family, the single-parent family, the weekend-parent family, and the two-working-parents family. Many parents are frustrated. They want to have better health habits themselves, and they want to teach them to their children as well. These parents need practical, effective, enjoyable guidelines for nutrition and exercise. Parent and child alike are faced with a combination of the mass media, advertisers, and a culture that attempts to poke and prod all of us from fad to fad and from product to product. Endorsements from such icons as Michael Jackson and Michael Jordan to the expert medical intervention of Michael DeBakey further confuse us. Celebrity product endorsements imply that health and family happiness are practically guaranteed by the purchase of a particular product. This vicarious association with celebrities and experts becomes a substitute for active participation in a more healthy and family-oriented lifestyle. When the substitutes don't work well they run to the health professionals, begging for help. We are not criticizing the media, the advertisers, the product manufacturers, the celebrities, or the well-known experts for offering what they do. Music, sports, and medicine play a vital role in our lifestyles, but they are only remotely associated with our personal health and personal happiness.

Perhaps one of the most significant problems that affects our personal health and happiness is that many parents are often no better informed about good eating and exercise practices than their children are. Others don't put into practice what they know, but still preach the "shoulds" and "should nots" to their children. It is little wonder their "do as I say, not as I do" philosophy means nothing to their children.

Taking Charge

As we settle into the last decade of this tumultuous century, we constantly hear the same refrain: "Life is out of control!" It seems that each of us is buffeted by outside forces that affect us every day. We have experienced massive political change in America. Shifts in world politics control our everyday choices as resources we take for granted become scarce and expensive. Population growth in our cities forces us to endure extra hours of commuting as well as gridlock traffic. Economic cutbacks, tax increases, and socially controversial governmental decisions have an impact on the entire family. While we could make monstrous lists of all the things over which we have no control (and get very depressed doing it), we'd rather take a more positive stance and consider some of the aspects of our lives that we can control.

First and foremost we can control our own health and the health of our children. Think of it this way: By taking charge of this primary responsibility, we can actually lengthen our lifespans and increase our vigor and do the same for our children. Considering all the other things we can't control, this is one of life's major victories!

Helping you establish a healthier lifestyle for yourself and your family is the goal of this book. Although it's going to take some work on your part and on the part of your children, the rewards will be incalculable. And the biggest bonus of all is that your family ties will grow stronger.

Let's Meet the Fosters

It is a sunny Saturday afternoon in Mapletown Groves, USA. Jim, the husband and father of the Foster family, is a thirty-eight-year-old service supervisor at the largest auto dealership in town. Jim completed two years of college and has made it as far as he has the hard way. He's managed to quit smoking. He still enjoys an occasional beer. And Jim is fifteen pounds overweight. Phyllis, Jim's wife, is thirty-five. Recently she returned to work as a receptionist after getting the three children semi "grown up" and off to school. She's thirty pounds overweight and she finds it somewhat difficult to balance her new life now that she is a working mother and a working wife. Jimmy Jr. is fifteen and has just made the junior varsity football team. Lori is thirteen and has just entered puberty. Her biggest concerns are her figure and her complexion. Lori and Jimmy Jr. haven't spoken a civil word to each other in two years.

■ *WHY ARE WE WRITING THIS BOOK?*

The youngest child, Tommy, is eight and still seems to be made of "frogs and snails and puppy dogs' tails."

What are they doing on this sunny Saturday afternoon? Papa Jim has just finished mowing the lawn and is resentful that his boy Jimmy Jr. wasn't there to help him. Mama is huffing and puffing, trying to "catch up" in the laundry room and grumping that no one appreciates her. After all, she's keeping the household together while holding a full-time job. Jimmy Jr. didn't help mow the lawn because he is warming the bench at his football game and feeling bad because his parents are not there to watch. Lori has been pressed into service by her mother to help with the housecleaning. She is angry she can't be with her friends at the Mall. Tommy, God bless him, the "Huck Finn of the nineties," is doing his best to dirty his clothes. He is rolling in the leaves his dad has raked up.

Welcome to America. Welcome to the 1990's version of the "Adventures of Ozzie and Harriet." In real life things are very different from the ways they are presented on television.

Tell-tale signs of health problems are surfacing at the Foster home. Dad is stressed and overweight with borderline high blood pressure. He avoids getting his cholesterol measured. Mom is overweight and overstressed, and diabetes runs in her family. Both parents feel frustration when they deal with their children. They have a sense of being out of control. Lori is worried about her weight and her complexion while she teeters between parental control and peer influence. Young Jimmy gets a good bit of exercise, but he has the normal "average kid" eating habits—he loves junk food. Even though he finds it difficult to communicate with other members of the family, for Tommy, at his blissful age, the world is still his oyster.

All over America there are families like the Fosters. And there are other families that are very different. There are single-parent families, his-hers-and-ours families, weekend- or part-time-parent families, and extended families that include grandparents and in-laws. But all these families, even with their differences, are struggling with very similar problems—how to achieve and enjoy good health and keep the family together.

Everywhere we see articles and programs that tell us how to manage situations, kids, money, and chores, how to be the best mother or father, how to help the children with their homework, how to communicate with our teenagers, how to survive divorce, how to do, be, or enjoy almost anything we might be interested in doing, being, or enjoying. We are a country of families trying to do our very best to survive to the best of our abilities. Some of us are doing fairly well; others are just struggling along.

From outward appearances the Foster family is doing quite nicely. But are they really? And what about your family? By your outward appearance, you may be the envy of your neighborhood. But, the neighbors may not see that within your family there are major lifestyle stresses that threaten your health and the harmony of your home.

The Better Life Institute Family Health Plan is a practical guide to improving the lifestyles of both parents and children as the practices of our daily lives relate to our eating and exercise habits and the unity of the family. This plan can help the Fosters. It can help your family too.

The Loving Centripetal Force

Those of us who know just enough about physics to know that we don't know very much, may remember that certain forces bring things together and other forces pull things apart. The bring-together forces are centripetal; the pull-apart forces are centrifugal. Most families are in continual motion with a constant barrage of outside forces pulling family members centrifugally in various directions. Work, peer pressure, school, PTA, community, friends, personal time all pull at individual family members. Since there are only twenty-four hours in the day, no family member ever has enough time to shoe-horn in every available opportunity.

To counteract this lifestyle centrifugal force—the tendency for many outside factors to pull the family apart—we believe you can initiate a loving *centripetal* force that will pull the family together. *The Better Life Institute Family Health Plan* will help you use nutrition and exercise so that it becomes a very loving centripetal force. If you think of your family life as cake, this centripetal force will be the icing. So, whoever said "you can't have your cake and eat it too" obviously hasn't read this book! Besides building better eating and exercise habits for you and your children, following the guidelines you'll find in this book will bring to your family a sense of solidarity, a feeling of mutual belonging, and the joy of working together toward a mutual goal. We want the Better Life Institute Family Health Program to set in motion the loving *centripetal* force that will generate health and will bring your family closer with more purpose and greater love and respect for each other.

Who Are We?

We are the Zifferblatts, Steve and Pat. Between the two of us, we have ten children, all from former marriages. Steve was married for twenty years and has one child who is now twenty-one. Pat was married for thirty years and has nine children ranging in age from twenty-two to thirty-eight. You can easily identify the "yours" and "mine." The "ours," however, is not a child. It is the joy we feel in bringing "yours" and "mine" together and building toward a strong family unit.

We think it is important for our readers to know about us, for like others, we have reveled in the joys of marriage and family life and have, sadly, borne the pain of divorce and family separation. The majority of the years of our adult lives have been wonderful family years. But, at some point there were serious breakdowns which led ultimately to divorce. Our children are now on their own. Some are beginning their own families, but all of us, together, are trying to build new connective tissue within the family. We know, we've learned through the years, that it's hard work to keep the family unit strong within a happy marriage. It is even more difficult in divorce.

Although we're very grateful we eventually found each other to build a new life together, our experiences have made us realize some basic truths about families. *Close, loving families don't just happen.* In the same way that a marriage license

■ ***WHY ARE WE WRITING THIS BOOK?***

doesn't mean the participants will know how to operate their sometimes unwieldy vehicle called marriage, birth certificates don't offer any kind of guaranty that new parents will be successful parents. Whether related by blood, marriage, or re-marriage, it takes determination, sweat, faith, understanding, and lots of prayer to build and constantly reinforce familial relationships. Making a commitment to improve family health makes it more of a challenge.

We do not claim to be experts that can solve your problems. An engineer is an expert you can employ to build a bridge for you. If you need a bridge, you can give the engineer the measurements and materials, and he will solve your problem by building the bridge you need. But alas, there are no such experts for health and health-habit change. We can't build your bridge for you. But we can help you build your bridge yourself.

We come from different worlds and have different strengths (and weaknesses—which you'll learn about as you read this book). Pat, by virtue of thirty years spent in the kitchen over a hot stove preparing family meals and another ten as a professional helping families to make heart-healthy low calorie foods, knows how to take the "un-healthy" out of food and keep the "healthy" in, how to make healthy food delicious, and how to prepare healthy, delicious food on the run, quickly and easily. Steve spent over half his career in academic and medical research settings before deciding to apply his skills directly to the practical health challenges that families face. He takes the "gobbledy-gook" out of scientific discussions and talks in a way everyone understands.

For a time we worked together at the Pritikin Longevity Center in Santa Monica with Steve as Associate Director and Pat as Program Services Director. When we realized a more practical and enjoyable, as well as more effective, program could accomplish the same health goals, we co-founded the LaCosta Lifestyle and Longevity Center near San Diego, California. There we worked with many families and helped them adapt our program to their individual needs. Ultimately, we decided to try to reach people from all over the country by moving beyond expensive residential and spa programs to more affordable programs.

We founded the Better Life Institute (BLI) in Grand Rapids, Michigan. At BLI we provide thousands of families with books, audio and video tapes, foods, workshops, and face-to-face educational programs. We now consider Grand Rapids our home, and we are touched by the warmth, hospitality, tradition, and honesty that we experience by living in America's heartland. We have tried to incorporate these solid time-honored values into our family health programs for nutrition and exercise.

Down to Earth and Back to Basics

While some people have achieved fantastic results on certain diet and exercise programs, we are experienced enough to know that the majority of people usually abandon these programs after two to four weeks. The Better Life Institute Family Health Plan is not a two-week "wonder program." It contains no diet cookies, pills, fat-eating liquids, or wonder foods. We don't support fads or a "diet of the month." We have been using this medically safe, scientifically sound nutrition and exercise program for years, and we know it works. We've worked personally with over eight thousand individuals over the years—eyeball to eyeball! Our program is safe for family members of all ages—the young, the not-so-old, and the mature. (Steve is fifty-one and not-so-old, and Pat, who is a few years older than Steve, qualifies as being not-so-old-approaching-mature.)

Our combined experience always brings us back to three basic components that are always found in a successful program: the program has to be *effective, livable,* and, above all, *enjoyable* in order to work. We don't believe in complicated, overly restrictive programs that require lots of planning, note-taking, and changes for the participants. We're not going to ask you to chant, to visualize the pounds melting away from your waistline, or to send your kids to school with lunch boxes filled with alfalfa and tofu. We're not going to compel you to memorize the calorie count of three-and-one-half ounces of chicken breast or how many grams of fat there are in a Big Mac. All our lives are already too complex to start overloading those magnificent God-given computers we have between our ears with lots of excess information. And we've known too well and too often that wiped-out feeling we all get when we've reached an information overload or have just too many "dickey-doo" things to keep up with.

We know that many people are becoming more aware of and interested in improving their eating and exercise habits and those of their children. They want to take responsibility for their kids' health and well-being. But, they just can't seem to get started. They think only of the "short term" instead of the "long haul." They need a sensible and enjoyable plan of action. They need something that will end the "we'll start tomorrow" mindset, the perpetual beginnings and inevitable endings, and the finger-pointing failures. They need to stop the seemingly infinite see-saw of start and stop, success and failure, pride and humiliation, self-worth and self-doubt. They need the Better Life Institute program.

Good health is far more than what the family eats or whether the family members exercise. There are many, many other factors that influence the length and happiness of our lives. Our experience has taught us, as yours has taught you, the importance of practicality. We all learn that the way to meet any challenge is to cut it down to a size we can work on. We feel the same way about family health. Our program focuses on eating and exercise habits because of their importance to your health and that of your children. This is not the last word on family health, but it is a very practical and important place for your family to begin.

Within this book is a chapter on family spirituality. Our purpose is neither to preach to you nor to convert you. We only want to point out that you can reach deep into your spiritual values, try to live more closely by them, and translate them into a program for daily living. This step often brings peace of mind, enhances self-respect, reduces stress, and improves health. Central to all spiritual thought is the value of the family to individuals and to society.

There is no magic in this book that will instantly turn your bodies into lean, mean machines or that will guarantee you will enjoy perpetual health and strong family ties. Fifteen years of experience have taught us that what works is the long

■ *WHY ARE WE WRITING THIS BOOK?*

haul. And we want you and your children to *practice what we preach* for the rest of your lives—*healthfully ever after*.

Common Sense and the "Lulu Factor"

We have a down-to-earth system that's based on a wonderful human commodity called *common sense*. We believe gradual realistic change is the only basis for developing a healthy way of life. One of us created a mythical lady named "Lulu" who represents the "nuts and bolts," "down to the nitty-gritty," "yes—but will it really work" moms and dads in our country. Any time we think of revising our program or adding a new technique, we always ask, "Will Lulu do this?" New ideas have to pass the Lulu-factor test. Lulu usually keeps us on solid ground because if Lulu thinks it will fly, it generally does.

A New Adventure

Let's think of the journey we're about to begin together as an adventure. Slowly your attitudes and behavior will change as you and your family travel down this new road. You'll see people, places, and things as you've never before seen them. A very wise man, Marcel Proust, once said, "The voyage of discovery is not in visiting new places or seeing new things, but in seeing the same things with a different set of eyes." To prepare for this trip we ask only that you have an open mind to hear what we're saying and to see certain aspects of your life "with a different set of eyes." Your common sense will motivate you and, perhaps, you will make a permanent improvement in your family's life—*healthfully ever after*.

How to Use This Book

All too often we pick up books, glance through the first and last chapters, see that the middle section is mostly filler, and then put the book back on the shelf to collect dust. We all have many $20 "dust catchers."

When we began to write this book, we intended to make it different. With that in mind, we have tried to bring to you a living, tried-and-true program complete with concepts and practicalities. We wanted to give you a "user friendly" book, as well.

This is a reading, discussion, and "how to" book all rolled into one. Every chapter can stand by itself. Although the information might flow a bit better if you go through all the chapters in order, you don't have to read them in order. For example, if you are interested in learning how spirituality contributes to family health, just skip ahead to that chapter. Move around the book as you please.

You will find that we inject short "truisms" in the text every few pages. They're placed for interest and to break the routine of continually reading pages. Most chapters have a "thought" section at the end consisting of "Yes, I can" statements and "Family Circle Suggestions." These are simple practical activities that everyone in the family can do.

We have also included several "Help" sections at the end of the book. There is a "Words to Know" section that makes the "what does this word really mean?" aspect of a health book much easier. And we have included some suggestions on where to continue to get health information for your family in the "Where to Go for More Information" section. These are solid, tried-and-true resources. We don't believe in fads.

Finally, we have included sample "Guardian Angel" letters for you and your family to use. We suggest that a "buddy" approach might lend motivation and support to new eating and exercise habits. Let us help you. Use the "Guardian Angel" letter idea so that we can be part of your support team.

Remember, we're here to help you and your family. You can always phone us for information or advice on where and how to get help right where you live—in your "neck of the woods." Try us!

PAT AND STEVE ZIFFERBLATT

Just Between Us

> *To be what we are, and to become what we are capable of becoming, is the only end of life.*
>
> **Robert Louis Stevenson**

The Challenge of Change

Thousands of years ago man sat by his fire with his family, looked at the stars, and dreamed of a better life. Just like us, he might have been dreaming of a better place to live, of better food and clothing, and perhaps of having another child. The challenge this man faced thousands of years ago is exactly the same one facing you today. It is to assume the responsibility to make your dreams come true—the challenge of personal change.

The nomadic hunter of prehistoric times, the farmer in Mesopotamia, the Roman pottery maker, the feudal serf, the Renaissance cobbler, the Age of Enlightenment printer, the Revolutionary War soldier, the Industrial Revolution ironworker, the pre-World War II auto assembly worker, the modern computer programmer—all have faced the challenge of personal change.

DO YOU REALLY WANT TO CHANGE TO MAKE THINGS HAPPEN?

We've all heard people say, "I want to change." We all know also that there's a vast difference between saying we will do something and actually doing it. If you really think about it, however, most of our challenges are not lofty ambitions, but very attainable goals. Few of us dream of piloting the Space Shuttle, doing by-pass surgery, or running a three-minute mile. We think about what we'll do tomorrow or next week.

Remember, when we discuss *change,* we are talking about thinking differently about ourselves, getting more closely in touch with our needs, eating broccoli and chicken instead of Twinkies, and wearing sneakers for exercise instead of making a fashion statement. To improve the quality of your family's health, you really don't need any new skills or college degrees. Initially all you need to do is change some of the foods you put in your mouth, get up off the couch, and begin to listen, talk about, and participate more in your self-improvement.

EXCUSES, EXCUSES, EXCUSES!

Ask anyone you know, including yourself, why they overeat or don't exercise regularly, and you will be treated to an all-expense paid trip to Excuse Land. Everyone has a pet theory that explains it: deep-seated psychological problems, hormonal changes, number and size of fat cells, genetics, "Mommy and Daddy loved me with food," stress, television and advertising, "food comforts me," no time for anything healthy, work, kids, an existential crisis . . . and on and on. What's your "theory"?

All of these theories suggest that *you* are not the cause of your health problem. Instead, the fault lies with your genes, your childhood, psychic forces, the economy, or other people in your life—but *never* with *you!*

America now has a population of 100 million overweight people, and the number is growing. But it excludes the increasing number of children ages 4–12 who are over-weight. All this fat simply can't be blamed on genetics, physiology, moms and dads, or even lifestyle factors. There are now too many countries in Western Europe and Asia with similar lifestyles, but their overweight statistics are much "slimmer."

Face the facts. Your eating and exercise concerns are entirely within your control. To put it more bluntly, your biggest problem with food and exercise is you stuff your face too much and are too lazy to get out of your chair and exercise! Sorry to be so blunt, but we have too many years of close, personal experience with parents and children who have struggled with the frustration of repeated failure to change eating and exercise habits. And both of us, Steve and Pat together, have known the pain of being overweight in our younger and middle years. Therefore, we're not going to pull our punches and sugar-coat the difficulty of changing your personal habits and those of your family members. There are, of course, costs involved in personal change, and you can't avoid paying them. The good news is that this book will help you to be smart in your approach to change—to do it in an effective, livable, and enjoyable manner. But remember, you're facing a change which will last not for a day, week, or a month, but for a lifetime!

TAKING THE EASY ROAD

Maybe you've thought about making changes for years, but you haven't done it be-cause you don't want to suffer by paying the price. M. Scott Peck, M.D., author of *The Road Less Traveled,* points out that all our maladaptive or neurotic behavior is simply our attempt to avoid suffering and having to face the consequences of doing things the right way. That's what the "diet of the month" is all about. It's sold with the seductive message that something external is going to make all the necessary changes for you. Everything is made easier for you . . . there's no sweat . . . you just take this pill . . . follow this seven-day program . . . drink this liquid . . . listen to this tape. . . .

The old adage about leading a horse to water but not being able to make him drink is applicable to trying to change your lifestyle. You can put the best diet in the world in front of people, but if they won't use it, it won't help them. You can contin-ually show people that smoking is dangerous to their health, but if they continue to puff away, the information doesn't help them. Wouldn't the world be different if we all took action when we receive rational advice? But, alas, we human beings don't always do things rationally. Tried-and-true habits, comfort, immediate pleasure, past history, childhood experiences, and emotion all play a critical and possibly the deciding role in your eating and exercise habits.

Please Step into Our Office

By reading this book, you have stepped into our office and are asking us, "What will it take to make the personal eating and exercise changes needed to improve my health and that of my family?" Our reply is that you have to face the good news and the bad news. The bad news is that if you're hoping against hope someone else will lead the way or something will work like magic, it won't happen. However, the good news is that if you want to take charge of and be responsible for your life, you can. You must decide if you are willing to roll up your sleeves, dispel your illusions and false expectations, and get on with the business of personal change.

REVEALING THE SECRET

For as long as you can remember, you've probably been searching for something magical that will change your life. Now, here is the humdinger! The secret to personal change is *there is no secret*. It just takes hard work, staying power, believing it's important enough to be worth the effort, and remembering you have to do it yourself. Of course you have to be smart too. When trying to make changes in eating and exercise habits, most people select programs that are very restrictive and turn out to be impossible to continue after only a few weeks. These programs have a built-in failure factor.

It takes time to build a successful business, and in the same way, you must change eating and exercising habits gradually. This kind of change doesn't happen overnight—hardly anything worthwhile ever does. Magic Johnson didn't perfect his jump shot in a week. You don't buy a tennis racket and step out on the court with Steffi Graf. The key words to successful change are: *slow, steady, livable,* and *enjoyable*.

Like us, you've probably survived decades of the repeating cycle of success and failure. Besides being harmful to your health, this on-again-off-again syndrome tends to erode your confidence level and your feelings of self-worth. We want you to dispel your fantasies and knuckle-down to business. You and your family are at a crossroads. You have the opportunity now to give yourself and your family a very precious gift while discarding old "die hard" habits. That gift is a positive "can do" attitude toward change.

Life is all about examining options and making decisions. When the proverbial push comes to shove, it all boils down to deciding whether or not you chose to do something. We hope that this book with its Better Life Institute Family Health Program will give you more than information and practical tips. We want it to motivate you toward good, solid personal changes that will remain with you and your family throughout your lives.

Personal Change

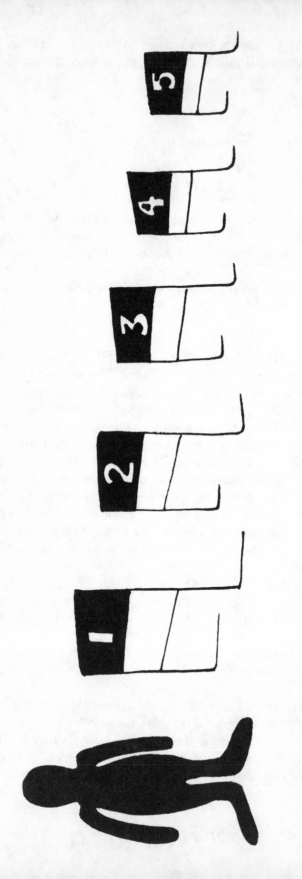

1. Exactly what is it you want to change? And why?

2. Do you truly realize how much personal respect and happiness not changing has caused you?

3. Do you want to change very badly?

4. Are you prepared to "pay" for it with immediate short-term inconvenience and discomfort?

5. Are you willing to change for "the long haul"?

ALL ABOARD—THE JOURNEY'S ABOUT TO BEGIN

From our own personal experience and from years of working with adults and families, we know that changing habits requires more than learning scientific facts and pragmatic methods. It would be unfair for us to imply that by reading this book, "family health is yours." The real issue is whether you truly want to change. Now's a good time to ask yourself that question, and only you can answer it. If the answer is "yes," welcome aboard! We're on a journey toward a life that's lived *healthfully ever after*.

Let's Hear It for Families!

■ ■ ■ ■ ■ ■ ■ ■ ■ ■ ■ ■ ■ ■ ■ ■ ■ ■

Wanted: A Parent

TRAINING: None
SALARY: Grossly underpaid
DATE NEEDED: Whenever you have the courage
JOB DESCRIPTION: The applicant will be responsible for creating and insuring a child's proper physical and mental health. The parent will be a psychologist with a comprehensive understanding of human nature and the uncanny ability to read the minds of children who can't speak, who won't speak, or who don't say what they mean or feel. The parent will have good domestic skills, a thorough background in nutrition, be able to delegate tasks and responsibilities, and serve as a referee able to negotiate the toughest problems. The parent must be a spiritual leader, a cheerleader, and a handyman able to fix whatever breaks, including the tiny hearts of seven-year-olds.

The applicant must be willing to work long hours under great stress (including double and even triple shifts with no extra pay) and be able to sustain interest in bedtime stories even when they put you to sleep. Most of all, the applicant must be prepared for a job that is highly unpredictable and comes with only one guarantee: *You'll never be the same again!*

We Are a Family

The old adage "blood is thicker than water" simply means that when the going gets tough, you can usually depend on your family for support. Instinctively family members trust one another more than they trust outsiders. Family trust goes back to the times, centuries ago, when clans huddled together for mutual protection.

Whenever anyone asks an American about his or her family, out of a wallet or purse come battered photographs and there begins a lengthy and detailed description of all the family members, what they are doing, and how they are getting on. As a nation, we're mighty proud of our families. And why not? The family gives each of us a strong sense of belonging. It's a warm, intimate and generally positive feeling that cannot be duplicated by our jobs, by outside activities, or in any other sector of our lives. Our families are important to us.

We both come from immigrant families. Steve's ancestry is Russian and Rumanian while Pat's folks came from Northern Italy. We both remember the stories our parents and grandparents told us about their early lives. And they told us their very good reasons for coming to America. Interwoven in those tales was one common rationale: they all wanted better lives for themselves and for their children. They went through terrible hardship to achieve their dreams. It reminds us of the wonderful lyrics of Neil Diamond's "America," that describes immigrants never looking back but only looking forward to coming to America. When our families came to the United States, they were like your families. They knew the way to survive is to support one another. Of course there were the normal family squabbles, but they still managed to see the big picture—the dream, togetherness, children, peace, and security. In our families the word *family* meant *acceptance, security, I belong, I am loved, I am needed.* These people took pride in what their families stood for and who their families were. Their children were taught to take pride in their families, and that gave them a strong sense of identity. The family provided a code of conduct. Through the years it gave us our personal "bill of rights and shoulds." It taught us there is a pride and a tradition of which we are a part.

The word *family* means different things to different people. To some it's a warm place with good smells and good feelings and people who care about one another. It's a port in a storm. It's a group of people that accept you as you are. You may not be the apple of their eye at any given moment, but you know that you are accepted as a part of the clan. To others, *family* produces mixed feelings. Not all families are warm and nurturing, and not all kitchens have good smells, inviting you in to sit down, relax, and talk. Regardless of your interpretation of the word, we'd like to begin our journey with the definition of family that we will use throughout this book.

To us the word *family* goes beyond the traditional sense of the word. We know that people who live together as parent and child obviously are a family. But, from our point of view, regardless of

THE BETTER LIFE INSTITUTE FAMILY HEALTH PLAN

whether you are parent and child, grandmother, great aunt, or cousin twice removed, the real meaning of family is that all the members are willing to pull together toward a common goal. For most of us, this is what family means, parents, grandparents, children, extended family members all leaning on one another, laughing together, crying together, working together, and arguing together. The key here is *together*.

THE "OZZIE AND HARRIET" FAMILY

That golden oldie TV show, "The Adventures of Ozzie and Harriet," portrayed the ideal family of the 1950's. And there are still a lot of "Ozzie and Harriet" families around. Despite the comedic overtones, the Nelsons were a solid family where together parents and children worked out their problems and differences. Ozzie, the bread winner, and Harriet, the homemaker, were always available to their sons. They were at home with their children in the evening. Saturday always included a family activity. Conversation was plentiful, not only around the dinner table, but before and after. And the nation got to watch the Nelson children grow up on television. In a way, we all grew up with them. The Nelsons of television represented the kind of family most people wanted to have, but very few actually did have.

Let's take a look at some of the different types of families we've worked with over the years. We've selected several "common varieties" with the hope you will be able to see yourself and your family among these types of families. There are countless variations, as we note every evening on television. One sometimes gets the feeling when watching "Knot's Landing," re-runs of "Dallas," or some of the daytime soaps that the definition of family has been extended to include everyone in the neighborhood.

And, let's not forget the relatively new yet increasingly prevalent families made up of several adults who live together because of economic necessity or because they are single or widowed. These "new wave" families are reflected in our mass media with films like *Three Men and a Baby* or television shows such as yesteryear's "Odd Couple" and "The Brady Bunch," and today's "Golden Girls."

Whatever the arrangement, whether the connection is by blood, marriage, economic necessity, convenience, or emotional need, our definition of family simply includes people living together who care about each other and want to share each other's lives. We don't mean to make a social statement about what constitutes a good family, a traditional family, or a family living with strong spiritual values. We are merely observing that today for many the term *family* encompasses something more than mom, dad, and the kids.

We will provide you with very specific and livable suggestions for how you can improve both family health and family unity. The

LET'S HEAR IT FOR FAMILIES! ■

3

fact that you are reading this book points to either interest and, likely, need. Please hear us out. We think we can help you and your family live longer and live better. And remember, as we must continually remind ourselves, your family is made up of individuals—each with different priorities regarding health. The Better Life Family program is designed for families, but it has specific components for each individual's health or weight loss needs.

WHAT EVER HAPPENED TO THE NORMAN ROCKWELL FAMILY?

Until a few decades ago, our perception of the family was illustrated with images of people laughing and breaking bread together, of intimate moments in counsel and support of one another, of hugs and kisses at bedtime. We've all seen the delightful Norman Rockwell paintings that often graced the cover of *Saturday Evening Post*. They reflect the ideal American family working, playing, praying, and celebrating together. As an artist, Rockwell captured the loving looks and connectedness between all generations of everyman's family.

If Norman Rockwell were alive today, how would he paint the typical American family? Does this seemingly rare entity still exist? Or should we ask what is typical today? Times have changed. Some folks may inappropriately call the changes progress, but we look at it as merely the reality of modern times. Society has changed and so has the unity of the American family. Economic necessity has diminished the cohesiveness and quality of family life. Dads spend more time on their careers and over half of married moms work. And that description doesn't include single parents. Remember, about 30 percent of children live in families with a single parent. Moms and dads no longer have separate, stereotypical roles. They share responsibilities. They all cook, chauffeur, shop, do the laundry, babysit as practical necessity dictates. Daycare centers and pre-school nurseries are where many children spend a large part of their childhood. And school seems to be the place where kids acquire their values instead of getting them at home. With so many mothers in the workplace, there is the new troublesome phenomenon of "latch-key kids" who are completely unsupervised between the time school lets out and their parents come home from work.

We could never invite Mr. Rockwell to paint our 1990's American family in the evening because he would have few people at home to paint. If he were to paint the typical American home in the evening it would be a dull painting—just furniture and empty rooms. Dad might be working at his second job. Mom might be taking a class at the adult education center to improve her job skills. The teenage daughter might be babysitting for the neighbor down the street. And most likely there would be two boys soaking up the Simpsons on TV

■ *THE BETTER LIFE INSTITUTE FAMILY HEALTH PLAN*

while eating a microwaved TV dinner. The Norman Rockwell family has just about disappeared. To paraphrase the French philosopher Voltaire, it seems that the only thing permanent in life is change.

Divorce, something that unfortunately we've experienced first-hand within our own families, was less common during the era when Norman Rockwell painted rose-colored portraits of the American family. And with the growing epidemic of divorce, we now have more single-parent families, extended families, absentee mothers, and weekend fathers. It is quite likely that most families in America, if not all, have experienced the pain of divorce, either directly or indirectly. Today, it may seem to many that the typical two-parent, blood-related family is a rarity.

Instead of painting a portrait of a large family enjoying a relaxed dinner together, Rockwell might paint a different dining table scene today. It could be a harried mom serving dinner to her children while talking on the phone and looking at the clock. Near the front door is mom's briefcase ready for her quick exit, and on the nearby desk are her checks and latest bank statement showing us she'd been trying earlier to balance her check book. The kids would be doing their thing around the table, which is teasing each other, while the family dog sits on his haunches begging for a table scrap. And don't forget that the TV is blaring in the corner.

We no longer spend as much time together as a family. Most of us lead very busy, hectic lives. Usually both parents work outside the home, which means that their children don't get to interact with them as much as children used to do. With more competing activities and less time for casual contact, parents now find it difficult to provide the deep nurturing, loving, and guidance each member of the family needs, including mom and dad. Mom has no time to show her children how to bake cookies, and dad can't find the hours needed to teach children how to fix things and build things. Children often spend more time with friends than with their parents—not to mention the countless hours they spend in front of the television.

In the United States today, over half of all married couples divorce. One out of every 3.5 parents is a "single parent."

Rounding Up the Kids (and Their Parents) for Health

All of us try to set goals for our lives. The purpose of this book and the Better Life Institute Program is to help you set the goal of a more healthful life for your entire family. With some work this goal is attainable, and it will set in motion that *loving centripetal force* which will make your family closer.

LET'S HEAR IT FOR FAMILIES!

Having a goal of health provides the basis for sharing values and purpose within your family. It helps to foster better communication and stronger relationships. And best of all, you and your family can build or improve mutual self-worth, confidence, and personal character.

Now you could be thinking that this goal might be achievable in other families, but it can never work in *your* family. Your family is different. Well, as different as all families are, they are all composed of people. And we've spent a few decades observing how people act and react within the family setting. Since our program has been successful in thousands of families, we know it can work for yours as well. All we ask is that you give it a try!

Exposed to the stresses of daily life, parents with the best of intentions are probably having a tough time with their eating, exercise, and weight control habits. Often the challenge is compounded because their children are not aware of, or have any interest in, living a more healthful lifestyle. As we said in this book's introduction, todays' kids are too worldly wise to fall for the old "Do as I say, not as I do" routine. The days of Nan, Babs, Junior, and Beaver saying, "Yes, Mom; Yes, Dad" without a question are gone.

A Potpourri of American Families

THE TYPICAL 2.3 CHILD—TWO PARENT—TWO INCOME FAMILY

Say Hello Again to the Fosters

Although nothing is truly typical anymore, we define the typical family as one with two adults who are biological or adoptive parents of the children they are raising. This is still the predominant family of America. Both Jim and Phyllis know that as they are losing their youth, they are gaining pounds and cholesterol points. Jim has begun to dream of a little red sports car for himself, but he'd probably hurt his back getting down into it, not to speak of getting out. Jim and Phyllis are both aware that they and their children should be leading a healthier lifestyle. But, they keep putting it off. They don't want to endure the discomfort of personal change.

Their kids put up the usual resistance to change, and these parents simply cave in, being too exhausted to fight them one more time about something they've fought about before. These parents are not abusive or thoughtless. They are cognizant of the importance of their family's health, but it's something that's "on the back burner." After all day-to-day life is pretty exhausting just as it is. And it requires too much effort to get this new priority moved to the front burner.

■ *A 15-year-old girl writes:*

I've lived my entire life with people reminding me it isn't okay to be fat. I have to accept the fact that I gross people out—even including some members of my family. My life is a Catch 22. I'm lonely and don't have friends because I'm fat, and I eat because I'm lonely. I have dreams about what it would be like to be thin. There is nothing I would not give to be thin. For me, living is literally hell. The insults I must endure, the pity, the loneliness, the self-hatred, and the loathing all seem to be punishments.

■ *THE BETTER LIFE INSTITUTE FAMILY HEALTH PLAN*

Most troubling of all, Phyllis and Jim are aware that heart disease and diabetes are in both sides of the family! But they tell themselves those things happened to their relatives, and maybe, just maybe, none of those terrible things will happen to them.

It seems bad enough that Phyllis and Jim aren't paying attention to the health habits they practice for themselves and demonstrate to their children, but that's not the whole story. The kids' grandparents complain regularly about getting older and how much they hate to take their high blood pressure medication. Just like their adult children, these older folks lack the motivation and the desire to take some action.

This whole family needs help!

THE "FAST TRACK" FAMILY

Let's Meet the Parduccis
Tony and Terri Parducci are in business together. Both are teachers in the local public school system and they have a successful evening school where they teach English language classes for foreign-born adults. Their workday begins at 6:00 A.M. When their daytime school duties are finished, they take care of routine family business at home. They have a quick dinner with the kids (eating whatever is easiest to prepare) before rushing out to their evening school jobs. Afterward it's not unusual to find both of them at a coffee shop at 10:30 P.M. eating cheeseburgers and pie à la mode and drinking diet sodas just to unwind. The kids, bless them, try to help out at home. They are good kids and understand their parents' responsibilities. They don't understand, however, what their parents' daily routine is doing to their health. Neither do Tony and Terri.

Tony's father, the children's granddad, has high blood pressure. So does Tony. Tony is smart enough to know that a good portion of what he is working for now will be spent in the future on doctor and hospital bills if he doesn't make a radical change in the way he lives. He wants to share more "quality time" with his kids, but he can't work it into his daily schedule. The thought of a proper family health program has indeed crossed his mind, but he hasn't had time to think about what it should be or how to go about doing it. Terri's not as conscious of family health risks, but she'll do anything to keep her husband and children around for a long time.

Like the Fosters, the Parducci family needs help!

THE SINGLE-PARENT FAMILY

Now a Nod to the Rothbergs
Diane Rothberg is having difficulty making ends meet despite the fact that her former husband, Jerry, contributes to her income. Conse-

Many parents find it very difficult to attend all their children's functions, such as games, class parties, recitals, and birthdays. When a parent is out of town, can't get away from work, or is a single parent, problems arise in communicating to the child that Mom or Dad can't always be there and making the child understand and appreciate the reasons rather than feel let down and resentful. These are some ideas to help keep communication alive:

■ Call or speak to
your child be-
fore the big
event. Explain
the circum-
stances without
laying blame on
anyone. Teach
your child that
life is not always
perfect and
there will
always be situa-
tions and solu-
tions. Together
you'll deal with
this situation.

■ Call or speak to
your child after
the big event so
that he or she
shares the spe-
cial time with
you.

■ Write your child
a note. Tell him
that you love
him; that you're
proud of him;
that he's always
in your thoughts
and prayers.

■ Make a date to
celebrate the big
event at another
time, either
before or after
the scheduled
time. Every
child needs to be
recognized and
loved. This
builds character
in both parents
and children.

quently she holds down two jobs. She is personal assistant to an account executive and receives a paycheck. Her other job is to be both
mother and father to her three children, ages six, ten and fourteen,
and she does not receive a paycheck or have regular, established
hours. She's fifteen pounds overweight, and it seems that each extra
pound adds about one year's age to her appearance. She knows a
good exercise program will not only help reduce her weight, but will
reduce her stress too. Family meals are a challenge for Diane because the kids don't care for the "diet food" she always tries to eat.
In her heart of hearts, neither does she.

Jerry, Diane's ex-husband, tries to help, but is having a difficult
time of it. Whenever he is with the kids, he feels very guilty. It really
hurts him to be around them. He finds himself being less a discipli-
narian and instructive father and more a pleaser and entertainer for
his kids. Having them on an occasional weekend is wonderful, but he
avoids any type of confrontation with them because of his guilt feelings. Junk food, movies, and fun, fun, fun are the agenda when he's
with the kids. This doesn't help Diane very much, since she gets to
play the tough-guy role all the time. Jerry knows that and feels
guilty about it too, but he thinks he can't do anything about it.

Like the Fosters and the Parduccis, this family needs help.

THE REMARRIED "CHEAPER BY THE DOZEN" FAMILY

Introducing the Brinkerhoffs

A hybrid style family is on the rise. Many divorced parents with children at home are remarrying. The resulting situations could, at
times, be good TV sitcom material—a wide range of ages and interests and habits that can be either good news or disastrous for family
life. Collectively the Brinkerhoffs have five children, ranging in age
from four to nineteen, and all five live at home. Dates, corsages, pim-
ples, barbells, dolls, dump trucks, and tricycles flourish side by side
in their household. Although both parents work, John is the career-
oriented parent while Sheila only "works for extra money." John's
second chin and spare tire and Sheila's cellulite and thighs are definitely going through a time of expansion. Even fourteen-year-old
Debbie is showing the psychological strain of an adolescent with ten
extra pounds.

Sometimes it seems that Superbowl Sunday, when everyone
knows about the game and either watches enthusiastically or stays
out of the way, is less chaotic than a typical Sunday in the
Brinkerhoff house. With five kids running in and out, countless
friends coming and going, the telephone ringing, the TV blaring,
meals to be fixed, laundry to be done, shopping, a few arguments,
and perhaps a non-custodial parent or two dropping by for a "visita-

tion," life can be hectic. As the dust settles, John and Sheila are now ready to do something for themselves and for their children—whether both generations like it or not!

The Brinkerhoffs want help!

EXTENDED FAMILY

Let's Welcome the O'Neill-Fuentes-Chang Clan

A United Nations banquet is child's play in comparison with these three women and their assorted ten children having dinner. While they represent three ethnic backgrounds, O'Neill is an African American, Fuentes hails from Guatemala, and Chang's family comes from Hong Kong, their meals are pure "Americana"—fast food, TV dinners, and anything that's frozen, freeze-dried, microwavable, and easy to assemble. It's not that they don't care about good meals or proper nutrition, it's just that work, daycare centers, nursery school, math homework, and football schedules make life an act of juggling opposing schedules. The one time they all get together is Sunday morning at church and Sunday school. There are no fathers or "father figures" to assist with childrearing or repairing the faucet or anything else. Including one sixteen-year-old aspiring nurse, there are four women and at least two different diets in progress for a day, week, or month at any given moment. There is an exercise bicycle in the dining room, but presently it is being used as a clothes drying rack. These women know the kids should be doing more to help, but as always, they play "catch up" daily to just stay on top. They need help.

What's a Body to Do?

SOME PRACTICAL GENERAL GUIDELINES

All of these families—the Fosters, the Parduccis, the Rothbergs, the Brinkerhoffs, and the O'Neill-Fuentes-Chang trio—have a great deal in common. They're committed to each other, they care and love one another, and all of them are needy in the better health department and want to do something about it. They just need to know what to do and how to begin.

We feel that family health and unity do not require anyone to go back to college or to get a Ph.D. in nutrition and psychology. You already have the knowledge and common sense to improve your own health and your children's health and to strengthen your family unity at the same time. That's the beauty of what we will suggest to you. You know all of it already; you just haven't used what you know in the way that is most beneficial to you.

■ *For many children, watching television has become a full-time job. According to a 1989 Neilsen survey, two- to five-year-olds watch TV about 25 hours a week, six- to eleven-year-olds watch about 22 hours, and twelve- to seventeen-year-olds watch about 23 hours.*

■ *During Prime Time television hours, your child will witness a fictional person drinking once in every twenty minutes. The average for popular crime and sit-com shows is once in every fifteen minutes. An average of thirty people are murdered individually on television every evening.*

LET'S HEAR IT FOR FAMILIES! ■

Let's look at some simple rules for building family strength. They're not new to you. Your grandmother taught them to you many years ago.

Never More Say, "Do as I Say, Not as I Do." Instead Try, "Do as I Do and Let's Do It Together."

Parents should serve as models of correct behavior for their children. We feel strongly about this principle. It is non-negotiable! However, we may disagree as to how we define *correct behavior*. We're not talking about perfect behavior. We want you to be parents who try to do things right and still have the option of trying to improve when you do things wrong. Making mistakes is a specialty of the human race. When a mistake happens, we should consider it an opportunity to learn to do better.

If you said to your children, *I'm really having difficulty getting enough exercise and maintaining my weight—I could sure use your help and support,* you might be surprised to see how your kids would rally to your side.

Let's think about this. You could find that your biggest pals and allies in solving the family's fundamental health problems are none other than your own kids!

When you make this kind of statement to your children, you get past the typical parental need to present yourself as perfect. You may get away with pretending to be perfect for the first five years of your child's life, but after that your children are really "hip." They know what's up. They realize you've got "raggedy edges." When you ask for their help and support, they also begin to recognize that you need them and respect them enough to ask them to be a part of your personal team. And you've added a component of reality to the situation by presenting yourself as a person who needs help and is smart enough to ask for it. The lesson in life is obvious since truly independent people are the ones who recognize that they need help to steer a happy and healthy course through life.

In addition you've added the component of *because you are important to me, I'm asking you to help me.* There is nothing as gratifying and as psychologically important to children as a parent who, by his or her actions, tells them *you are important to me and I need you.* Your children's self-esteem and confidence are helped more by their understanding that you actually need their support and help than by your merely telling them that you need them.

Most importantly, you've made a best friend for life, and the nicest part is that your newfound "buddy" is your child. Your child will feel the same way about you. Your simple *I need help* statement opens an entirely new dimension to family relationships. It will probably lead your child to become more receptive to your guidance in health and other matters.

If You Scratch My Back, I'll Scratch Yours

Many parents are exhausted on workday evenings. They feel they don't have the energy or interest to do the things their children like to do. The weekend should be a time to recover from the week before or prepare for the week ahead. It's also the only time most of us have to do the errands that constantly hang over our heads. However, on weekends children *should* make some demands upon their parents' time. That's what a family is about. When your children stop making demands on your time, you shouldn't be relieved; you should be concerned. Soon they'll be filling the time they should spend with you by spending it with people outside the family.

Children (and, we hope, parents) do have a strong sense of fair play, but using it well is a technique that has to be taught and modeled continually. What, actually, is fair play in a family? It is consistent, loving give and take. Many family tasks can be shared if the give-and-take principle is applied. For example, make a pact with your children to do something they want to do on Saturday if they help you with a weekday task. You might believe that they should do something simply because you tell them to do it. But discipline is taught best by your own example, which builds mutual love and respect for both parent and child.

You should expect your children to make some demands on your time. It is their right—after all, they are *your* children! In your quest to get through your own daily hassle, you may overlook the special needs your children have in relating to you. Let them know in a meaningful way that you do have time for them even though it may not be immediately.

"One on One" Is Great Basketball—It's Great Family, Too!

Many families are squeezed for family time because of outside commitments. In addition to their work time requirements, parents may belong to organizations that require their time during evenings and on weekends. And the kids are usually saturated with after-school activities—athletics, clubs, hobbies, tutoring, and so forth. The occasions when parents can spend "quality time" with their children are rare. Often what time is available is spent with as many members of the family as possible, for the "best coverage."

If we stop to think about it, we will realize that we have our children for just a short time, and the time goes by too quickly. That means our children should become a high priority on our list of "life's precious gifts." While it is important for the family to spend time together as a group, you mustn't forget the preciousness of spending time one-on-one with each child. These are some important benefits of one-on-one:

• All of us remember those special private moments when we had our parents all to ourselves. All children have a number of different types of family relationships that make an impact on their lives. However, the one that leaves the strongest impression on a child is the special private relationship with the most significant people in his or her life—Mom and Dad. It is always there etched indelibly in the memory throughout childhood, adulthood, and eventual parenthood. Don't forget to give this wonderful legacy of time to each of your children.

• The personal, individual relationship you forge with your child by spending time together creates an environment of "impressionable time." Personal time is likely to result in more lasting impressions from an instructive and educational perspective than will result from any other time you spend with your family.

• Remember, being one of many in a family provides a wonderful sense of belonging. However, each child is an individual and regularly needs a personal and private relationship with a parent as well as with brothers and sisters. It is this one-on-one experience that tells each of us a great deal about ourselves and about the other person.

• Many children from larger families may remember the feeling of not having a special, private relationship with every family member. There's always too much going on at any given moment for meaningful relationships to develop. It tends to color their family experience in a different way. One-on-one adds a valuable dimension to the benefits of growing up in a large family, and you must make the time to have these times with each of your children.

Tradition . . . Tradition
The farmer, Tevya, in the film *Fiddler on the Roof,* says it all with his song "Tradition . . . Tradition!" A sense of roots and of belonging through tradition provides psychological security and comfort for you and your family. Many of us remember practicing our faith alongside other members of our families, and usually we associate the memory with comfort and peace of mind. Grandparents are ideal sources of providing your children with a link to the past, to their roots and traditions. Family routines, whether accepted or rejected, are often

remembered more fondly as we grow older. You now have an opportunity to strengthen family life and family ties by encouraging family routines and providing opportunities for yourself, your spouse, and your children to forge closer, more supportive links to their grandparents and other family members. When you do, several important things will happen:

• By fostering closer ties with your extended family—particularly the older members—you continually remind your children that you were and still are someone's child. They will have a better understanding of how you got to be you.

• Close and ongoing relations with grandparents and other seniors extend the size of your family beyond Mom and Dad. Children get to interact with family members who are not always there every day to discipline them or be a part of a routine. They make "family" more exciting and interesting. The experience leads to closer ties.

• Grandparents usually don't have a custodial relationship with their grandchildren. They often provide fun and good times, and since grandparents don't see the kids every day, there's a degree of specialness that they express toward their grandchildren. Their grandkids are the apples of their eye—a thought weary parents usually don't express. And finally, grandparents tend to spoil their grandchildren. They can tell great stories about life before television, video games, and the Super Bowl. This special doting relationship provides children with a sense of being special that parents can't regularly provide.

• Family routines are important ways to keep parents bonded with children. We all remember family routines even if some were not liked as much as others. As the years pass, we become more objective about these routine parts of our early lives, but we still recall our parents asking us to clean our rooms, take out the garbage, walk the dog, go to the hardware store with Dad, shop with Mom, have brunch after church on Sunday, spend various holidays as a group. These traditions and routines provided a sense of family to you that you can pass on to your children and that they will pass on to their children. (Then you will be the grandparents and can spoil your grandchildren without feeling any guilt.)

• There are many reasons why a strong daily sense of spirituality can add meaning, joy, and strength to your family life. The family is a base upon which to practice and live spiritually. Whether you at-

Children develop coping skills from real life situations. When a child learns to work through difficult times, he is preparing himself, with your help, for real adult life.

tend church or synagogue or simply forge your relationships with spiritual dictates, living spirituality can add much to your family unity and health. We'll talk about that more in the following chapters.

• Tradition, routine, grandparents, and a strong spiritual life can partially offset the loss of a parent. The continuum of this family structure provides enormous support for children in a broken or widowed family.

Now I Lay Me Down to Sleep . . .

Remember the old adage "don't let the Sun set on your anger"? Well, we'd like to refocus it a bit to say, *don't let your kids go to bed until you've spent a few minutes with them.*

• Every evening until Steve's son, Jon, was fourteen, Steve took the time to lie on Jon's bed with him for a few minutes just to talk. (By the time Jon was fourteen, there was not enough room in his bed for both of them; Steve got kicked out and had to sit on a chair. But the talks continued.) If Steve was out of town, he would call his son before bedtime. Both father and son looked forward to this daily time together, and it became a very meaningful family tradition. It was a time when they talked, not of "shoulds" and "oughts," but of whatever came to mind. There was an exchange of feelings, such as "I wonder if . . ." or "Why does the. . . ." Both parent and child need such quiet moments together after the hectic hours of the day. It becomes a time when the most important thing is your mutual thoughts and feelings. Many parents tuck their children in at bedtime and give them a kiss. They should also take a few minutes to talk quietly. And, the habit shouldn't be stopped at some arbitrary age. We loved this time as kids, and your children will also love it. We loved this time as parents, and you will love it too. This tradition helps to nurture a special relationship with people you love. Naturally, it can become a bit difficult when your kids get married. But, it's not impossible; it just doesn't happen as often.

• Don't forget the power of a short "how are you doing?" telephone call. Frequent contact among family members tickles the "I love, I care, and I think about you" button. Pat's children check in with one another at least once a week, and they're scattered throughout the country. (The officials at AT&T *love* us.)

• Write or send a card to someone in your own home on special occasions or for no reason at all.

■ *THE BETTER LIFE INSTITUTE FAMILY HEALTH PLAN*

You Can *Do It*

A warm, close family life cannot be bought nor does it automatically arrive when you become a parent. Pat always says, "You don't get an owner's manual when your newborn infant is placed in your arms." Being parents doesn't give you any guarantee that your family members can all live together with joy, security, and health. We think it takes a *can-do, trial-and-error* attitude. You can never go wrong in your family if you honestly try to improve family life. Of course you should try to go about it as sensibly as possible. The practical guidelines offered above can go a very long way toward improving your family's life, unity, and health.

We have deliberately left the best for last. Communication among all family members—talking, laughing, arguing, negotiating, instructing, educating, correcting—is the mechanical or structural basis of family unity and health. The following chapter will describe the communication core of the Better Life Family Health Program: the *Family Circle*.

The Family Circle

Chapter 2

■ ■ ■ ■ ■ ■ ■ ■ ■ ■ ■ ■ ■ ■ ■ ■ ■

How to Make a Family

2 or more willing and able people
1 cup each friendship, understanding, and mutual trust
1 cup support
1 cup patience
1 cup wisdom
4 cups love

Take the people and place them in the right spot, at a gym, at an exercise club, in school, or at home. Add friendship and mix well. Spoon in understanding, support, and patience as needed to keep the family mixture pliable and workable. Knead gently as you would knead bread. Sprinkle in wisdom, and stir just until blended. Allow to rise. Bake slowly in a warm friendly oven—forever. Frost generously with love.

Senator Paul Tsongas, former United States senator from Massachusetts, retired for a time several years ago when he learned he had cancer. The disease was detected early enough to be treated successfully. The senator, who has now returned to the political arena, decided to take some time out in order to spend more time with his wife and two daughters. He said, "I used to walk them to school and think about re-election. Now I think about their homework, their smiles, and the sunrise." Someone once wrote to him and said, "When you're on your deathbed, you won't think about how much more time you should have spent at the office." We all need to look at life the way Senator Tsongas learned to do. His new philosophy is

"You need to take time out and smell the roses." Enjoy your family members as if they were roses.

The Legacy

Those of you who studied Roman history will remember that the Roman Empire provided many legacies to Western civilization that still greatly influence our lives. Roman engineering—bridges, roads, aqueducts—and Roman law are the foundation of many of our modern public works. A walk through our nation's capital or a visit to many major public buildings throughout the country reminds us of the majesty of Roman architecture.

Rome also paved the way for the use of discussion, debate, and negotiation in making decisions for the welfare of the public and the state. Even today, the ruins of the spectacular Roman Forum is one of the great showplaces of the Western world. The Forum was the place where city leaders could speak and where citizens could be heard. Important civil and judicial proceedings were often held in the open Forum, allowing participation and discussion by the people.

Other cities throughout the Roman Empire adopted the concept of the Forum, and it proved to be a valuable means of communicating with the people. Assembling at a forum also allowed people to speak out and settle their differences.

Both the Greeks and the Romans left a legacy of democratic and participatory governmental interaction which is still very much alive in America. New England town meetings are based upon equal participation and representation as is our bicameral legislature, the House of Representatives and the Senate. Equal representation, equal voice, one individual-one vote are all inalienable rights of Americans. We are now going to introduce you to the family branch of a participatory tradition that extends back in time to over two thousand years ago.

The Family Circle

Just as the Romans needed opportunities to exchange ideas with each other, family members need a time to talk to each other. Each of us needs to be able to state our viewpoints as a basis for negotiation, discussion, and compromise. In addition parents and children need to air their feelings regularly, to "let it all hang out." Too often family members get bottled-up with emotion and then later explode when barely provoked.

■ *THE BETTER LIFE INSTITUTE FAMILY HEALTH PLAN*

In order to start a family health program and keep it going, you need to provide a forum for your family—a Family Circle. We're not going to ask you to wear togas and sandals and go down to City Hall. Instead we're going to ask you to form a special circle in the privacy of your home.

Circles are quite amazing geometric forms because they have no beginning, middle, or end. They just go around and around infinitely. And when you form a circle with human beings, literally and figuratively, it has the potential energy of linking one family member to another—all of whom become part of the whole circle, the family.

There is no one aspect of the circle that is more important than any other part. That is why round tables are so democratic. Legend has it that back in Camelot, King Arthur devised the Round Table to allow all of his knights an equal place and to guarantee that no one person would ever consider himself in a place of special influence or honor. King Arthur didn't even want his royal self to sit at the head of the table.

Similarly, your Family Circle should never allow one family member more authority than another. When the Circle convenes, everyone present, whether five years old or forty, has an equal voice. We are asking fathers and mothers to pay special attention to this. We are not suggesting that you relinquish your parental responsibility for your family; we are only asking that within the Family Circle, you give equal attention and respect to the voice that represents someone five years old and weighing 40 pounds that you give to the voice of another who is forty years old and weighs 150 pounds. There has to be a place in family life when all family members feel they are equally represented. Every family member, whether big or small, has thoughts and feelings that should be acknowledged. Your responsibility and authority, whether you are a king or a parent, is not challenged by allowing your children an equal voice at the Family Circle. Arthur's knights knew who was the king, and your kids know who is in charge. If they don't, it's time they learned.

GETTING YOUR CIRCLE ROLLING

All right, we can already hear the moans and groans about everyone barely having enough time to take a breath and relax, let alone time for a weekly family pow-wow. We can sympathize with that since most of us do lead overly scheduled lives.

Why?

Family Circle must become a high priority on your "Things to Do" list since it serves many functions—all of them positive and essential to decisions and support of better health. It will be the vehicle that initiates and maintains your family health program. It gives everyone the opportunity to participate in fiddling with and fine tuning the eating and exercise program that suits them best. It allows each person to select and consent to others' requests for support and help in keeping the family health program together. And, most importantly, the Family Circle allows each family member, child and parent alike, a safe place to blow off steam, ask for advice, criticize constructively, and build help and support systems based upon belonging and caring for and loving each other.

How?

The best way to start the Family Circle rolling is to plan a time when the family is together without interruptions. Don't drop the idea on everybody like a bomb at an inconvenient or rushed time. Plan to discuss it at a time when everyone can pay attention. Perhaps a good time would be right after Sunday's breakfast or just before a weekday dinner when everyone is available.

When?

Introducing the concept of Family Circle correctly requires that everybody have the time to think about it and react without being rushed. Announce that you'd like to set aside some time each week with everyone in the family present. Decide together when that time will be. Explain that the purpose of these weekly meetings is to allow everyone the opportunity to help improve their own health and help other family members improve theirs as well. Be sure to say that the meetings will be short and will have time limits.

Why? (Again)

Emphasize that there will also be times at these meetings when the family plans activities that are lots of fun. You might even plan to go out for dessert afterward or ask Mom to prepare something really tasty to eat during Family Circle. It's important that each family member give consent for this family project. Take time to ask each person individually for any thoughts, ideas, and concerns.

FAMILY CIRCLE BASICS: THE NUTS AND BOLTS

Family Circle works only if everyone is comfortable and relaxed and feels it is all right to speak freely. Family Circle is not a free-for-all or an opportunity to take cheap shots under a so-called flag of truce. You will have a wonderful opportunity to show your kids democracy in action.

One of our family's habits that has always made us want to scream is the constant arguing and name-calling that often go on among brothers and sisters. Continual disciplining or a plea to stop

20   ■ *THE BETTER LIFE INSTITUTE FAMILY HEALTH PLAN*

was usually ignored. The Family Circle should serve as a model for your kids to learn better discussion, negotiating, and problem solving techniques. It should give everyone the opportunity to learn and continually practice new communication skills. Your kids may even find replacements for arguing and name-calling outside the Circle.

Differences of opinion within the family and with outside friends and workers are inevitable. But children need opportunities to learn the value of give and take. It will help them in all aspects of their lives because all of us encounter differences of opinion. Some parents as well need practice in responding to someone else's passionate point of view. Everyone needs to understand that strong feeling, even anger, is okay. What is most important, however, is how you express your anger and other legitimate feelings.

Disagreements between most parents are a fact of life. To hide or deny them to your children implies that disagreements are bad or if they can't be avoided they should be kept secret. Most likely your children will sense a disagreement, even if you try to hide or deny it. Disagreements, or different points of view, happen in all relationships. The issue is not whether you have them, but how you resolve them. An argument that is settled by the loudest shouter teaches a lesson to children about shouting. The same holds true for using cursewords or name-calling. Consider a disagreement an opportunity for everyone involved to learn a valuable lesson. Mutual respect, a calm voice, and negotiation are all part of arguing. Don't be afraid to acknowledge at Family Circle the disagreement you had with your spouse.

The number one rule for your Family Circle is to have an agenda—a list of things the family wants to talk about. It doesn't have to be elaborate. A brief outline of points to discuss is all you need. We suggest you poll the family a few days before and collect the items each person wants to talk about. Or put a memo pad for the agenda on the refrigerator, and ask everyone to write the topics that interest them. When all family members participate in planning the meeting, Family Circle becomes more relevant and interesting to everyone. If you haven't had time to prepare the agenda, then postpone the meeting. Children need structure to absorb new thoughts and ideas. Adults do too. Never "wing it" without a plan of what is going to be discussed at the meeting.

Next, you need to schedule a time when people aren't itching to race off elsewhere. You may think this is impossible, but just ask each family member for the most mutually convenient time to meet together as a family. It may be a weekday night, or it might turn out to be early Sunday morning. Although you should be flexible for vacations or special school and recreational events, it's important to establish a consistent time *each week* when everyone is expected to be present.

You should also impose a time limit for each meeting. Open-ended meetings become unwieldly and ultimately turn into time-wasters or what we call "yawners." Also, you'll need to consider the relatively short attention span of children, although we are amazed at how long they can keep their eyes glued to a television program without losing interest. We suggest you limit your Family Circle to thirty minutes in the beginning, and depending upon success and need, later you may want to expand it to an hour. When the participants know they have only a specified amount of time, they will stick to the items for discussion.

The meeting should have no interruptions. Turn off the radio, stereo, and TV. Take your phone off the hook or turn on your answering machine. Everyone has set aside precious personal time to do some positive personal and family work. You can't allow outside factors to break the focus of the meeting.

Either Mom or Dad can lead the first few meetings just to get the program off the ground. Once Family Circle has been launched and is meeting regularly, you can end each meeting by asking a different volunteer to lead the next one. That individual will be responsible for collecting the discussion items that will comprise the agenda and preparing in other ways for the next meeting. You'll be pleasantly surprised at your children's ability to lead the meetings once they find Family Circle worthwhile and are shown the necessary skills.

WE'RE ALL IN THIS TOGETHER

If your family is like ours, we can guarantee that everyone is going to feel a little self-conscious at your first Family Circle. A great way to break the ice is to have everyone join hands in a symbolic gesture of family unity and caring and repeat an affirmation like, "We're going to work together as a team because we're a family." This suggestion came to us from a number of our families, and it often works. These words may not be your style or "cup of tea." But if you decide to use an opening statement, make sure it's positive and uplifting. Holding hands as a family is the most important part. You may want to just hold hands and observe a moment of silence, a method which seems to suit some families.

The Family Circle should not be run like a corporate board meeting. It should be informal and fun. At the same time, it is not a whining session where everyone sits around and complains about something or someone. And it is not a time to punish, to teach your kids a lesson, or to manipulate members of the family. No one should ever feel like a scapegoat or be the butt of criticism and jokes at Family Circle. Family Circle should be an uplifting experience. It should capture people's interest and allow everyone to feel cared for and supported. Affable and positive communication is the fuel that propels Family Circle and will keep it chugging along for years.

Every day of our lives, we all play different roles. Adults can be husbands and wives, parents, children themselves, brother or sister, workers, and parishioners. Kids' roles range from student to playmate, to son or daughter, to pet care provider, to an expert in sports or comic books. These varying roles usually depend upon individual experience, age, and ability. But during the time allocated to Family Circle, every member of the family should be present and playing the same *supportive* role. Everyone has an equal place and an equal voice at Family Circle. And each person has the same stake in achieving and enjoying a healthier life.

Ten Commandments of Family Circle

(Suggested Guidelines)

Unlike the original Ten Commandments, these guidelines are not etched in stone. They are flexible, and you will need to judge how to use them based on the mix of personalities and ages and the number of people in your family. There is, however, a *spirit* about these recommendations that can help improve the enjoyment and effectiveness of your Family Circle.

I

SPEAK QUIETLY.

Family Circle is not a shouting match; each person should speak quietly. Some of us grew up in families that allowed "the squeaky wheel" to get the most "oil." We learned that people tend to pay more attention to you when you raise your voice.

What happens in Family Circle when you raise your voice? You are trying to get your way or to emphasize your point. How does that affect the others in Family Circle? They feel you are being intimidating and confrontative. The fact that in the past when you raised your voice people listened and possibly you got your way doesn't mean "out talking" the others is useful. People don't feel good about being intimidated by a raised voice. You don't feel good about it when someone shouts at you, either. Winning points is not what Family Circle is about.

Insist that everyone speak in a quiet voice. When you talk quietly, all the others can listen to what you are actually saying. They can hear the substance of the issue instead of just being accosted by the tone of voice. Many families are used to an environment where the person with the loudest voice commands the most attention. But teaching yourself and your children to speak quietly about important things is a very mature and civilized measure in a sometimes uncivilized world.

II

ALLOW EVERYONE TO SPEAK WITHOUT INTERRUPTION.

Communicating your point of view is a key element of Family Circle. Sometimes, though, emotions may run high when someone disagrees with what is being said. Those who disagree have a natural tendency to "jump the gun" and interrupt the person who is speaking. This cuts off the communication before it is finished. And, interruptions tend to sidetrack the matter being discussed.

Insist that no one interrupt another. All members of the Family Circle have the right to be heard in their own words and on their own terms. Discouraging interruptions also means that family members will listen more carefully to what is being said. Because they know they have to wait until the person who is speaking has finished, they will be motivated to show more respect for each person and for what they say. Since each person knows that whenever they have the floor, they can speak without someone jumping in on their words, every one learns a valuable lesson in give and take.

III

MAKE ONLY POSITIVE COMMENTS AND GIVE ONLY CONSTRUCTIVE CRITICISM.

Think how uncomfortable you are when people criticize you or put you down with inappropriate derogatory remarks. Even when they are correct with the intent of their criticism, you are usually hurt by the comment and may even feel you have been attacked. It is also unlikely that you truly listen to what they say because the way the criticism is spoken unleashes many negative emotions.

THE BETTER LIFE INSTITUTE FAMILY HEALTH PLAN

Insist that Family Circle support each family member and never blatantly criticize anyone. Rather than concentrate on what's wrong, show them how to offer constructive suggestions instead. The family will appreciate this while feeling protected and respected. And this type of protection will encourage open communication and the freedom to admit mistakes.

IV

LISTEN TO CONTENT AND FEELINGS. REALLY LISTEN!

There are two messages to which everyone must pay attention at Family Circle: the substance, or *content*, of what is being said and the feeling, or *emotion*, of the person saying it. Older children and adults can easily pick up on feelings, but this may be a bit abstract for small children. Still it's easy to say to one of them, "How do you think Debbie feels about what she is saying?" Little kids just need to practice being sensitive to what a person says and how that person feels. When your family does this regularly in Family Circle, each one will respond to the person who is speaking with a great deal more caring and sensitivity.

If someone forgets the rules and "steamrolls" a family member, don't criticize, but use it as an example. Ask the guilty party how he or she senses that the attacked person is feeling. You might say, "If someone said to you what you just said to Debbie, how do you think you would feel?" And then you might say, "Look at Debbie. Do you think that is the way she feels now?" Your family will appreciate your caring when you insist on protecting the individual feelings of each member of the family.

V

TRY TO UNDERSTAND THE OTHER PERSON'S POINT OF VIEW.

You may disagree with what another family member says at Family Circle. However, opposing points of view are often just as rational as the areas with which you do agree. It's just that you see the matter differently. Always ask yourself and the others at Family Circle to try to see the point of view of the person who is talking. Remember, there's always another way of doing anything. No one person has a lock on common sense.

VI

ALWAYS HAVE THE SPEAKER ASK WHAT OTHERS THINK ABOUT WHAT IS SAID.

What you say to others and what they hear you say and understand that you meant may be very different. It is extremely important to make sure that the person talking and the people listening are all on the same wavelength. It is also important for everyone to have an opportunity to react constructively to what was said. This allows the talker to be sure communication is on target and allows the listeners to react in a supportive manner.

VII

BE HONEST.

Honest open discussion is a very important aspect of family health and unity. Of course, what a family member says is important. But *equally* important is that everyone be honest when they talk in Family Circle. Teaching yourself and your children the value of honest discussion is itself a valued experience. Make a special effort to recognize and support honesty in communication whenever it occurs—regardless of what is actually said. Remember, it is very easy for you or your children to hide thoughts and actions with evasive answers, but being dishonest in Family Circle damages the family unity you're trying to nurture.

Let's think for a moment on why we lie. Usually it's a defensive reaction and often it is motivated by fear, whether real or imagined. And the consequence of lying is guilt, which usually makes us feel even worse. So, when you think about it, why should we do something that will ultimately make us feel bad?

Teaching your family members to express themselves honestly is one of the cornerstones of Family Circle. They must learn to trust that they are in a safe place where grudges and bad feelings are never harbored.

VIII

NEGOTIATE AND COMPROMISE TO FIND SOLUTIONS.

Think of your family as a kind of United Nations of Opinions. It certainly would be easier to reach a consensus if there were no differ-

■ *THE BETTER LIFE INSTITUTE FAMILY HEALTH PLAN*

ences in views and opinions, but it would also be dull as dishwater. A diversity of opinion will often lead to different ways to do things. There are two simple common-sense rules to follow when the time comes for decisions. First, all must be comfortable and in agreement with what they are going to do healthwise. If any are luke-warm about it or feel it was pushed down their throats, they will not do it well nor will they do it on a long-term basis. Second, the basis of Family Circle is mutual respect and family enjoyment. You may have the *power* to get another person in Family Circle to do something he doesn't want to do, but he will resent you and Family Circle for having been subjected to this type of emotional extortion. This is not the basis upon which to build a good family relationship or teach others how to make decisions.

When differences of opinion occur in your family, it is a reflection of each family member's individuality. Now is the time to teach the effectiveness of negotiation and compromise. Point out that there is always a middle ground where solutions can be found. The first step is to negotiate a new action that is satisfactory to everyone:

- The kids don't like the tuna salad without mayonnaise. How about using lite mayonnaise or no fat mayonnaise?
- How about using soft drinks made with Nutrasweet or Equal instead of sugar?
- How about riding the exercise bike while watching TV instead of just watching TV?
- How about using food products with salt in them, but not having a salt shaker on the table?
- The morning is too early for exercise. Select your own time, even if you break it up into two time periods.
- One hour of exercise 4 days a week is too much effort. How about half-an-hour 4 days a week?
- Let's mix half of your cold cereal with half of mine.

Another strategy is "if you do it this way now, we'll do it your way the next time." A little give-and-take goes a long way:

- We'll alternate between turkey-burgers and hamburgers.
- We'll use your music for aerobic dance this week and mine next week.
- We'll eat dinner at home four nights this week and eat out three nights.
- We'll have your favorite dessert tomorrow, and mine the next night.
- You'll lead Family Circle this week and she'll lead it next week.

- I'll be home at 5:00 at least three days this week.
- I'll wash the dishes this week, if you'll do them next week.

IX

ALL SUGGESTIONS MUST BE LIVABLE AND ENJOYABLE.

Deciding *whether* to do something is one issue. After that, deciding *what* to do is the "payload." In their enthusiasm, however, most people try to do too much, too soon. It is important that a "reality check" be made on each and every change suggested by family members. Encourage everyone to be realistic in what they would like to do. A typical reality check, for example, would be to look at a new exercise program and encourage the family to do a little less, but do it well and enjoy it. That's being realistic.

- Is it an action that is worth doing?
- Is it a practical and livable activity? Or is it something that requires unrealistic effort, a lot of deprivation, or too much time?
- What do you need to learn or practice to do it correctly?
- Is it going to inconvenience or annoy anyone else?
- Is it something very specific and observable and not merely a thought or a feeling?
- Is it *enjoyable?*

Health habit suggestions coming from Family Circle should be easy to implement and do. The path to better family health should be filled with livable and enjoyable steps that don't require enormous willpower or deprivation to sustain.

X

LIGHTEN UP!

What is life without a sense of humor? Family Circle is a wonderful opportunity to teach the whole family they can have fun as a family and do something important for themselves. Family Circle has to be light, not confrontative. It should be dessert, not vegetables. Try to avoid heavy sessions that leave people with a somber I-must-take-my-medicine attitude. Sometimes you can serve the family a treat at Family Circle, but always try to keep the conversation cheery and upbeat. Ask if anyone has heard a good joke, what's going on in school sports, or if there are suggestions for a good movie to see. Give the family an opportunity to relax with each other, have some fun, and get some business done at the same time.

Remember, Family Circle should be part of family life. If our ten suggestions (Commandments) are followed, the family will enjoy this time together. There is no better way to strengthen family unity than by providing positive and edifying discussion. In the years to come, the warm moments within your Family Circle will create wonderful memories for you and your children. And perhaps your kids will re-create the same experience with their children. And who knows, one day, you may be invited to one of their Family Circles—as a grand-parent!

The Family Circle: A Circle of Solidarity

Besides implementing your own clan's program for better health, the weekly Family Circle gathering creates a deep-seated feeling of belonging. It demonstrates that families can share openly while caring for one another. It teaches your children the art of compromise and negotiation while refining your own abilities. It will help everyone in your family work together—something they truly may want to do, but may lack practical experience in how to do it—the mechanics. And we hope your Family Circle will start a chain reaction that results in your family beginning to feel like a solid, unified whole. It's a tradition that will warm the hearts of all of you for generations to come.

Now that you know the techniques for making Family Circle a safe place where everyone feels comfortable discussing their concerns, we want to make suggestions to help you with the meeting's procedure.

1. SITUATIONS AND SOLUTIONS
We suggest you begin each meeting with a "How Do We Solve This One?" activity. Keeping it light and upbeat, ask a volunteer to suggest a "situation" and the family to suggest "solutions." If there is no volunteer, the person leading Family Circle should always be prepared with an opening situation that calls for a solution. For example:

The Situation—
DAD: "Every day my assistant brings in doughnuts at coffee-break time. I know I should say "no thanks," but it's tough. How can I keep from pigging out?"

The Suggestions—

DAUGHTER: "Just eat them and then eat less during the rest of the day."

SON: "Why don't you take a walk around the block during your coffee break? That way you'll get some exercise and might even burn off some calories, and you'd get away from the doughnuts."

MOM: "Why don't you ask your assistant to pick up some bran muffins and fruit along with the doughnuts?"

The Solution—

DAD: "You're all more than just pretty faces. You've given me some great ideas. How come I didn't think of them? I like both ideas about a walk and a better snack. Lori, I appreciate your idea, but I know myself well enough to realize that I can't go through the whole day eating less without getting into big trouble. Thanks for the thoughts. I'll let you know next week how it's going."

The Situation—

DAUGHTER: "When I come home from school, there's nothing here to eat. And that's why I buy candy on the way home."

The Suggestions—

MOM: "I usually leave last night's leftovers in plastic dishes in the fridge. It only takes a minute to warm them in the microwave."

SON: "Yuuck! Who wants to eat leftovers?"

DAD: "How about keeping sliced turkey, rolls, and fresh fruit on hand this week for after-school snacks, and next week we'll change it to something else that we've all agreed on?"

The Solution—

SON: "Great idea! I love sliced turkey and how about getting some of those new fruit yogurts?"

2. THE DISCUSSION

Each person has the opportunity to discuss their past week's eating and exercise program. There must be total support and no criticism—only situations and solutions. And don't forget to:

- Encourage everyone to share their situations and solutions.
- Thank everyone for sharing at Family Circle.

■ *THE BETTER LIFE INSTITUTE FAMILY HEALTH PLAN*

- Compliment people on being open and honest.
- Compliment people on being supportive to others at Family Circle.
- Compliment others for being positive and constructive.
- Compliment the group for allowing no jeers from the "peanut gallery."

How's Everyone Doing?

The discussion part of Family Circle focuses on how family members are handling concepts and projects from previous meetings. It's a way of taking the temperature and finding out the status of everyone involved. For example:

The Situation—

MOM: "I'm not exercising every morning before work like I should. I keep finding excuses. What should I do?"

The Suggestions—

SON: "If you're too rushed in the morning, why don't you exercise before dinner?"

The Solution—

DAD: "Good idea, Son! We can all pitch in, set the table, and get things going for you. Just give us some directions. And maybe we'll try to eat out a few days during the week."

The Situation—

SON: "I'm really tired after my morning workouts. They're no fun anymore . . . just boring old endless exercise."

The Suggestions—

MOM: "I've never felt better or slept better than since we started our dawn routine. Let's keep the time slot and change the exercise. We could try some different things to make it more interesting."

The Solution—

DAUGHTER: "Why don't we try some fast walking? My teacher said that race walking is an Olympic sport. I bet we could make it to Logan Square and back in less than an hour."

SON: "Can we take Bruno? I promise I'll keep him on his leash."

3. CLOSING THE MEETING

Ask each family member if there are any other concerns he or she wants to bring up. These can be problems (situations-solutions) or suggestions to other members of the family that someone thinks will help.

- Ask if everyone knows what they need to do in the following week.
- Ask for a volunteer to lead the next Family Circle.
- Confirm the date of the next meeting and ask if anyone has a conflict.

Family Circle should be simple, natural, educational, supportive, and *fun*. Don't try to make Family Circle into "family group therapy." It is not! Family Circle is just a family gathering that is organized to help each family member and have some fun doing it.

Family Circle activities will vary depending on the ages of your family members. If you have children below eight years of age, it is difficult to give them a great deal of responsibility at Family Circle. You always have to use your judgment concerning what your children can do. But, whatever the ages, it's important for your family to plan to have some enjoyable and supportive time together. Develop a new tradition in your family. Your youngsters will fall into the habit very easily, and it will give them a very special sense of closeness at an impressionable age. It will help them develop a "Yes, I can!" attitude.

YES, I CAN!

- I can try to exercise on a regular basis.
- I can try to include other family members in my exercise program.
- I can try to taste new foods to see if I like them.

FAMILY CIRCLE SUGGESTIONS

Discuss inevitable setbacks—weather, schedules, illness, surprises—and how each person will handle them. Get each person involved in helping each other.

Discuss the term *dependability* and what it means to each person.

Start to get some suggestions for some fun weekend activities. Keep a list.

State of the Nation: The Healthy and the Unhealthy

■ ■

Chapter 3

The Ambulance Down in the Valley

'Twas a dangerous cliff, as they frankly confessed,
Though to walk near its crest was so pleasant;
But over its terrible edge there had slipped
A Duke and full many a peasant.
So the people said something would have to be done,
But their projects did not at all dally;
Some said, "Put a fence round the edge of the cliff";
Some, "Put an ambulance down in the valley."

Well, the cry for the ambulance carried the day,
For, it spread through the neighboring city;
A fence may be useful, or not so they say,
But each heart became brimful of pity
For those who had slipped over the dangerous cliff;
And dwellers on highway and in alley
Gave pounds and pence, not to put up a fence,
But an ambulance down in the valley.

"For the cliff is all right if you're careful," they said
"And even if folks slip and are dropping,
It isn't the slip that hurts them so much
As the shock down below when they're stopping."
So day after day as those mishaps occurred,
Quick forth would the rescuers sally
To pick up the victims who fell off the cliff
With their ambulance down in the valley.

Then an old sage remarked, "Tis a marvel to me
That people give far more attention
To repairing the results than to stopping the cause,
When they'd much better aim at prevention.
Let us stop at the source of this mischief," cried he
"Come neighbors and friends, let us rally,
If the cliff we would fence, we could almost dispense
With the ambulance down in the valley."

"Oh, he's a fanatic," the others rejoined;
"Dispense with the ambulance? Never!
He'd dispense with all charity, too, if he could.
No! No! We'll support them forever.
Aren't we picking up people as fast as they fall?
Shall this man dictate to us—shall he?
Why should people with sense stop to put up a fence
While an ambulance waits in the valley?"

Anonymous

THE BETTER LIFE INSTITUTE FAMILY HEALTH PLAN

Anyone landing on our soil for the first time is impressed with the physical stature of Americans. Not only are we generally tall, but we're relatively big people compared to others who inhabit our planet. Since foreigners expect most of our men to look like a Tom Selleck or a Robert Redford and our women to resemble Meryl Streep or Madonna, they are often surprised to see us as we really are. Some of us have ample thighs, chins, bellies, and rear ends, which clearly proclaim that we're a "land of plenty" in more ways than one. We Americans have been blessed with a bounty that ranges from sea to shining sea—and most of us show it! Regardless of age or financial status, we have become victims of overabundance.

In addition, modern technology, which has given us lasers, disk players, cellular phones, and exotic surgeries, has also created an entirely new lifestyle for adults and children. Walking to work or school is almost unheard of these days, and most parents even end up driving their kids to Little League practice. American lifestyles have changed radically since the days of our forefathers. Instead of chopping, farming, or lifting, our work days often consist of sitting and watching a computer screen. We don't get our dairy products from local farmers, nor do we buy our produce freshly picked from the field. On holidays we fly or drive to family reunions instead of trekking "over the meadow and through the woods to Grandmother's house." Our evolving sedentary, overfed lifestyle has made us prime targets of a new deadly enemy called *degenerative disease*.

Paying the Consequences

As a nation, we pay the proverbial "piper" with a high occurrence of degenerative disease. This alarmingly high rate is directly related to our overflowing dinner plates and lack of regular exercise. The following chart reflects the number of Americans now suffering from these different forms of degenerative disease:

Heart Disease	40,000,000
High Blood Pressure	60,000,000
Adult Onset Diabetes	8,000,000
Overweight	100,000,000
Liver and Kidney Disease	40,000,000
Cancers	10,000,000
Stroke	15,000,000

these categories overlap

These categories overlap one another, which means, for example, we can simultaneously be overweight, have high blood pressure, and be a victim of heart disease. How's that for a triple threat? We're one of the most educated and affluent nations in the world, but we still have one of the highest percentages of life-threatening disease in the Western world. We may look great on the outside, with our designer jeans, expensive athletic shoes, and suntans, but as we all know, looks can be deceiving.

THE MANY FACETS OF MODERN MEDICINE

As John Naisbitt notes in his book *Megatrends,* "We live in a time of transition." Naisbitt refers to the current challenge to America's dominant role as the leading political and economic power in the world today. But we face a similar challenge in the areas of disease prevention and health. This is a time of transition from the old days of "cut and bleed" to the "medicine" of food and exercise. We now hear about alternative medicine where many people, those with high blood pressure, adult onset diabetes, or high cholesterol, for example, are using exercise and diet to control their illnesses without using medication.

Unquestionably we have the most effective, advanced medical treatment system in the world. But the challenges facing you and your family may be different from what you think. Modern medicine cannot cure all the diseases you and your children can have today and may face tomorrow. However, even as medical science rapidly progresses, it is in our best self-interests to stay as healthy as we can in order to be around to take advantage of the improvements and techniques of the future. The subject of this book is "take charge"— you can take the responsibility to keep yourself and your family healthy by putting primary emphasis on diet and exercise.

The Way It Was vs. The Way It Is

Modern science and medical technology have virtually eliminated our traditional killers. We no longer suffer and die from most infectious diseases, malnutrition, and unsanitary drinking water. Improved sanitation, public health programs, drugs, and vaccination and inoculation programs have wiped out smallpox, typhoid, typhus, tuberculosis, intestinal diseases, and countless other infections. We live longer now with an average life expectancy of 75 (men) and 82 (women) years, quite a change from a hundred years ago when life expectancy averaged 55 to 65 years. But, there are other aspects to the story which you will soon understand. When you do, you'll see

THE BETTER LIFE INSTITUTE FAMILY HEALTH PLAN

why a turkey-burger and a pair of sneakers are important players in "high-tech" preventive medicine.

Although it sounds like science fiction, some experts now agree we have the biological potential to live to the ripe old age of 100! But most of us want to live that long only if we can lead full and active lives. Remembering there are no guarantees in life and that anything that's worthwhile requires effort, we want to help you get started on the road to a fulfilling old age.

GETTING TO KNOW THE NEW ENEMY

The major killers and cripplers in America are now heart disease, high blood pressure, stroke, diabetes, liver and kidney disease, and cancer. They are very different from tuberculosis, typhoid fever, smallpox, polio, and all the other infectious diseases that troubled our society a few years ago. These "new" diseases are not caused by little microbes attacking our systems. And, they are not treatable by drugs that kill the germs or viruses that cause them.

These new illnesses are degenerative or "aging" diseases. They actually age, or *degenerate,* your body, and whether it's premature or not, aging can't be cured. But, IT CAN BE SLOWED DOWN! Our new enemy must be treated differently from the way past generations treated the old enemies. The length and quality of the lives of all of us depend on it.

Some Things You Need to Know About Degenerative Disease

Let's pretend you just bought a shiny, new compact car. But, when they deliver it, you realize they made a mistake on the assembly line. They put the chassis (the entire body including the seat and roof) of a mid-sized car on top of the frame of your little compact car. What do you think will happen to your compact frame, suspension system, tires, engine fuel pump, fuel lines, and shock absorbers? All the parts especially designed for a compact are going to wear out and age, or *degenerate,* very quickly with supporting a chassis that is too heavy to carry. You won't get much mileage on your new car.

BIG POUNDS CAN LEAD TO AGING PROBLEMS

That's exactly what happens to your body when you put forty extra pounds on a frame meant to carry a smaller or compact load. It simply wears out and ages, or degenerates, and you won't get even decent "mileage" on it! You can trade in your car, but unfortunately,

The great publicity given to such spectacular medical procedures as open heart surgery and organ transplants tends to make us forget that many of these patients would not have been hospitalized if preventive measures had not been severely neglected.

John Knowles, M.D.
Rockefeller Foundation

We are left with the same roster of common major diseases which confronted us in 1950. The accumulation of knowledge is not yet sufficient to permit the prevention or outright cure of any of them.

Lewis Thomas, M.D.
Memorial Sloan-Kettering
Cancer Center

you can't trade in your body. That's why being overweight is considered a degenerative disease. It's not just a cosmetic problem, especially since the wearing down of your body often doesn't show on the outside. It happens *internally*. It's a health problem because you'll age and wear out before your time!

Suppose you put sugar or fat in your gas tank. Your fuel lines would clog and crack. The chemical change would age the rubber, and it would harden and crack under the constant pressure. Your car would not run, or if it did, it would always cause you problems.

In your body the blood vessels deliver nutrients and life-giving oxygen to your cells. They are your body's fuel lines. When these fuel lines get clogged or cracked, the target organs and tissue to which they deliver nutrients and oxygen do not get the right amount of fuel or the correct octane level. That is why it is important to keep your fuel lines healthy, which means maintaining the proper levels of cholesterol, fat (triglycerides), and sugar (glucose) in your bloodstream. If these values are too high, they lead to premature clogging and cracking of your body's fuel lines, your arteries. If your blood vessels age prematurely, even though you may be only forty you'll have the arteries and the organs and tissue of a fifty-five year old.

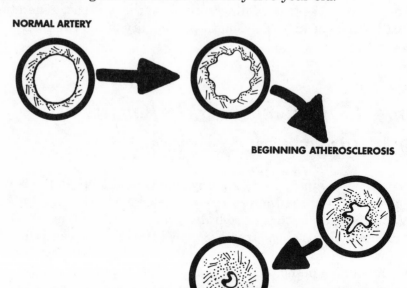

NORMAL ARTERY

BEGINNING ATHEROSCLEROSIS

ADVANCED ATHEROSCLEROSIS

EXACTLY WHAT IS DEGENERATIVE DISEASE?
Very simply, degenerative disease is "fuel-line disease" that results in your body parts aging or degenerating much more quickly than

THE BETTER LIFE INSTITUTE FAMILY HEALTH PLAN

they should and, usually, too early in life. When fuel lines from your heart harden or get stopped up, we call it heart disease. (Atherosclerosis is *clogging* of the arteries, while arteriosclerosis is *hardening* of the arteries.)

If fuel lines to your brain are clogged, you are at risk for cerebrovascular disease, known as stroke or transient ischemic attack (TIA). Adult onset diabetes is a disease that weakens the large and small blood vessels. Diabetics usually suffer from poor circulation to the eyes, major organs, and extremities such as arms, fingers, legs, and toes. Liver disease and kidney disease are manifested when the blood supply to those vital organs is diminished. Sight, hearing, even the wrinkling of your skin are all related to the basic and common process of aging or *fuel-line delivery disease.*

If your "engine," your heart, is not being fueled correctly, it has to work harder. When the fuel lines harden and get cracked or clogged, your heart is forced to pump with greater pressure. We call this *hypertension,* which is also known as high blood pressure. If your body is too big for your pump and fuel lines, your blood pressure is likely elevated.

Thus, our bodies' fuel lines go to and from our hearts delivering the essentials for life to all organs, muscles, and cells. When these vital vessels aren't working properly and aren't doing an efficient job, the cells, muscles, and organs will wear out and age, or degenerate, thus the term *degenerative disease.*

Do you take better care of your car than you do of your body?

Your car will eventually wear out, no matter how well you take care of it. But you would feel cheated if you bought a new car and got only twenty-five thousand miles on it before it broke down permanently. If you had known that would happen, you probably would have taken much better care of your car. You might have used a better grade of fuel or oil and you would have paid more attention to maintaining the brakes, plugs, pistons, and shocks. Or you just might have traded it in at twenty thousand miles.

This comparison is important to remember when you think about your body. We've already established the fact that your body is one item in your life you can't trade in. As a practical wise man would say, "What you've got is what you've got" and all you've got. Of course, you can repair it, but it would be better to think about preventive maintenance. "Take care" is better than repair.

Many of the degenerative diseases we suffer, and our children will likely suffer, are caused by fuel-line delivery disease. The chart below describes the aging process and the array of biological consequences. In some ways you should consider your body a network of blood vessels searching for a disease.

■ **Car Maintenance**

■ *Use correct fuel?*

■ *Keep your mileage low?*

■ *Maintain tire pressure?*

■ *Use the right oil and get regular oil changes?*

■ *Check brakes?*

■ *Check fluid levels?*

■ *Clean and wax regularly?*

■ **Body Maintenance**

■ *Fill up with nutritious food?*

■ *Take opportunities to slow your pace?*

■ *Maintain the proper blood pressure?*

■ *Keep your weight at a healthy level?*

■ *Exercise regularly and wisely?*

■ *Care for your skin?*

■ *Get proper rest?*

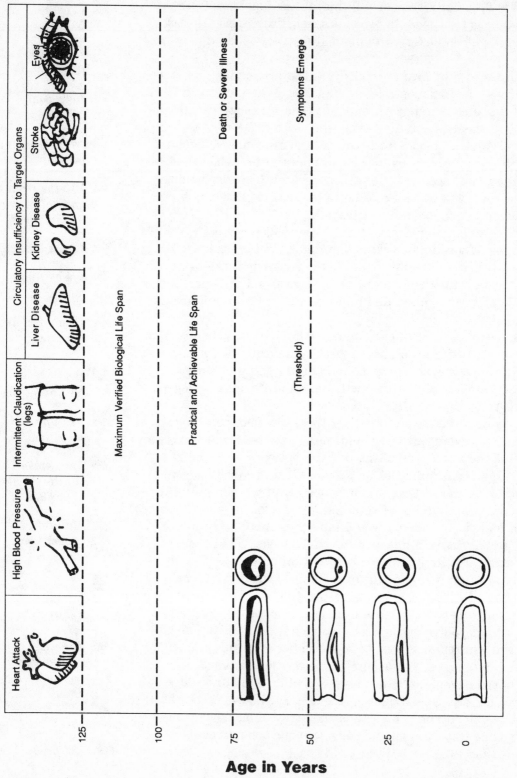

Blood vessel disease, Circulatory disease, Degenerative disease, Cardiovascular disease - are all diseases of premature aging...They're all essentially the same!

YOUR CHILD AND DEGENERATIVE DISEASE

It is often said, "The child is the father of the man." What we are taught as children often sets the course for the rest of our lives. We all agree that parents provide their children with their basic values: the difference between right and wrong, honesty, morality, humility, compassion, charity, and courage. We also learn from our folks other important social values such as the importance of family, community, achievement, and friendship.

But what about health? Isn't a child's current and future health as important as any of the other areas of parental concern? If nutrition had been given more attention when you were a child, you certainly would have acquired a very different set of eating habits.

We look at our slim, active children and think they are pictures of health. Yet inside their bodies are the beginnings of blood vessel or degenerative disease. Now, we don't want to strike fear in your heart, but this is a fact that must be recognized and accepted. It's true. Children's eating habits have changed considerably over the last few years, and you'd be surprised, well, *alarmed* by some of the scientific assessments of the status of their health.

Some studies suggest that one in four children, ages five to sixteen has at least one elevated risk factor (cholesterol, triglycerides, or weight) for heart disease. One of the reasons is that the number of children engaging in regular exercise programs has decreased significantly. Gone are the "good old days" when kids came home from school every day and "chose up sides" for a game of baseball, football, or basketball. Everybody played, brawled, or did something active in the rain or sunshine, summer and winter.

We estimate today that by the age of twelve only 12 percent of our kids engage in regular athletic activity. Instead they're usually inside watching television. Our children consume too much sugar in cereals and soft drinks and too much fat in the fast foods that are so popular. We parents did not grow up with Ho-Ho's, Dippy Do's, Slurpee's, and Whoppers. But today's children are, and their cholesterol levels are on the rise. A recent survey of Louisiana children revealed that at twelve years of age 25 percent have fatty deposits in their arteries. Other studies estimate that as many as 35 percent of our children of all ages have an elevated cholesterol (above 140 mg/dl) and predict that most of these kids will carry it into adulthood.

In the mid 1950s, the Framingham Heart Study established that blood vessel disease occurs in our youngsters. In other studies doctors had the opportunity to examine the blood vessels of American soldiers aged eighteen to twenty-seven who had died in battle during the Korean War. Blood vessel disease among G.I.'s was compared with that of a similar number of Korean soldiers in the same age range. The investigators were surprised to find that about 75 percent of the young Americans had significant blood vessel deposits while the Korean soldiers' blood vessels were clear. Ironically, our young men appeared to be fit and strong, but actually they were well on the way toward premature death due to degenerative disease. Our children could well be on the same unfortunate track unless we decide to take some action.

BLI and many other health organizations recommend a maximum blood cholesterol of 190 mg/dl. beyond age sixteen, regardless of age or sex, and below 150 mg/dl. for children under sixteen.

NATIONAL BLOOD CHOLESTEROL LEVELS

AGE RANGE	RECOMMENDED GOAL LEVEL	MODERATE RISK LEVEL	HIGH RISK LEVEL
2–19	180*	200	220
20–29	200	220	240
30–39	200	240	260

*Mg/dl.

Source: National Heart, Lung, and Blood Institute

The recommended cholesterol values shown in the adjoining chart are national goals suggested by the National Heart, Lung, and Blood Institute. We suggest a more aggressive approach given the wealth of information that documents a powerful relationship of blood cholesterol and fat with blood vessel disease. The Better Life Institute along with many other health-oriented organizations recommends a maximum blood cholesterol value of 190 mg/dl. beyond age sixteen, regardless of age or sex, and below 150 mg/dl. for children under sixteen. The lower your blood cholesterol values the "safer" you are from increased risk of blood vessel disease. The values we recommend seem safe and practical for most Americans. We have solid evidence from Mediterranean countries with similar eating habits that these levels of cholesterol are achievable from a practical point of view. There is too much evidence concerning the effect of blood cholesterol values and health for you to be "easy" or casual about the eating habits of your family. New evidence suggests that in the future the problems of blood vessel disease will be more complex than assessing only your cholesterol level. Genetics and many subtle chemical indicators in your body will play an increasingly important role in diagnosing and treating blood vessel problems. But for the time being altering your eating habits in order to control your blood cholesterol levels is a practical and important place for your family to start. With the Better Life Institute program you and your family will eat more plant food and less beef, lamb, pork, veal, and whole milk dairy products. The payoff will be less dietary fat, lower cholesterol, more fiber, and fewer calories. You can't go wrong!

We all know the pain and difficulty of trying to change our eat-

THE BETTER LIFE INSTITUTE FAMILY HEALTH PLAN

ing habits. Changing these patterns of behavior is as difficult for adults as it is for children. You can't change the past, but you can change the present and ultimately the future. Since good eating and exercise habits start at home and not in school, parents (not teachers) need to set an example for healthy living. There is no better way to improve your own health than by showing your children how they can live better!

CANCER IS ALSO A DEGENERATIVE DISEASE

Cancer is described as a degenerative or aging disease because it usually occurs in the later stages of life. Medical researchers think that repeated exposure year after year to cancer-causing agents, called *carcinogens,* and free radicals and the resulting damage to body organs and tissue, increases our risk of cancer. At this time we don't know the true causes of cancer, but scientists agree that reducing exposure to known carcinogenic "triggers" is an excellent way to diminish the risk. The accompanying chart describes the general lifestyle factors related to cancer.

WHAT CAUSES CANCER?

PERCENTAGE OF CANCER DEATHS FROM VARIOUS FACTORS

Food	35%	Alcohol	3%
Tobacco	30%	Pollution	2%
Occupation	4%	Food Additives	1%

Source: American Institute of Cancer Research, 1986

Food is related to cancer risk in several ways. All cancer research organizations suggest that high-fat foods increase cancer risk. They also assert that foods high in fiber reduce cancer risk. In general, plant foods are higher in fiber and lower in fat content; animal food has no fiber, contains cholesterol, and usually has high fat content. That's why we have begun to emphasize the role that fruit, vegetables, whole grains, beans, and peas play in reducing the risk of all blood vessel diseases as well as certain cancers. By emphasizing plant food in your diet, you get a two-for-one pay off! You get a three-for-one with dark, leafy green, orange, and yellow foods. Their antioxidants help prevent cancer.

You've Come a Long Way, Baby!

For many years research suggested that women have lower heart disease rates than men. The joke went that if you want to reduce your risk of heart disease, be a woman! However, recent scientific evidence runs counter to this previously well-accepted assumption. Several major medical groups—the American Heart Association, the University of Massachusetts, Rochester University, and Duke University—have conducted studies which show that while men do suffer more heart attacks than women, women who have had heart attacks are more likely to die or suffer a repeat attack than men. We have had "Women's Lib" in the work place, now we seem to be having "Biological Lib" in the area of health. With increased rates of smoking, obesity, and stress and a decrease in exercise activities, women now have the privilege of having a lot of the "good things" that men have!

LONGEVITY AND VIGOR WHILE SLOWING THE AGING PROCESS

Yes, eventually your body will degenerate. But, remember, some scientists believe that you can have 100 vigorous years before that happens. Most Americans are lucky if they can get seventy vigorous years from their bodies and when they do, it's a biological miracle if they can remember their own address! We believe that if you take proper care of your body by observing a preventive maintenance program, you'll be around to enjoy productive and fulfilling senior years. You should be able to remember your address and even recall your grandchildren's names without stuttering when you're over 100 years old.

ESTIMATED PROPORTIONAL CONTRIBUTION TO PREMATURE DEATH

	LIFESTYLE	GENETICS	MEDICAL SERVICES
Heart Disease	63.0	25.0	12.0
Cancer	61.0	29.0	10.0
Stroke	72.0	21.0	7.0
Liver Disease	79.0	18.0	3.0
Diabetes	34.0	60.0	6.0

Source: Stanford Heart Disease Prevention Program Newsletter

Several years ago, the Stanford Heart Disease Prevention Program Newsletter published a table that provides an estimate of what factors contribute to premature death. You'll notice the incredible influence that *lifestyle* has on health. (A nearly 35 percent effect on diabetes is still pretty effective.) You may be surprised at what the table reveals about genetics and medical services. While geneticists are making breakthrough discoveries splicing and identifying faulty

THE BETTER LIFE INSTITUTE FAMILY HEALTH PLAN

genes in the laboratory, at this time there's not much we can do about our genetic disposition. Physicians, hospitals, and other medical services are very important when you get one of these diseases, but generally we can't cure them. Usually we can only patch things up. The real trick is to avoid getting one of them in the first place.

Overhauling Your Eating Habits

ALL SYSTEMS GO

It's not as confusing as it might seem. Actually it's very simple since there are no inconsistencies. There are some easy nutritional guidelines that cover *all* the degenerative diseases. The nice part is that even if you are concerned with just one health problem, for example, overweight, you get the bonus of reducing your risk for all other degenerative diseases that you or your family may encounter.

Because a child's digestive system is much smaller than an adult's, you should encourage your child to eat a healthy diet with fiber in it, but not in the amounts that an adult eats. Ask your pediatrician for guidance.

SOME VERY BASIC GUIDELINES

- Eat chicken, fish, seafood, and lean meats in moderate portions.
- Use lower fat dairy products, such as cheese or ice cream, made with skim milk.
- Use monounsaturated fats (canola, olive, and peanut oils) in cooking whenever possible and tub-type spreads only when absolutely necessary (in our opinion they never are).
- Use snack foods that are calorie, fat, and sugar reduced.
- Use fat and sugar reduced products whenever possible.
- When in doubt, eat a plant!

Don't be frightened by what appears to be a complete overhaul of your family's eating habits. Fortunately for Mom, gone forever are the days of preparing the family's food while slaving over a hot stove. It is no longer necessary to spend hours boiling, baking, grinding, and chopping. You probably won't even find the family cook using a rolling pin or flour sifter to make home-baked goodies. Using the Better Life Institute program, the key skills for family nutrition are knowing how to shop properly, read a food package label, combine prepared foods healthfully, and become both an efficient and healthy cook. A considerable portion of this book is devoted to showing you the practicalities of "Better Life" eating. (See Chapter 9.)

We encourage you to prepare simpler, faster meals. We are not dedicated to making you an award-winning nutritional "chef de cui-

TO IMPROVE YOUR HEALTH

	STROKE	HIGH BLOOD PRESSURE	DIABETES	OBESITY	LUNG CANCER	BREAST CANCER	LIVER DISEASE
Reduce Dietary Intake							
Total fat	X	X	X	X		X	X
Saturated fat	X	X	X	X		X	X
Cholesterol	X						
Salt or sodium		X					
Alcohol	X	X	X	X		X	X
Sugar	X	X	X	X			
Calories	X	X	X	X (if overweight)		X (if overweight)	X
Meat, dairy, eggs	X	X	X	X		X	X
Increase Dietary Intake							
Fiber	X	X	X	X		X	X
All plant foods	X	X	X	X		X	X
Aerobic exercise	X	X	X	X			
Smoking cessation	X	X	X		X	X	

As you can observe for yourself, many of the health actions recommended by scientists are common to the prevention and treatment of all the major killer diseases. It's no coincidence that by helping yourself in one area, you're improving your health in all areas.

sine." We are planning only to help you cook easy, fast, tasty, healthy meals for the entire family.

Good eating habits will reduce the risk factors for degenerative disease for every family member—from child to grandparent. That is why we place so much emphasis on the nutrition-related factors that are associated with good health: proper weight, healthy blood pressure, and lower levels of blood cholesterol, triglyceride, and sugar. Along with regular exercise, it's an unbeatable program to reduce risk for degenerative disease.

Besides having different taste preferences, each member of your family has different health needs. Whether high blood pressure, diabetes, or many excess pounds, The Better Life Institute Family Health Program is scientifically sound and medically safe no matter what your health needs. We invite you to make this plan the map for your journey toward better family health and effective disease prevention.

YES, I CAN

- I can change what I mean when I say "mess up" to "what do I have to do to improve?"
- I can say "I've decided," rather than "I have to."
- I can help prepare at least one family meal during the week.

FAMILY CIRCLE SUGGESTIONS

Everyone has "tough days." So will everyone in your family. Rather than have a "feel sorry for me" attitude, ask them exactly what went wrong and what they think they can do to improve or how to avoid the situation the next time.

Sometimes someone in the family is in a bad mood and is grumpy or negative to others in the family. If this happens at Family Circle ask the person to just tell everyone "I'm in a bad mood, please be patient with me." Have the one who is feeling moody tell others that they are not to blame and say "It's not you, but me, and I apologize for the mood."

Ask your spouse whether he or she is getting the support needed from the rest of the family. Make sure your spouse is specific and phrases any concerns or comments in a positive way.

Nutritional Recommendations for Good Health and Weight Control

Chapter

4

■ ■

If life is a journey, then life's greatest tragedy is not having enjoyed the trip.

God, motherhood, and apple pie are the symbols of all that is good in America and certainly part and parcel of family life and health. In this section we'll set God aside for the time being (He needs a separate discussion), and concentrate a little on motherhood and a lot on apple pie.

You can't turn on the TV or radio or read a newspaper or magazine without someone telling you more about nutrition and health. Whether the topic is weight control, cholesterol, fiber, fat, sugar, or salt, we are knee deep in nutrition education and ways to cook healthy. We have become almost immune to ads touting the miraculous transformation of pouting husbands and children into beaming ecstatic converts after they are exposed to a breakfast cereal that snaps or crunches and "doesn't taste like breakfast cereal." The media assault us with statements like "makes you regular," "lowers your cholesterol," "good for the kids," "the right thing to do," "ask any doctor," "Mama says, 'It's good—eat it!'" "you can be both wonder mom and wonder wife," and "Bo, Bubba, and Bif know."

Actually, Bo, Bubba, and Bif don't know, but *you* should take the time to find out. The nutrition information explosion has helped make you aware of the need to improve your own and your family's eating habits, but how can you make sense of all the nutrition recommendations and product claims you hear about? All you want is a "pathway" of eating that is more healthful, easy to prepare, and tastes good. *It's a challenge!*

Parents Are the Best Teachers

For better or for worse parents will always be the most significant influence in their children's lives. It's a role you just can't ignore.

There are certain responsibilities in life that are biologically and culturally destined. Mothering and fathering are such roles. We recognize our parental responsibilities in certain areas without much effort. We never doubt our responsibility to provide food, clothing, and shelter for our children. And most of us accept our roles as "shepherd" and counselor. In general, most parents would agree that their children's health is a concern.

We never doubt for a moment our responsibility when our children are sick. We're right there with doctor visits and medication for colds and sore throats. But as parents, it's also important to teach our children good eating and exercise habits, to check out what the kids eat at school, to make sure they are getting all the vitamins and minerals they need for growing bodies. In a nutshell, health is part and parcel of how we all live every day.

Better Eating: It's Come of Age!

America is crossing a new frontier in its commitment to the relationship between food and health. Until now food was merely "food." Today, due to a rather substantial research base, food is something you put in your mouth and if you are not careful, you'll wear it tomorrow around your mid-section or in your arteries. New, more health-oriented foods are pouring onto grocery shelves. Truth in labeling laws are now being crafted. The restaurant industry is trying to keep up with a more health conscious customer. Vitamin and mineral research and food supplement use have reached unprecedented heights. Our food scientists are now starting to genetically alter plants and food molecules to create more healthy foods for us to eat. We are living in a new age!

THE HEALTH NUT BECOMES THE HEALTH CONSCIOUS CONSUMER

Ten years ago if you made a decision to improve your eating and exercise habits, your friends would place you in the "strange health nut" group. You had to buy special foods in health food stores. Supermarkets had special "health food" sections. The foods were lackluster, had exotic ingredients, cost a lot, and were packaged as if they were to be sent to institutions and convalescent homes. Ten years ago if your exercise was recreational—tennis, golf, racquetball—you raised no eyebrows. If you jogged or used aerobic equipment, people thought you were either verging on the fanatical or had special physical rehabilitation needs. Any use of vitamins and minerals over and above a one-a-day multivitamin and mineral was deemed "eccentric," perhaps dangerous.

WHERE IS THE HEART-HEALTHY FOOD?
Today, the supermarket is the only place one needs to go for more healthy foods. It is hard to find a supermarket that does not have hundreds of the new health conscious foods on the shelves. They are merely part of the regular products for sale. They are tasty, attractively packaged, easily prepared, and competitively priced. The abundant and ever-growing selection available makes acquiring better eating habits routine, enjoyable, and adventurous. Whether young or old, gourmet cook or take-out-food addict, there are thousands of wonderful foods available to you and your family. It's a "field of flowers," and all you have to do is go out there and "pick 'em"!

The Chinese from the province of Canton say that eating is the only source of pleasure man can enjoy throughout his entire life. Eating is also a wonderful family activity. There is no need today to sacrifice the pleasures of eating at home or in restaurants for either parent or child. We have progressed to the prepared-food phase for health-oriented foods and side dishes. Lines of "lite" seasonings and salad dressings, mayos, jams, cereals, and desserts are matter of fact. And the word that people used to associate with "junk food," *carbohydrate,* has been redeemed and placed at the top of the health list.

At the same time, fast food businesses are also making a healthy change. You can walk into any fast food emporium and sample from the salad bar or the taco bar and have a baked potato and a chicken sandwich as well. Pasta, turkey sandwiches, low and nonfat yogurts, and diet drinks can be ordered without anyone raising an eyebrow. Restaurants carry heart-healthy low calorie and low fat selections, or they will prepare your dish to your specifications without sacrificing taste. Kids can have just as good a time eating out as parents, and still choose from an array of heart-healthy selections.

THE CHALLENGE OF CHANGE
We, as parents, need to teach our children better eating and exercise habits. If you start with your kids early in their lives, you'll find it's easier. The best way to teach your children is to set the example yourself.

■ *50% of all leading deaths in the U.S. are lifestyle related.*

Source: National Institute of Medicine, 1987.

■ *Diet is the key to wiping out the epidemic of heart disease in this country.*

Today I eat defensively. Fish, pasta, vegetables, fruits, and cereal grains are the staples of my diet.

William Castelli, M.D. National Heart, Lung, and Blood Institute, 1986

DO AS I SAY; DO AS I DO

There are some easy ways to sift through the maze of nutritional recommendations, products, and recipes and provide healthy and enjoyable eating for everyone. It's not as confusing or overwhelming as you might think. Our experience with people who are interested in changing their eating habits suggests they have accepted its importance, but they really don't know enough specifics about food, health, and weight control. We are here to help you learn. That's what this book is all about.

We want you to know why you are taking this journey and what your destination is. We want the trip to be an enjoyable and meaningful one. And the journey can be one that brings your family closer together. An important thing to remember is the best way to teach your children is to show them.

The following section should give you a clear idea of why food is extremely important to health. In it we will describe in detail the approach to nutrition we take. We will discuss our nutrition strategy from several points of view that include parent and child, specific health, and weight loss concerns.

Family Eating: The Better Life Point of View

A healthy diet is of no help to you and your family unless you use it on a *lifelong* basis. The "best diet," from the Better Life Institute point of view, is one that is effective, livable, and enjoyable. Overly restrictive, unpalatable diets, no matter how healthful, are short-term and practically useless. What do we mean by "effective, livable, and enjoyable"?

EFFECTIVE

Effective nutrition means "it hits the nail on the head." Whether your needs are weight loss, blood pressure control, lower cholesterol, fat reduction, or all-around healthy living, your new program can do the job in a reasonable amount of time. Effective nutrition also means that the nutritional content of your eating program is medically safe: You do not expose yourself to new risks because you are eating differently. With the BLI programs your new health plan will be *effective*.

LIVABLE

The comment from our graduates that gives us the most pleasure is, "I can live with this." If you or your children can't live with the eating program you select, it is of no use. Many people make the mistake of selecting a diet or an eating program that is overly restrictive and very aggressive. In their enthusiasm to lose weight or improve their health, they want "the best." If you can afford the best, you can buy the finest TV, car, or vacuum cleaner on the market. There's no obligation other than to pay for it. But, the best diet or eating program has far different consequences. You pay for it, but you cannot buy it. You have to shop for it, cook it, and most important, *eat it!* You can't pay anyone else to eat it for you!

Livable means using the Better Life Program at home, at work, and at play. *Livable* means it's easy to prepare. *Livable* means you can go out to eat with your friends in any restaurant in the country and not order steamed vegetables and a piece of broiled fish. *Livable* means your children have variety in their school lunches and they can eat at their friends' homes without being self-conscious. *Livable* means nobody has to take special foods, books, scales, calculators, or other weight control paraphernalia with them wherever they go. *Livable* means that when you are out with your friends, you will not attract their attention or make them uncomfortable. No one has to do anything out of the ordinary that makes the dining experience an evening they'd "rather forget."

If you follow the BLI programs, your family nutrition plan will be *livable*.

ENJOYABLE
Lulu says, "If it ain't fun or real tasty, it ain't worth eatin'!"

Everyone looks forward to food. We find food to be one of life's highlights. There is no reason why you and the kids should not truly enjoy your food and a healthy family life. All the recipes and food hints provided in this book are designed for your complete enjoyment because we don't believe food should be merely acceptable. We believe it can and should be healthy and enjoyable.

Most people associate "eating more healthfully" with a boring, lackluster diet, something like charging outside to eat your lawn. Nothing could be further from the truth. But you have to know how to shop intelligently and prepare foods that tickle the palate and tantalize the taste buds. It's getting easier every week as new, more easily prepared foods appear in the grocery stores.

Eating out is one of the most enjoyable occasions for the family. Once you learn how to "survive and thrive" in a restaurant or fast food store, you'll be able to eat anywhere you choose, with no exceptions.

And you'll find the food as well as the experience *enjoyable*.

Effectiveness, livability, and *enjoyment* are the three conditions that must be met in your new family health program. There must be no compromises. Your program is for a lifetime, and it is designed to improve family life. It can do this only if everyone looks forward to it and enjoys the experience.

OURS IS A 60 PERCENT SOLUTION

Think of your BLI plan as a practical, effective 60 percent solution! In your impatience you may be thinking that only doing 60 percent is not enough. Our experience with thousands of families over the years has shown us that 60 percent of success with a plan that brings pleasure is far better than the frustration of 100 percent of nothing. Going for 60 percent for a lifetime instead of 100 percent for three weeks will keep you on your program for good. Be smart about your health program and keep it *effective, livable,* and always *enjoyable*—forever.

The Facts of Diet-Health Relationships

There is absolutely no doubt that the food you eat every day directly affects your health and that of your children. A wealth of scientific evidence has established that heart disease, high blood pressure, diabetes, stroke, certain cancers, and being overweight are diet related. You read about it every day in the newspapers, and you hear about it regularly on television.

■ **A Nation of Dieters**

■ *65 million of 240 million people are on a diet.*

■ *47% of women and 25% of men claim to be on a diet.*

■ *27% of women and 24% of men are overweight.*

Source: Food Marketing Institute

Weight Control: The BLI Lower-Calorie Program

There are no special nutritional secrets for weight control. We will not try to convince you that any special combination of foods known by the names of cities, states, prominent physicians, celebrities, universities, or letters of the alphabet will do something magical for you. For those of you who have been a "professional dieter," we want you to know that there is only one way out of your weight problem. You simply must change the foods you eat and the way you exercise for the rest of your life. Your native intelligence should have told you that the special "quick and easy," "down and dirty" claims and promises made by diets, pills, and gadgets are hype and nothing more. But some of us want to believe those claims simply because we want to believe there is an easy way out.

■ *THE BETTER LIFE INSTITUTE FAMILY HEALTH PLAN*

GETTING OUT OF THE GET-SLIM RACE

The most important measure of a dietary program is not how much weight you can lose in the shortest amount of time. Still many people need to get that immediate gratification of having their friends compliment them on taking off so much weight "in no time flat." Sometimes they starve themselves thinking they're in some kind of race. Generally, when you take off weight too fast, your program is unhealthy and unrealistic, and the weight will return at the same rapid clip. Sometimes it will come back faster. On the other hand, you are just being smart if you adhere to a low-calorie (not lowest-calorie) plan that is safe, livable, enjoyable, and *works* throughout your life.

The Better Life Nutrition Program lays no claim to any special nutritional and scientific wizardry. No one can claim that, and you should know it by now. What we do claim is to make eating and exercising "sing," to make them an enjoyable part of your life. Kids and parents can eat together and enjoy the same food. Everyone has the opportunity to learn safe, healthful, delicious ways to eat—for a lifetime!

1990 ACCEPTABLE WEIGHTS FOR MEN AND WOMEN

HEIGHT*	19 TO 34 YEARS**	35 YEARS AND OLDER**
5'0"	97–128	108–138
5'1"	101–132	111–143
5'2"	104–137	115–148
5'3"	107–141	119–152
5'4"	111–146	122–157
5'5"	114–150	126–162
5'6"	118–155	130–167
5'7"	121–160	134–172
5'8"	125–164	138–178
5'9"	129–169	142–183
5'10"	132–174	146–188
5'11"	136–179	151–194
6'	140–184	155–199
6'1"	144–189	159–205
6'2"	148–195	164–210

*without shoes   **without clothes

I'M STARVING, SO WHAT'S FOR DINNER?

Starving yourself to achieve maximum weight loss guarantees that in a short time you will return to your old eating habits. Severe re-

■ *Heart attacks are twice as likely for overweight people as for normal-weight people.*

■ *Excerpts from magazine advertisements regarding new "technology" for dieters:*

■ *Tablets made of pond scum*

■ *Capsules made of the urine of pregnant women*

■ *Small whips to hit yourself with when you eat too much*

■ *Coffee enemas (caffeinated)*

■ *Plastic suits to suspend yourself upside down to "displace" fat*

■ *Pills that "eat fat" while you sleep*

striction of your caloric intake is also unhealthy from a nutritional point of view. You need a certain amount of protein, fat, and carbohydrate to sustain your biological needs. Repeated weight loss from fad diets is merely an attempt at "cheap" shortcuts to avoid facing what you truly know you must face: lifelong change in eating and related health habits.

How many calories should you eat? All basal metabolism calculations are "guestimates." Rather than dealing with the complexities of basal metabolism calculations, we suggest a *daily minimum* of 1200 calories for women and 1500 calories for men beyond age sixteen.

And you don't need an exercise physiologist to design your exercise program. Just walk about twenty to thirty minutes a day at a brisk pace. Do it at least four times a week. You can buy a fancy pair of jogging shoes, color coordinated with aerodynamic heels, or you can use a comfortable pair of shoes. The result is the same. If you want some variety in your exercise, there are lots of different activities which we'll discuss in Chapters 7 and 8. It is important that you discuss your or your children's exercise program with your physician and select a safe, but effective, one together.

CALORIE INTAKE AND KIDS

Kids are "growing up." Too many of us are "growing out." A child's nutritional needs for full growth potential are different from an adult's. What children need nutritionally for proper growth and development is an appropriate amount of healthy, well-balanced calories. It is absolutely mandatory that you consult your pediatrician before ever putting your child on any kind of a nutrition program that is calorie restrictive.

Before the age of two, children need more fat in their diets for the maturation of their nervous systems. That is why mother's milk is 50 percent fat. After age two, your kids can eat the same foods you eat and remain in the 20 percent fat range. Kids need calories to grow; just give them *healthy* calories. The major point to remember when preparing meals for young children is *balance*. Kids need a balance of healthy things to eat even though they may personally desire to eat only "pink" food or refuse to eat things that are "mixed up."

LIKE PARENT, LIKE CHILD

Parents, set the right example for your children! The earlier you expose children to the proper eating habits, the healthier they will be. A slow and steady development of eating habits is most effective. Remember, your child did not come out of the womb with a hamburger in one hand and a piece of cake in the other. Why is it that

Mexican children like tortillas, tacos, and beans and Italian children like pasta and sauces? These "likes" were learned from their parents. This is why we advocate that the entire family eat the same food. All the recipes and food preparation tips in the following sections can be used for your child's weight and nutritional concerns, as well as your own.

WEIGHT GAINS OF AMERICAN CHILDREN

Between the years of 1963 and 1980, the following percentages of children weighed more than the average weight of their age groups.

AGES	PERCENTAGE OF GAIN
6–11	54% increase
12–17	39% increase

The weight control challenge that we usually face with our children, as with ourselves, is *too much of the wrong stuff*. We cannot overemphasize the value of your children seeing you eat as healthfully as you ask them to eat. Experts may argue with the simplicity of this approach, but it is practical and safe. The key is to provide your children with eating habits in their youth that will carry them safely into adulthood. Concentrate on providing them with eating habits that will make their adult lives enjoyable and very, very long.

Better Life Lower-Calorie Eating Habits For the Entire Family

HERE COME THE "CARBS"

The "name of the game" is a *heart-healthy diet*. The way to play the game is to eat more fruits, vegetables, whole grains, beans and peas, chicken, fish, low fat dairy products, fiber, and less sugar. These foods are lower in fat and calories than the usual mix of foods. They will provide more than enough volume while ensuring an intake that is low in calories, fat, cholesterol, sugar, and salt while being high in fiber. This program is generally called a "high complex carbohydrate diet." We're sure you've heard that name before.

Scientifically, it is the best dietary approach available. It is completely safe for all the family. It is also an effective, livable, and enjoyable way to reduce and control your weight and reduce risk factors for degenerative disease at the same time. When you reach your target weight—*slowly and healthfully*—you can increase your caloric intake to approximately 1500 calories or more for women and 1800 or more for men, depending upon individual experience. Just eat a little more of the higher calorie foods. See Chapter 9, Section 4, for caloric values of common foods. And always maintain your regular *aerobic* exercise regimen.

The following chart will aid you in planning your daily food intake:

NUTRITIONAL BREAKDOWN, LOWER CALORIE EATING PROGRAM—1200-1500 CALORIES

- 60% of total calories from carbohydrates
- 20% of total calories from protein
- 20% of total calories from fat
- up to 200 mg cholesterol daily

Colon and prostate cancer are more frequent in overweight men. Uterine and breast cancer occur more often in overweight women.

If you eat more than 1200–1500 calories, you can decrease your protein to 15 percent and increase your carbohydrates to 65 percent of your total calories. This approach is not only safe, it is practical, livable, and enjoyable on a life-long basis. Major medical organizations such as the American Heart Association, the American Medical Association, and the National Heart, Lung, and Blood Institute use similar general guidelines.

HABITS TO PROMOTE WHEN LOSING WEIGHT

- Always plan to eat regularly three times a day. Plan a snack in between meals. Your goal is permanent, lifelong eating habits. This is not a "crash diet" for two weeks.
- Review all the foods we suggest and use the lower calorie items for your weight loss program.
- Never, never eat foods you don't like. You're wasting your time if you do. The trick is to adapt our recipe suggestions to your taste if you don't like them. If your program is to be a permanent one, your food must be enjoyed. But remember that tastes change. What was "yukky" to you when you were twelve might be ambrosia to you at thirty!
- Select very low calorie snacks that you like. Use desserts or beverages with non-sugar or fruit juice sweeteners. Try half a piece of fruit as a snack. There are countless lower calorie snacks on the supermarket shelves and in our recipe section. The trick is to have them available at the right time for the family.
- Always avoid hunger and skipping meals. You tend to be "out of control" if you are hungry. That meal you skipped will be more than compensated for at your next "feeding frenzy."

THE BETTER LIFE INSTITUTE FAMILY HEALTH PLAN

- Once you learn the Better Life Institute food basics, you'll be able to select foods and portion sizes without counting calories. Many people feel they have to count calories to lose weight. You don't have to be that exact about it. When you learn to take the fat and calories out of your food and keep the healthy part in, your caloric intake will be in the correct general "ballpark." That's all that's needed—along with regular exercise.
- A regular aerobic exercise program is absolutely essential for weight loss and lifelong weight control. Do not think "whether," think "must."

The Better Life Institute Family Health Program: Nutrient Composition

RECOMMENDED EATING PLAN
(percent of calories)

	PRO-TEIN	FAT	CARBO-HYDRATES	CHOLES-TEROL	TOTAL FIBER
Typical Diet	18%	42%	40%	500 mg.	16 gms.
Good	15%	20–30%	55–65%	150–200 mg.	25–30 gms.
Better	15%	20%	65%	150 mg.	30+ gms.
Weight Loss (1200–1500 cal.)	20%	20%	60%	150–200 mg.	25 gms.

LAND OF THE CHEESEBURGER WITH FRIES

There are several national guidelines we considered before choosing the one we recommend. We prefer a more aggressive approach than the ones most often recommended. Our guidelines usually mean a lower fat and a greater plant food content. Although most experts agree this is the best approach, our plan's reliance on plants rather than meat and dairy products appears to make it less appealing to many Americans. Eating meat and cheese seems to be one of Americans' inalienable rights. We usually think our kids are immortal, that they can eat anything. But children's eating habits become adults' eating habits. Welcome to the world of degenerative disease. It is unfortunate that we have encouraged our own unhealthy eating habits in our children. This trend in eating needs to stop, and the best place to stop it is with you at the family level.

We do not presume to ask you to prepare food no one will eat.

We have created an eating plan that has been tested for ten years on all types of families. Our program emphasizes plant food—fruits, vegetables, whole grains, beans, and peas. But, the difference is that it is very tasty and very flexible and easy to adapt to your palate. We want you to provide the healthiest possible meals for your family. We do recognize the importance of complete enjoyment of your food. We ask the same for ourselves. Try it—you'll like it!

I CAN LIVE WITH THIS

The old saying, "If it tastes good, spit it out," is just that—old, out-dated, no longer true!

Today's food products make it possible to eat a heart-healthy diet that tastes delightful.

There is general agreement among scientists, nutritionists, and doctors concerning the safest and most healthy eating programs for adults and children. All groups suggest lower fat, sugar, salt, and cholesterol intake and higher dietary fiber intake (children cannot eat as much total dietary fiber as adults). There is no disagreement as to what comprises a healthy diet. Differences do exist, however, among health professionals concerning what is feasible and tasty. Generally, the lower the fat content of the eating plan, the less it resembles typical American eating habits. We love our meat, fried food, cheeses, and fatty desserts!

The Better Life Institute dietary approach is on the leading edge of the nutritional guidelines recommended by major national associations. Every dietary health trend is toward reduced fat intake, and we're there already! There is complete consensus regarding the health merits of the BLI eating plan and health point-of-view. This eating program is one that will provide you with "health insurance" and "weight control insurance." It will reduce all heart and blood vessel disease and cancer risk factors related to nutrition.

It's the tastiness of reduced calorie, reduced fat meals that's the issue. We agree that by lowering the fat content, preparing tasty meals for the family becomes a challenge. But, as you will see, the Better Life Institute's recipes and program flexibility will perform a little "magic" in this area.

Our suggested well-balanced dietary program can help to prevent problems. Be sure to check with your family doctor and/or pediatrician before you begin any new diet and exercise program. We doubt that any health professional will argue with the weight control or health promotion aspects of the Better Life Institute Diet.

THE TUMMY RUMBLERS

Some changes will occur in your body as you start to eat more carbohydrates. The one that affects almost everyone is gas. People become very flatulent (a fancy term for gassy). They say that their bellies "rumble." This is all normal and natural as your digestive process starts to change and adapt to more plant food. As your body adjusts to this kind of eating program, you'll notice the gassiness and rumbling diminish. At the same time you may find out who your friends really are!

Vitamin and Mineral Supplements

We suggest the entire family use a multivitamin and mineral supplement on a daily basis. While recognizing that scientists have not, as yet, been able to agree on the advisability and level of supplementation, BLI feels that, at present, there is sufficient scientific evidence suggesting the protective and preventive benefits of a higher vitamin and mineral intake. Physicians are lined up on both the pro and con sides of the fence. The issue is an emotional one with some.

There is a growing body of evidence supporting their *potential* contribution to health. There is little, if any, possibility of adverse effects unless you take excessive, irrational amounts. That's why we suggest the general use of quality food supplements. Particularly you don't want to appreciably exceed the recommended daily amounts of vitamins *A, D, K,* and *E.* There is growing evidence, as yet inconclusive, that suggests anti-oxidant supplements such as *beta carotene* and vitamins *A, C,* and *E* have some protective effect against heart disease and cancer as well as many other diseases. We won't give you the dark-leafy-green and yellow-and-orange lecture right now, but make friends with these vegetables. They are high in the anti-oxidants recommended for cancer prevention.

Furthermore, the methods used in food production, storage, and processing may deplete the vitamin and mineral content of foods, especially fresh fruits and vegetables. Unique lifestyles, skipping meals, dieting, and high stress levels along with increased emphasis on plant rather than animal food may present some potential vitamin and mineral sufficiency challenges as well. Therefore, we feel taking a daily vitamin and mineral supplement is an excellent "insurance policy." We suggest you speak with your physician concerning the use of children's vitamin and mineral supplements.

And, we must make it perfectly clear that *vitamin and mineral supplementation should not be used as a substitute for proper nutrition.* They are only an *addition* to proper food selection. For those of you using the Better Life Institute Nutrition Program at home to reduce your calorie and fat intake, particularly at the 1200 calorie level, there is always the risk that a lower calorie diet will not provide 100 percent of the U.S. RDA of each nutrient. Therefore, if you or your children (in consultation with your pediatrician) decide to restrict caloric intake, a multivitamin and mineral supplement should be considered by both parent and child to avoid possible nutritional deficiencies.

■ *Dark, leafy green, yellow, and orange vegetables are high in anti-oxidants. Eat lots of them at every meal, if possible.*

■ *The take-home message of this conference, shared by the outstanding group of experts we've assembled, is that micronutrients (vitamins and minerals) can modify the disease process. That's a striking new thought.*

Dr. William Pryor at the Antioxidant Vitamins and Beta-carotene in Disease Prevention Conference, London, 1989

WHAT VITAMINS AND MINERALS DO

NUTRIENT	US RDA	BLI PREFERRED SOURCE	FUNCTIONS IN THE BODY
Vitamin A	10,000 I.U.	Fruits, vegetables	Essential for vision in dim light; plays a role in the formation and maintenance of skin, mucous membranes, bone growth.
Vitamin D	4000 I.U.	Fish	Essential for normal bone growth and maintenance.
Vitamin E	30 I.U.	Whole grain cereals	Helps form red blood cells, muscle and other tissue.
Vitamin C	60 mg	Citrus fruits, melon, berries, leafy vegetables, tomatoes	Necessary to form collagen, the binding substance needed for tissue strength, bone and teeth formation, wound healing.
Folid Acid	0.4 mg	Fruit, yeast, leafy vegetables	Assists in forming body proteins and in the formation of hemoglobin.
Thiamine B_1	1.5 mg	Dry peas and beans, whole grain enriched breads and cereals	Helps obtain energy from food, promotes normal working of the digestive system, growth, digestion.
Riboflavin B_2	1.7 mg	Lowfat or skim milk, dark leafy greens	Helps cells produce energy essential to many chemical changes in body tissues and to the absorption of carbohydrates, proteins, and fats. Also important to the maintenance of mucous membranes.
Niacin	20 mg	Whole grain	Needed by cells for the utilization of

THE BETTER LIFE INSTITUTE FAMILY HEALTH PLAN

NUTRIENT	US RDA	BLI PREFERRED SOURCE	FUNCTIONS IN THE BODY
			oxygen to produce energy, therefore important for the health of all cells.
Vitamin B$_6$	2 mg	Meats, lowfat or skim milk, beans	Helps in the absorption and metabolism of protein, the use of fats, and the formation of red blood cells.
Vitamin B$_{12}$	6 mg	Lowfat dairy products	Essential for normal development of red blood cells and the functioning of the nervous system.
Biotin	0.3 mg	Multivitamins & minerals	Present in the formation of fatty acids and the utilization of carbohydrates.
Pantothenic Acid	10 mg	Whole grains, legumes	Essential for the intermediate metabolism of carbohydrates, proteins, and fats, and the formation of hormones.
Calcium	1 g	Lowfat or skim dairy products, leafy greens	Important for structure and growth of bones, and teeth; assists in blood clotting; important for proper functioning of nerves, muscles and heart.
Phosphorus	1 g	Present in almost all foods	Works with calcium to build bones and teeth, helps utilize fats, carbohydrates, proteins.
Iodine	150 mcg	Seafood	Necessary for the proper functioning of

NUTRIENT	US RDA	BLI PREFERRED SOURCE	FUNCTIONS IN THE BODY
			the thyroid gland; contributes to proper growth and metabolism.
Iron	18 mg	Poultry, fish	Combines with protein to make hemoglobin, the blood substance carrying oxygen from lungs to cells. Helps release energy from food.
Magnesium	400 mg	Whole grains, nuts, seeds, dark green vegetables	Plays a role in the metabolism of calcium and potassium; contributes to normal functioning of nervous and muscular systems; aids in maintaining acid-alkaline balance; is essential for the utilization of protein and is an essential part of many enzyme systems.
Copper	2 mg	Oysters, dried peas and beans	Aids in the formation of red blood cells and is necessary for the absorption and utilization of iron.
Zinc	15 mg	Whole grains, beans	Essential for proper growth, plays a role in good appetite, is an important constituent of enzymes in many major metabolic pathways, functions in the repair of tissues.

Fat and Cholesterol

In the United States our main concern should not be undernourishment, but rather *overindulgence*. Because our diet is so rich in meat and dairy products, we eat far too much fat. And, as we discussed in a previous section, we pay a dear price for our nutritional excesses: illness and early death.

The role of fats and cholesterol in early death is a detailed story in itself. Only a few highlights will be mentioned in this section. But reducing your fat intake and using the proper fats and oils in your diet are extremely important. For this reason, the entire "fat story" will be told in a separate chapter, Chapter 6.

The challenge is to learn how to select and prepare more healthful foods. Cholesterol is only found in animal foods: meat, chicken, fish, and dairy products. Plant food does not contain cholesterol. In addition, all beef, lamb, pork, and veal contain a substance called *saturated fat,* which elevates your blood cholesterol. We suggest you learn to prepare delicious dishes using fish, seafood, chicken, turkey, and very lean meat. Prepare them baked, broiled, poached, stir fried, or by any other method so long as you use a cooking spray and other seasonings instead of oil or butter. Use nonstick cookwear. Egg whites are almost all protein, contain no fat or cholesterol, and are quite tasty when properly prepared. Egg yolks are very high in both fat and cholesterol and should be restricted (or avoided if possible).

Fats have more than twice the calories of carbohydrates (plant foods). In addition, when used in excess, fat plays a far more harmful role in the occurrence of heart disease, obesity, and certain cancers than other foods do. In the past, polyunsaturated fats such as corn, sunflower, and safflower oils have been touted as "good fats." However, recent evidence suggests a high intake of polyunsaturated fats is associated with an increased incidence of colon cancer and gallbladder disease. We suggest you use monounsaturated fats, such as olive, peanut, and canola oils. These fats seem to moderately lower cholesterol and triglycerides and reduce your LDL cholesterol level, which you will later learn is your "bad" cholesterol level.

> *It's not only the level of cholesterol in your blood that counts, but the amount of cholesterol you eat, regardless of your blood cholesterol level.*
>
> Drs. Jeremiah Stamler and Richard Shekelle, Northwestern University Medical School

Sugar and Sugar Substitutes

Sugar in small amounts is not a major dietary concern. Fructose is a slightly better choice; it is sweeter than sugar, which means that you use less. Fructose also may not "challenge" your body's insulin reaction as does sugar. Consequently, you may not have the highs and lows with fructose that you do with sugar. The adult-onset diabetic may be able to handle fructose better than sugar. In either case, fructose or sugar used sparingly will not be a problem. All diabetics should consult their physicians on all dietary considerations and monitor their blood sugar levels due to the change in dietary intake and the potential need to adjust insulin dosages.

A ROSE BY ANY OTHER NAME IS STILL A ROSE

Sugar comes in many forms and it's all *natural*. Honey, molasses, raw, brown, or turbinado sugar and concentrated fruit juice sweeteners are still sugars of one kind or another. Enjoy them in moderation.

People have been using sugar in small amounts as a spice for thousands of years. The problem is that you eat too much of it either directly or in processed foods. Recently several studies in England have possibly implicated high levels of glucose and insulin with increased damage to small blood vessel walls. The average American eats about 140 pounds of sugar a year in contrast to 13 pounds a year a hundred years ago. The best way to deal with sugar is to change your taste preferences so that you need less of it, whether natural or artificial. Eat more fresh fruit for the satisfaction that comes with a sweet taste. But don't eliminate sweets or artificial sweeteners completely. These "all or nothing" cult-type recommendations cause people to throw up their hands in disgust and chuck their entire eating programs out the window, rejecting some of the good things they'd tried to do because going all the way seems so unpleasant. That's not what the Better Life Institute Program is all about.

ASPARTAME (NUTRASWEET™ OR EQUAL™)

Aspartame is a sweetener that is 180–200 times sweeter than sugar. It is made from two amino acids (building blocks of protein) identical to amino acids found naturally in foods. Aspartame has been investigated in over 100 separate scientific studies to assess its effectiveness and safety and the FDA approved Aspartame over a decade ago. Other agencies approving Aspartame are the American Medical Association, the Canadian Department of Health and Welfare, the European Economic Communities, the World Health Organization, and the regulatory agencies of more than fifty Western nations.

Since 1981 there have been a number of reports of adverse reaction to Aspartame. Several studies were launched to investigate the basis of these concerns. Based upon studies at Harvard, Duke, and the University of Minnesota Medical Schools and the Center for Disease Control in Atlanta, Aspartame has been deemed totally safe. FDA Commissioner Frank Young stated that "Aspartame is safe for use by adults, children, pregnant women, including carriers of the Phenylketonuria gene, for the overweight in a weight loss program, and for the diabetic." Please consult with your physician if you have any questions.

There are label warnings because Aspartame contains phenylallaline. This and aspartic acid are the amino acids found in Nutrasweet™ and Equal.® They are also found in most common foods. Since Aspartame is a synthesized substance and has a higher amount of phenylallaline than is usually found in natural food, it requires a warning label for a very small group of people called "phenylketoneurics." Their level of blood phenylallaline is influenced by the amount of phenylallaline they eat (unlike the rest of us). If it gets too high, they are at risk for certain brain disorders. You would already know if this were a problem for anyone in your family.

Sugar substitutes are very popular today, and it's likely you use them. Just remember, sugar substitutes have not made the difference between normal weight or overweight in millions of people. Changes in food selection and preparation are the key—not sugar substitutes. We recommend that you limit the use of *all* sweets, whether artificial or natural.

Sorbitol

Sorbitol is a form of carbohydrate that does not produce the same glucose-insulin response as conventional syrups or sugars. It naturally occurs in fruits and berries and is used in a variety of foods, candies, and drug preparations. It is metabolized differently from sugar and the American Diabetes Association states it produces a "flatter" glucose-insulin response, thus avoiding rapid elevation and depression of blood sugar. With sorbitol you don't get the giant mood swings that you can get from sugar. This is also a favorable condition for either the pre- or actual diabetic. Sorbitol has about the same caloric value as sugar. When it is used in excess of fifty grams, the label must state its presence. At these levels it can act as a diuretic or possibly cause diarrhea.

Salt (Sodium)

Excess salt or sodium has been implicated in high blood pressure. Several recent studies suggest the ratio of sodium intake to calcium, magnesium, and potassium intake is more important in blood pressure control than sodium intake alone. Some people are also more "salt sensitive" than others. Practically speaking, it is important to reduce salt intake by not adding salt to your food and by reducing your use of food products made with a lot of salt. This will help control weight; in some cases, it will also control blood pressure and prevent future high blood pressure problems. An easy way to control salt intake is to not "salt the pot." Also, leave your salt shaker off the table. Using this formula, you likely will find yourself in the 2500 mg. per-day range. As an alternative, use salt-free spices and flavorings. You can't start early enough to build lower-salt tastes for your family.

The chemical formula for salt is sodium chloride. About 40 percent of salt is sodium, and it's the culprit. Sodium is found in many other food additives and it is still sodium, whether or not the additive is salt. As we said before, "A rose by any other name is still a rose," and sodium is sodium regardless of where you find it.

Monosodium Glutamate

According to the Joint Expert Committee on Food Additives, monosodium glutumate, known as MSG, does not pose a health hazard. This committee is a scientific advisory body to the World Health Organization (WHO). In fact WHO recently removed any limitations based upon body weight on the use of MSG. It also placed MSG in the "safest" category for food additives. The organization also reported that MSG poses no additional risk to infants.

NOT JUST AT CHINESE RESTAURANTS
The sodium in MSG is the problem. Therefore, since we're not in favor of salt, we also recommend you reduce your exposure to MSG, but it is difficult if you eat out. Historically Chinese and other Oriental foods have contained relatively large amounts of MSG. Consequently, some people have complained of "Chinese Restaurant Syndrome," a set of symptoms involving head and muscle aches after eating food heavily laced with MSG. Many people feel they have an allergic reaction to MSG, but few realize that any time they eat out, in any type of restaurant, they are probably eating MSG. It is a flavor enhancer and preservative for food. Very few, if any, adverse effects are associated with a small intake of MSG. When you eat at Oriental restaurants (Japanese, Chinese, Korean, Thai, and Indian), request that they eliminate the MSG. And don't deliberately add it to your cooking.

The Food and Drug Administration (FDA) allows food companies to use the term "hydrolyzed vegetable protein" on food labels. *Be*

THE BETTER LIFE INSTITUTE FAMILY HEALTH PLAN

warned. This substance contains a considerable amount of MSG. And MSG contains sodium. Remember, "A rose by any other name . . ."

Caffeine

A DRUG IN A CUP

Caffeine is a powerful stimulant and because of its acceptance and availability, you can get hooked on caffeine very easily. Its metabolic effects are well known. It raises the levels of blood sugar, fat, and insulin. It stimulates the production of adrenalin and thyroxin. It is a stimulatory drug! Periodic review of the relationship of caffeine intake to certain diseases sometimes implicates caffeine and sometimes lets it off the hook. Unfortunately, the jury is still out on caffeine since we just don't know if it's as dangerous as alleged. But we do know it is a stimulatory drug, and such a drug cannot be good for you except for certain medically diagnosed reasons. Your family will be exposed to less risk if you cut your caffeine intake.

Many experts feel excess caffeine intake (more than two cups of coffee, four cups of tea, and/or four 12-ounce soft drinks per day) is associated with aggravating existing heart disease and high blood pressure. However, there is no substantive research linking caffeine to illness and death from cancer. Tea has about 40 percent of the caffeine found in coffee. Chocolate has a small amount of caffeine too. BLI recommends reducing or eliminating your exposure to beverages high in caffeine. There are excellent naturally decaffeinated teas and coffees available. Read the labels on soft drinks and limit your intake of beverages that contain caffeine.

Periodic review of the relationship of caffeine intake to certain diseases sometimes implicates caffeine and sometimes lets it off the hook, except during pregnancy and lactation when coffee consumption should be limited to two cups or less per day.

Alcohol

If you so wish, we recommend that you drink no more than two ounces of alcohol a day. While some heart scientists point out that alcohol elevates your HDL level, the "good" cholesterol, we now know that even HDL has several fractions and that alcohol may not elevate the good part. Even if it did, the documented adverse effects of alcohol on the stomach, intestines, liver, pancreas, arterial walls, and blood pressure outweigh its advantages. We recommend that you never drink to improve your health. Drinking to relax should be replaced with behavioral changes in your lifestyle. Try to limit your alcohol intake to social occasions, and eliminate it completely if possible.

Crude Fiber

There is very convincing evidence that high fiber intake reduces your risk of gastrointestinal cancer. All unrefined or unprocessed plant-based foods (fruit, vegetables, whole grains, potato, beans, and peas) contain fiber. Usually when food is unprocessed, it contains more fiber. Animal foods have no fiber content. The fiber in food hydrates in your stomach and tends to give you a full feeling. Fiber also tends to reduce the absorption of fat and cholesterol in your bloodstream. Crude fiber can help control your blood sugar level. A high fiber intake also eliminates constipation, which ensures a miminum exposure-time for toxins and carcinogens in your digestive system. Finally, when you eat more fibrous foods, you are adding lower calorie bulk to your diet. Proper eating habits are best, but if you believe you do not get enough fiber in your diet, you may wish to consider the use of fiber tablets at each meal. Fiber tablets with a *full* glass of water can help provide noncaloric bulk in your diet and assist in weight control.

Water Soluble Fiber

Oat bran, beans, peas, lentils, and pectin (in fruit) can help provide noncaloric bulk to food and control blood cholesterol, fat, and sugar levels. These foods can also aid in avoiding constipation. And, as with crude bran-type fiber, they are excellent for weight control because they add bulk and not many calories. While a recent study suggests that oat bran may be only indirectly effective in lowering cholesterol (as a substitute for fatty foods), many more studies have demonstrated its effectiveness. More research with larger groups of people needs to be done. Oat bran cannot in any way harm you, and used minimally, it provides a lot of fiber and bulk for your diet that is lower in calories. So, go for it!

■ *Coconut and palm oils are usually used at very low levels to mask the taste of other oils used in food processing, and they probably are about 5% of the total amount of oil.*

Partially-Hydrogenated Coconut or Palm Oil

The bad news is these fats, which are known collectively as *tropical oils,* are highly saturated. They tend to elevate your blood cholesterol

■ THE BETTER LIFE INSTITUTE FAMILY HEALTH PLAN

level much more than foods high in cholesterol do. They are also key ingredients in many packaged food preparations because they enhance taste and texture considerably more so than other oils. Tropical oils also increase the shelf-life of many baked goods and common items like candy bars.

The good news is that recently many concerned consumer advocates and medical researchers have forced a number of major food manufacturers to substitute relatively safer fats for the tropical oils in packaged crackers, cookies, and other popular snack foods. Even though this is becoming a trend, please carefully read the labels of all packaged goods before making your selection in the grocery store. We suggest that you significantly reduce your intake of these fats.

Yellow Dye #5

The FDA has approved the use of yellow dye #5 on several occasions after it was studied. They estimate there is an adverse reaction in only 1 out of 100,000 people. The dye is still the only commercially feasible alternative to yellow food coloring. It is used extensively by all food producers and is probably in many of the foods you now eat.

The Meal in a Glass—A Word About Meal Substitutes

Most scientists agree that eating nutritious, readily available, high bulk foods on a regular and moderate basis is the best way to maintain good health. So do we. The logic is irrefutable. However, for many, the pace and individual needs of their daily living patterns are such that an easily prepared, well-balanced nutritious meal substitute is far more convenient.

This is certainly more desirable than a hit-or-miss, nutritionally inadequate diet. And as we have preached before, we do not advocate missing any meals. There are some excellent nutritionally balanced liquid meals and food bars available on the market. Just make certain they truly are "meal substitutes" and not simply very low calorie diet drinks. The advantages of a balanced complete meal substitute, when used intentionally with a heart-healthy, low calorie selection of foods, are obvious.

No Tricks in Our Apron Pocket

The nutritional suggestions of the Better Life Family Program are not faddish in any manner. Probably we are telling you what you already inherently sense, but don't necessarily want to hear. We have no gimmicks or special foods that can lead to *healthy, lifelong* weight control and proper nutritional eating habits. We have no nutritional tricks up our sleeves or in our apron pockets. We do, however, have some other "tricks and treats" for you.

As all major national groups do, we recommend you eat more plant food and less fat and cholesterol. Our specific meal plans and recipes for the entire family will follow in Chapter 9. We will not teach you to be a "calorie slave" or to use precise measures and strict menu plans. That would make no sense because you have to learn to think "lifelong," not "flash in the pan." We'll provide you with guidelines to a way of thinking about food that you and your children can use anywhere, any time. The table below describes the general characteristics of all foods.

NUTRIENT VALUES FOR FOOD GROUPS
(per 3½ ozs. cooked)

FOOD	PERCENT CAL/ PROT	PERCENT CAL/ FAT	PERCENT CAL/ CARBO	CHOLES- TEROL MG.	TOTAL CALORIES
Dairy (cheese)	20	70	10	95	350
Meat	25	75	0	75	300
Nuts (raw)	15	70	15	0	600
Fruit (raw)	2	8	90	0	45
Whole grains	15	10	75	0	85
Beans/peas	20	10	70	0	95
Vegetables	10	10	85	0	25
Poultry	80	20	0	70	150
Fish	90	10	0	55	110

We suggest that you "make friends with a plant." Plant foods are lower in calories and fat, have absolutely no cholesterol, and are higher in carbohydrate and fiber. Use smaller and leaner servings of meat, chicken, and fish and non or lowfat dairy products. It's that simple. We'll show you how in Chapter 9.

THE BETTER LIFE INSTITUTE FAMILY HEALTH PLAN

SUGGESTED SNACKS

- Raw vegetables—unlimited amounts
- Fresh fruit
- Skim or lowfat milk
- Nonfat fruit yogurt
- Vegetable or tomato juice
- Popcorn (hot air popped, seasoned with low-sodium flavoring)
- Shredded Wheat Nibbles™
- Dips and spreads
- Breadsticks and acceptable crackers
- Fruit sorbet
- Cold cereal with skim or lowfat milk
- Meal replacement drink with skim or lowfat milk (or any other balanced, low calorie meal replacement, not a high protein drink!)

Summary

We are drowning in diet and nutrition books, all professing new secrets for improved health and weight control. The marketing hype and claims of special secrets give the impression that selecting a correct diet for health and weight control is a complex matter. Actually, it is not. A few simple guidelines are all that you need. You do not have to devote a lot of time to the search. It's simple. You have to devote time to implementing and living with a common sense approach to family nutrition and health. Emphasize plant foods and limit fat foods. No one need become a vegetarian unless they so wish. When you live by this simple guideline, you reduce your risk of degenerative disease and can more easily control your weight on a life-long basis.

START PLANNING FOR LIFE

The major food related challenges that you and your family face today are related to excess calories, fat, cholesterol, and sugar and lack of fiber. The risks of obesity, heart disease, hypertension, diabetes, and certain forms of cancer far outweigh the potential risks of food additives. We might add that those risks have been extensively studied, reviewed, and re-reviewed by major research institutions and verified as a health hazard. We suggest you minimize all nutrition-related risks as much as possible. However, it is important to base your efforts on fact and adopt eating habits that will help you avoid major degenerative diseases that can strike you and your family. We suggest that you concentrate your efforts and select food for a life-long, moderate, enjoyable eating plan. The trick is lifelong control, not a two week, "fad of the day" control. The benefits with respect to weight, cholesterol, blood pressure, and blood sugar are well documented and should be obvious to you by now.

It is important that we remind you of our discussion pointing to the fact that we can't cure these degenerative diseases in the same manner as we can virtually wipe out most infectious or microbiologic-germ disease. We don't yet have the scientific and technological ability to do this. All that the best medicine can do is contain the damage and minimize the side effects. We do it better than any other country in the world, but it is a limited approach for the time being.

That's why we are taking the time to explain to you that your kitchen and the street on which you and your family exercise are wonderful tools in living long and living well.

TIPS

- Substitute plant food for animal food whenever possible.
- Eat whole grains instead of processed or enriched grains.
- Use salt substitutes and reduce your use of salt.
- Use monounsaturated fat instead of adding butter, margarine, or lard to your food.
- Reduce or limit intake of sugar, other sweeteners, and sugar substitutes.
- Use fruit for desserts.
- Reduce your intake of all caffeine and alcoholic beverages.
- Use lowfat or nonfat dairy products in place of whole milk and cheese.
- Try foods that are baked or broiled instead of fried.
- Take a multivitamin and mineral and fiber supplement daily.
- Have three meals per day and snacks in between to prevent feeling hungry. Never, never, ever starve yourself.
- Last, yet most important, if you have any specific health concerns, discuss them with your physician.

YES, I CAN

- I can eat vegetables at every evening meal and encourage the rest of my family to do so.
- I can start a hobby with one of my children that I share solely with him or her.

THE BETTER LIFE INSTITUTE FAMILY HEALTH PLAN

- I can take a healthy snack to work rather than use the "roach coach," the snack vendor.

FAMILY CIRCLE SUGGESTIONS

Have everybody stand up and give each other back rubs. It feels great!

Serve a "snappy" dessert during Family Circle. It makes Family Circle a little more interesting. Food always does that!

Try to spend a few minutes with each child at bedtime. Sit down on the bed and just talk about anything that interests the two of you. Don't use the time for lectures.

Let's Grow Healthy Kids!

■ ■ ■ ■ ■ ■ ■ ■ ■ ■ ■ ■ ■ ■ ■ ■ ■ ■

Too Thin, Too Fat, Just Right—It's All the Same!

WHAT DOES *DIET* MEAN TO YOU?

Let's talk about the term *diet* for a few seconds. The Better Life Institute definition of *diet* may be different from yours. You and many others think that *diet* means just *calorie restriction*—any way, any shape, any form. To us, *diet* has a much broader scope. BLI sees *diet* as *a nutritionally balanced way of eating*. It really doesn't refer to calorie counting or the use of special "trick" foods, pills, and drinks. If calorie restriction is your concern for your child, there is no need to sacrifice nutritional balance and healthful eating. This is a given. It is nonnegotiable!

What children need for proper growth and development is an appropriate amount of healthy, nutritionally balanced calories, just like adults do. There may be some exceptions, and if there are, your pediatrician will be glad to explain these exceptions. Before starting any new nutritional plan for a child under five years of age, consult with your physician. Please *do not make an independent decision* to place your child on a diet.

A Balancing Act

Your nutritional strategy for your children should be the same, whether you are concerned with weight gain, weight loss, or merely maintaining their proper weight. Proper nutritional balance and developing healthful eating patterns for life is the top priority, regardless of the weight of your child. Unless your child has a health problem, your concern about whether the child is too fat or too thin can be handled simply. You can introduce a proper exercise and activity routine along with a balanced nutrition plan. That's all that is needed.

Setting the Right Example for Your Children

If you expose your children to healthy eating habits early in their lives, you'll find these habits will last. Children acquire taste preferences and learn to like foods depending on their upbringing, their nationality, their culture, and most importantly, what Mom and Dad eat themselves. The best way to develop good eating habits is for the entire family to eat the same healthy foods. Instead of thinking "kid's foods" or "mom and dad's foods," think "family foods."

WHAT ABOUT VITAMIN AND MINERAL SUPPLEMENTS?

Life between the ages of one and sixteen is very different from life between sixteen and thirty-two even though they both cover a term of sixteen years. It's like comparing four years before World War II with four years during World War II! Children face unique developmental, biological, and growth challenges during these years. That's why we are so emphatic about balanced nutrition for children. We feel that a children's multivitamin and mineral supplement is a good idea even though there is no "across the board" agreement among pediatricians regarding the use of a children's vitamin and mineral supplement.

Insurance

Our suggestion to give your children a daily children's vitamin and mineral supplement (teens over sixteen can use adult supplements) is a practical and "fail-safe" one. If it can do no harm, and is likely to do some good, why not? It also relieves some of the pressure you feel trying to be sure your children get balanced nutrition. A vitamin and mineral supplement is *not* a substitute for good eating habits. When taken as directed, it is good developmental and growth insurance. Just consider a vitamin and mineral supplement a "helpful friend" and get on with the major challenge of providing good food and exercise for your children.

Parents of health-conscious children are more likely to be health-conscious themselves. It works both ways, folks. We don't care whether "the horse comes before the cart" or "the cart comes before the horse." It's all the same!

In the Beginning . . .

WHAT A BEAUTIFUL BABY!

When a baby is born, this beautiful little person is completely dependent on the parent for life. When the baby is fed a few hours after birth, it is introduced to formula or mother's milk. About 50 percent of the calories in mother's milk comes from fat. It also includes all

■ *THE BETTER LIFE INSTITUTE FAMILY HEALTH PLAN*

the nutrients necessary for proper growth and development. Formulas have been designed to imitate mother's milk as closely as possible. Your pediatrician will help you to decide whether breastfeeding or formula is best for both of you, depending on your lifestyle. Nature has its perfect way of showing us exactly what our babies need to thrive.

Before a child is two years of age, he or she requires a higher fat diet for proper growth and development than is needed after the age of two. As you wean your baby from mother's milk or formula, please consult your pediatrician for the proper general diet. We must re-emphasize the importance of putting your child on a well-balanced nutritional program that follows the guidelines of your physician.

Habits Begin Early in Life

Nutritionists agree that one of the largest sources of saturated fat in the American diet is whole milk. Quite often pediatricians recommend whole milk for children because of a concern about adequate fat intake for proper growth and development. However, there are "better fats" to use than milkfat and butterfat. A taste preference for whole milk is difficult to change after the early childhood years. We suggest that you discuss with your pediatrician some alternatives that will provide adequate fat in your child's diet and at the same time help establish proper eating habits for their adult years. You might discuss adding a "smidgeon" of canola or vegetable oil to your child's baby food to ensure proper fat intake and using lowfat milk after the baby is weaned. Discuss this strategy with your pediatrician. There should be no difficulty. Too many adults tell us they "can't drink that thin blue stuff." If you start your children on the "thin blue stuff" when they are young, they won't have any further taste difficulties with fat reduced milk. This will reduce their exposure to saturated fats in their earlier years and help get them started on the way to heart-healthy eating habits.

Beyond Nursing or the Bottle

GO AHEAD, RUIN MY APPETITE!

When your child begins to eat from the table, to have "real people's food," that's when the good-habit training begins. This time in your child's life is very special to both of you, and you don't have to compete with television and food advertisers for your child's palate. You'll have to deal with advertising aimed at kids later on, but right now those little taste buds are all yours to shape by yourself. And if you make meal-time fun for your toddler while you introduce her to good food, you'll lay the foundation of insurance against the barrage of advertising that's sure to come later.

Little bodies cannot and should not consume only three big meals a day. We encourage you to teach your child to "graze," not "gorge." This is the time to teach him to eat healthy snacks between meals. Years ago, children were discouraged from eating between meals because it "ruined their appetites" for their regular meals. Now nutrition scientists know it is better to eat smaller, frequent meals rather than three big meals a day. So you can go ahead and ruin their appetites. It's okay as long as you ruin it with healthy, nutritious foods!

In Chapter 9 of this book, you'll find a list of healthy and enjoyable snacks.

The Toddler Years

After the age of two, children become more active and more social. They are much more aware of what is going on around them. This also is a very impressionable age. And you, as parents, are the greatest influence in their lives. Your biggest competition is television, and at this stage in their lives *you can control the tube!*

DECLARATIONS OF INDEPENDENCE

About age two your child will begin to develop a mind of his or her own. "No, I don't want to sit on the potty seat. I want to sit on the 'big one'!" "I don't want to wear red socks. I want the purple ones!" So too, your child's taste buds will start to assert themselves. "No, I don't want carrots." Your little person always ate carrots before, but now refuses. This is all part of a child's first step toward becoming a grownup. He or she will begin to voice likes and dislikes about *everything*. This stage (sometimes known as the "terrible twos") is not the time to tell your kids they are bad or to try to force them to eat a specific food. How many of us have a dislike for certain foods because they were forced on us? And how many of us have done this to our own children?

KEEP IT LIGHT

The best thing to do at this age is to encourage your child to eat certain foods by saying, "I think these foods taste good. I like them, I'm going to have some. Watch how Mommy and Daddy eat them!" It also doesn't hurt to have a running monologue, which might go like

About 80 percent of the food ads shown on television on Saturday morning are for foods that have poor nutritional value. Most of the ads are for foods high in sugar and fat. There's new legislation in progress that will give you more accurate and understandable information. Watch for it.

THE BETTER LIFE INSTITUTE FAMILY HEALTH PLAN

this: "Oh, carrots are good! They grow in the ground. And they come up this pretty orange color. The little rabbits and horses eat carrots and grow strong. Mommy and Daddy eat carrots because they help us to grow big and strong. Look how strong Daddy is!" (Don't laugh. It worked with our kids.)

After the "Terrible Twos"

After age two, one of the most important things you can do to build proper eating habits is to control what your children watch on television. We're not going to go into a harangue about television because when used properly, television is a wonderful way to expand the visions and the world of your children. But, this mesmerizing "joy box" has the potential to influence your children's eating and living habits more than you do. Let's face it. We're only parents, and we can't compete with cartoon characters or puppets. But, you are the *parents,* and you have an advantage over television. You can turn off the television, but you'll still be there. You must assert your rights and your responsibilities as your child's first and most influential teacher.

Once your very impressionable child is exposed to television at the preschool level, they learn a great deal. Their little brains soak up information like sponges. We were constantly amazed at what our children remembered from television. Often we see children at the supermarket asking a parent to buy "Nerds,™ Pops, Zips, and Cracks." It will happen to you and your kids. Your little child might not be capable of speaking a full sentence, but he will know all about Nerds!™ And he'll ask you to buy them.

LET'S MAKE A DEAL!
You can't fight television, but you can be smart enough to make it work for you instead of against you. Rather than refusing to buy what your children see and want from television commercials, make a deal. You might say, "OK, you can have a box of Nerds,™ but we're also going to buy some other cereals that are more healthy for us. You can put a little Nerds™ in your bowl of cereal every day, if you want." As your children go through this stage, and you are continually exposing them to good eating habits, familiarity leads to tastiness and permanent eating habits.

A snack for a child will be a graham cracker, a slice of apple, and a glass of lowfat milk, rather than some more expensive junk food. Dinner can be a turkey-burger, baked potato with non fat

■ *Ingredients on breakfast cereal labels, as with all labels, are listed in descending order by weight. Check the label for the position of "sugar, honey, or other sweeteners." It should be near the bottom on the list, never one of the top two ingredients.*

cheese, and peas and carrots rather than fried chicken and french fries. These eating habits will become a part of everyday life when the child has very little else with which to compare it.

We must continue to emphasize the importance of YOUR influence on your child's eating habits. The correct formula is "Do as I do and do as I say," not just "Do as I say." Set the proper example and healthy family eating habits are born. Everybody wins, especially the family.

Let's Go to Kindergarten

Kindergarten is where your child "goes to work." But unlike yours, children's "work world" plays a far more impressionable role in their lives. They learn new social skills, and they're exposed to different children and lifestyles. Let's not forget that this is the first time children face an adult authority figure that's not in their immediate family. Of course, some children have already been exposed to other adults in nursery school or daycare centers. Nevertheless, kindergarten is a big step. It's important that you retain as much control as possible—no matter what your lifestyle. Our firm belief is YOU are the parent, and it is YOUR responsibility to teach YOUR child the basic rules for life!

NOTHIN' SAYS LOVIN' LIKE SOMETHING FROM YOUR OVEN

We suggest you pack healthy snacks for your children when they go off to school or other activities. An apple granola bar, graham crackers, Fig Newtons,(™) or a little individual pack of dry cereal and an aseptic container of fruit juice is easy for you to prepare and easy for your child to manage.

Pack healthy lunches for your children also. They may never have been exposed to a bologna sandwich on white bread in your home, but it looks very appealing in someone else's lunch. Remember how we used to trade lunches? We suggest, on occasion, that you give your children TURKEY bologna sandwiches on a healthy whole grain bread. Ask your children what they would like for lunch. This will teach them that you are ready to listen, compromise, and bring a balance to eating patterns. And, really, a bologna sandwich, every once in a while isn't going to kill anyone. We survived with a lot worse. Yet, the extra minute or two that you spend putting together something good and tasty for your children will be appreciated. It's a message from home that "somebody cares."

■ Do you know that the term en-riched bread has a different meaning from what you think? It does not mean increased nourishment. It usually means the bread was stripped of its fiber and processed so that 80 percent of its nutrients were removed. Then it was "en-riched." The nutrients were put back into the bread, but the resulting "en-riched" product usually has only 80 percent of the nutrient value of the original natural product.

(If you want to think about this same ratio in financial terms, we'll "enrich" you in the same manner. Give us ten dollars and we'll "enrich" you by giving back to you eight dollars.)

■ THE BETTER LIFE INSTITUTE FAMILY HEALTH PLAN

Speaking of Messages . . .

Every once in a while, include little personal notes to your children. That will please them and tell them that you love them. A note might say, "I'm so glad that you're my son/daughter," or "Just a note to say I love you," or "Always do your best, and it doesn't have to be straight A's."

I Want to Buy My Lunch

Many schools have a lunch program. As a parent it's your responsibility to check out what's for lunch. If your child wants to have lunch with the other kids who buy lunch, then together you must plan the days they're going to buy lunch. It takes only a minute, but it sends a powerful message, "I care. You are special to me."

Always, always ask if they liked the lunch, or what they had for lunch. Make sure Dad gets in the act also.

The Middle School Years

THE UNHOLY ALLIANCE: TV AND JUNK FOOD

As a child progresses in grade school, different things can happen. Many children become involved in sports programs, music and dance lessons, church, and community activities. Educators know that by the time a child is eight years old, his patterns are beginning to gel. They can be changed, but it requires more time and effort. The same can be said of your child's nutritional habits. It's during these years that we see a child's health problems begin to emerge. It's at this time also that kids start to become "couch potatoes," and if you're not attentive, they become "junk food junkies" too. Some recent studies have pointed out that children who watch television have a tendency to eat more junk food. Therefore, they develop more weight problems and blood risk factors than they do at earlier ages.

WHO'S THE BOSS?

Never forget who's really in charge. You just happen to be the boss. And you have to control the amount of time that your kids watch television. Encourage your children to become more physically active. It doesn't have to be in organized team sports. There are many individual physical activities that are interesting for your child. Some are at school. Some are at the "Y" or at a community center. And some are at home.

Be sure to keep healthy snacks around for your children. The kids can't eat them if they're not in the cupboard or refrigerator. It's

Pizza with extra sauce, a little skim milk mozzarella cheese, and parmesan cheese tastes good. I like the mushrooms and onions and hate the green pepper. I eat twice as much as I used to and still feel good.

Source: Ange and Marti Walters (Pat's twin daughters)

Your child's blood cholesterol should be around 120 mg/dl. After age 16, ideally it should be around 150 mg/dl. This is slightly more aggressive than national guidelines. But, we are on the "leading edge" at the Better Life Institute.

important to have enjoyable snacks. Healthy food should not be punishment just as unhealthy food shouldn't be a bribe. You will find many easy and tasty ideas for snacks in Chapter 9.

FAMILY CIRCLE IS A TIME TO CHAT

Use Family Circle to have regular talks with your kids about what's going on in their lives. This is the time to chat not only about food, but also about exercise, school, and friends.

The "Wonder" Years

As children approach puberty, life becomes a little more complex—for everybody! One of our friends whose daughter is approaching puberty comments, "At least once a week I consider putting her up for adoption!" Moody behavior, loud music, hair spray, zit remover, and clothes that you wouldn't wear in public become the most important topics of conversation. These subjects are "life-giving" because to kids they ARE life!

TEEN TURMOIL

It's at this time that many kids, especially girls, begin very unhealthy eating habits and behaviors that include starvation, crash diets, anorexia, and bulimia. Sometimes the boys go on "training table" and "iron pumping" diets. Most are also very weight and looks conscious. What makes life more complicated is that this is their developmental-crunch period. Rock stars and sports figures become their heroes and heroines, and they may have more influence on your teens than you do. It's important to stay in close contact with your teenagers as they go through these turbulent years. It's sometimes difficult for you, we understand that, but if you "hang in there" you can avoid a lot of unnecessary pain in the future. That's where Family Circle can really help you!

Once a teenager from Texas came through our program with his family. The father had had a heart attack before age fifty. They needed help, more so than most families. They paid attention and talked a lot to each other while at BLI and went back home as a family committed to living a healthier lifestyle. We received a Christmas card and the occasional telephone call, and they always said they were doing just fine. About a year and a half after they completed the program, they came back for a visit. We hardly recognized the fourteen-year-old boy. He had lost thirty pounds and grown five inches. The daughter had no need to lose weight. She was growing up to be a beautiful young lady. She was "sailing through puberty"—

a healthy survivor of hormonal and fatty-tissue changes that characterize that tumultuous period of time. We asked the kids, "How did you do it?"

United We Stand

The first thing they said was they did it together as a family. They worked together. They talked and negotiated together. They learned a lot about themselves together in the Family Circle. We asked the young man, "How did you lose the weight? We know how you grew." He said he ate breakfast and dinner at home. His mom always had healthy things around the house. His problem was when he was away from home—at school and with his friends. He learned how to compromise. When he was with his friends, he didn't want to be singled out as "strange," so he learned how to make compromises. If he had a hamburger, he had it with a diet soda. He put boundaries around his behavior and used common sense.

He got a lot of suggestions during Family Circle for his exercise. He joined the tennis club at school. And he and his dad play golf together and walk the eighteen holes. The nice part about it was that the family "normalized" his situation. They openly discussed what to do and made it practical, livable, and enjoyable, with lots of opportunities to "bend the rules." The beautiful part of the story is that the rules were bent but not broken. The young man is now in college. He is six-foot-two inches and still likes loud music, but he has found a way to "survive and thrive" despite the fact that heart disease runs in the family. His health history has changed from high risk to low risk, and he now has a "can do" attitude! This attitude is going to benefit him in every aspect of his life for as long as he lives.

There's a good moral to this story. Think about it for a minute.

Some Hormones Are Thin

Some teenagers go the opposite way. They don't gain weight. You can feed them continuously as if they have two hollow legs. Being on the thin side is not an excuse to pig out on unhealthy foods. Kids can get lots of calories from bread, pasta, cereals, potatoes, beans, big bowls of chili, and nonfat yogurt with fruit. They don't need an extra thick milkshake. Smart athletes gain weight healthfully by "carbo loading," not fat and protein loading. Extra calories, not excess protein and fat, are the issue. Be sure to make them healthy calories. That will lead to healthy habits as well.

Thin or Not So Thin, Make a Plan

If your teenager has a weight problem, is either too heavy or too thin:

■ *Cooking turkey or chicken with the skin on it and then removing it will not result in an increased amount of fat in the cooked chicken. It will result in a more juicy, tastier piece of chicken.*

■ *The "training table" should be a "carbo table."*

1. Consult your physician and arrange a physical exam.
2. Plan a nutrition and exercise program with your teenager that involves other members of the family for support.
3. Make the program fun.
4. Have the child participate in the program in a way that will work for him.
5. Encourage the child with many, many compliments.
6. Remember, "slow and steady wins the race."

The challenge is to make this program practical, livable, and enjoyable *for life*. Think lifestyle—familystyle, not diet and exercise. It's not "me, you, and us." It's "we—together!"

A Final Note on Cholesterol and Kids

Several years ago a study in Bogalusa, Louisiana, revealed that children around twelve years of age already had fatty streaks in their arteries. These fatty streaks are not dangerous at age twelve, but they are the "start of something big." Fatty streaks in arteries may be the forerunner of artery blockage in adults. Heart disease begins in childhood. It does not commence on the day before you have a heart attack. Fatty streaks at age twelve pose no immediate risk for children, but these children are at risk for the future. We recommend, as does the American Health Foundation, a cholesterol check for your child by age two.

If there's a family history of blood vessel disease, having your children's cholesterol checked is even more important. The national recommendation is a cholesterol level of 140–170 mg/dl. Since we provide you with the skills to provide tasty foods low in cholesterol and fat, we suggest that a cholesterol level of 120 mg/dl is an excellent target value. Be sure to discuss your plans with your pediatrician.

The American Heart Association recommends the following dietary guidelines for children:

- Beyond age two, children need between 20 and 30 percent of their calories from fat.
- Limit fast foods to 1–2 times a week and teach your children how to eat less fat and more salads, veggie pizza, pasta, beans, etc.
- Use lower fat foods such as tuna, turkey, and chicken.
- Serve more whole grains for dinner dishes.
- Use whole grain cereals and breads whenever possible.

- Eat fruits and vegetables daily and especially for snacks.
- Limit the amount of fried foods.
- Use lowfat or skim milk and dairy products.

Our children are our own personal extension into the future and our country's future. We want them to be able to give to their families, their community, and their country everything that they are capable of giving. The best way to influence your children's future and your own is to work on the present. The present then becomes the future.

If you want a glass of "whole" milk and mistakenly bought skim milk, don't worry. Add two pats of melted butter and mix, and you'll have the "whole" thing—fat and all.

YES, I CAN

- I can say "I want to" instead of "I have to." Teach your children to do the same.
- I can take my children to a fast food restaurant, and we can enjoy a healthy meal together.
- I can exercise on a regular basis and ask my children to do the same.

FAMILY CIRCLE SUGGESTIONS

Ask the family to suggest a healthier menu at an Italian restaurant than the one you usually order. It's a fun activity. Try it with other types of foreign food restaurants too.

If you or your family use headphones during exercise, make sure they do not block out the sounds of traffic when you are exercising outside. Talk about the danger during Family Circle.

Set an example by telling your children what you had for lunch at work and where you need to improve.

The Fat Story

■ ■

Nutrition is a complex area, and science is still unlocking the doors that lead to health and prevention of disease through better nutrition. However, we do have some general pathways that most scientists agree you and your family should travel. We don't want you to suddenly throw everything out of your pantry. The transition should be slow or else your entire family may start a revolution. Our goals at the Better Life Institute are nutritional excellence coupled with palatability. We are not satisfied with mere adequacy. We want to change the type and amount of fats you eat, but we still want your food to taste good. The earlier you and your family start to reduce the fat content of your diet, the easier it will be to control weight and to reduce risk factors for degenerative disease. And it's not as difficult as it might sound.

A New Age of Fats

In this decade you will witness a great deal of scientific activity related to fats. Americans are concerned about weight control, and fats are our main source of calories. The average American eats about 40 to 45 percent of his total daily calories in the form of fat.

Excess fats have also been proven to play a key role in all blood vessel (vascular) disease—especially cardiovascular (heart) disease and certain forms of cancer. You will see further reductions in recommendations for dietary fat intake from national medical groups.

The food industry is preparing for the decade ahead with a burst of new products to substitute for fats currently used in prepared or processed foods. Olestra,® Simplesse,® and a host of new gums and starches have either already been introduced or are about to come on the market.

Scientists agree that some fats are less harmful than others. New techniques in agricultural biology and biochemistry have made it possible for our food scientists to actually alter the harmful molecules in fats and oils. They can "re-engineer" the oil to be less harmful. You will see new oils on the supermarket shelf that have unusual names or numbers attached to their names.

New developments in genetic science will also allow farmers to grow plants for animal feed as well as consumer use that are genetically different and more healthful. Our corn or soybean oil in the future will differ in chemical structure. Best of all, Americans will soon be enjoying many of their favorite foods without having to ingest a high level of fat. We will also be able to use fats that will be less harmful to our health. It won't be long before all of us will have our cake, and contrary to the old adage, we'll be able to eat it too!

"PHONEY" FATS

Food companies have begun to substitute mono- and diglycerides for fats in baked goods. These chemical substitutes for fats act as emulsifiers and stabilizers that help ingredients combine and remain together. They provide the same texture and "mouth feel" without as many total calories because you need less to do the job. Even though mono- and diglycerides are metabolized by the body as fat and have the same caloric value on a fat gram per gram basis, they do not have the artery-clogging potential and other health risks of animal fat, and less is needed resulting in much fewer calories. We're just around the corner from a variety of new fat substitutes that will keep your interest in eating right up there in the "top 3" interests of your life. You figure out what the other two are!

FAT HISTORY

Ten years ago, many scientists were considered "on the fringe" if they discussed the role of fats in circulation, blood vessel disease, and general health. We agreed that fat was an important nutrient to restrict if weight control or weight loss was a concern. And many health professionals believed that reduction of dietary fat intake was a "good thing to do," but they did not consider it necessary to promote overall health.

The next ten years will be known as the "decade of fat reduction." More research is being conducted in this area, and at present, most research findings support our current concern that we and our children eat too much fat. The food industry is well aware of these trends and, for reasons of disease prevention and weight control, there are many fat reduced foods available. "New age" fats are replacing the old traditional corn, safflower, sunflower, and soybean fats used in most of our foods. Olive, peanut, and canola oils are high on the BLI list of preferred fats and oils. A bevy of engineered and genetically restructured oils will require you to have a "fat dictionary" to understand the foods you eat. The Better Life Institute recognizes these trends, and all our dietary and recipe recommendations reflect the "cutting edge" of fat consciousness.

In 1978 the recommended daily allowance (US RDA) for fat was 40 percent of caloric intake. One year later the McGovern Nutrition Report recommended a dietary intake of about 30 percent fat, including a reduction in animal fats and an increase or substitution of vegetable fats. Current dietary recommendations for fat have been amended as "not to exceed 30 percent" or "up to 30 percent." If you can reduce your daily fat intake to less than 30 percent and still enjoy the food you eat, you will be ahead of the game. Many may think this will affect the palatability of their diets, and initially it will. But, as we've said, *tastes are acquired,* which means *they can and do change.* Don't you think it's worth a change in taste to lower your family's daily fat intake? The big bonus is that they will be eating a lower calorie diet that is heart-healthy and could prevent certain cancers and other deadly diseases.

WHERE'S THE FAT!

ITEM (3 OZ. COOKED)	GRAMS FAT	TOTAL CALORIES	PERCENT CAL/FAT
Beef chuck (pot roast)	26	350	67
Lean ground turkey	6	143	39
Corned beef	19	251	68
Flank steak	14	244	51
Lean ground beef	12	256	57
T-bone steak	10.4	214	44

Source: USDA Handbook #8

Fat Facts

If you're motivated to stay healthy, you should know your *fat facts.* Fat research is the fastest growing area compared to any other aspect of nutrition. We want you to understand the terminology and concepts as you wend your way through the maze of foods and fat ingredients on labels.

THE BIOLOGICAL FUNCTION OF FATS

Fats are essential to maintain your life. They are one of the three major nutrients along with carbohydrates and protein. Fats are composed of two major substances:

1. *Fatty acids* are necessary for growth, metabolism, proper use of vitamins and minerals, and the synthesis and uptake of many hormones.
2. *Glycerides* are a secondary source of energy for activity and essential body processes.

Simple, isn't it? It's also very basic. Fats are divided into the three fat families.

1. Monounsaturated fats (monos):
   olive, peanut, rapeseed (canola), and vegetable oils
2. Polyunsaturated fats (polys):
   corn, safflower, sunflower, sesame, cottonseed, and soybean oils
3. Saturated fats:
   lard, animal fats, butter, and coconut, palm kernel and palm oils

There is no difference among fat families with regard to weight control. The only difference, visually and textually, is that polys and monos are thin (liquid) at room temperature while saturated fats are thick, creamy, or solid at room temperature. Many people don't realize that fat is high in calories. There are 100 calories in every tablespoon of butter or margarine, and there are about 120 calories in every tablespoon of oil. Compare those figures to a total of 75 calories in a hard roll, 80 calories for a whole orange, and 45 calories in a tablespoon of sugar. In general, excess fat intake poses a health risk. At BLI the phrase *excess intake of fat* means "in excess of 20 percent of total daily calories." We will, therefore, provide you with many ways to prepare your family's food with less fat and still keep it tasting good!

THE TYPES OF FATS IN OUR FOOD

Each of the three fat families is found in all foods, but one of them usually predominates. Fish and shellfish are high in a special type of polyunsaturated fat and have a little bit of the other two. Fish and shellfish contain about 10 percent of their calories in the form of fats. Fish fat, called "Omega 3" fat, has very different effects on our circulatory system than the typical polyunsaturated fats which will be discussed in another section.

Chicken and fowl are high in monounsaturated fats and also have a little of the poly and saturated fats. When the skin is removed

■ *In Japan the amount of fat consumed is only about 10 percent of total calories. The Japanese risk of cancer is much lower than in the United States where we get about 40 percent of our total calories from fat.*

after cooking, chicken and most fowl contain about 20 percent of their calories from fats. The exceptions are duck and goose which contain a great deal more fat. All meat and dairy products are high in saturated fats and contain about 70 percent of their calories from fats.

By contrast vegetables are high in monounsaturated fats and contain about 3 percent of their calories from fats. (The exceptions are coconuts, coconut oil, palm kernel oil, and palm oil which are the highest natural sources of saturated fats. They should be avoided all the time except as trees if you want some shade in the tropics. The only thing more dangerous than eating coconut oil or milk is being hit on the head by one.) Remember that the average plant contains about 10 percent or less of its calories from fats while the average meat and dairy product has about 70 percent of its calories from *fats*.

■ *An average peanut butter and jelly sandwich contains about 400 calories—50% fat, 15% protein and 35% carbohydrate. Try less peanut butter and choose whole grain bread and a low sugar jelly.*

PERCENTAGE OF FAT FROM CALORIES

	PERCENTAGE OF CAL/FAT	CAL/ 3½ OZ.
Meat	75%	300
Chicken	20%	175
Fish and shellfish	10%	160
Dairy (whole milk and firm cheese)	75%	375 (cheese)
Peanuts and all nuts and seeds	70%	600
Beans, peas, whole grains	10%	180
Fruits	2%	50
Vegetables	5%	25

It's obvious by the chart Percentage of Fat from Calories that plant food is far lower in fat and calories than animal food. Plants have fiber, which is not found in animals. Animals have cholesterol, which you won't find in plants. That's why we're always encouraging you to "make friends with a plant." If you eat more plant food and less animal food, you'll have fewer problems with weight and a lower risk factor for degenerative disease.

What Exactly Is Hydrogenation?
Have you noticed that you can buy a bottle of liquid corn oil (polyunsaturated fat) and can also buy a tub of solid corn oil margarine? Both are corn oil, but they come in either liquid or solid form. Other oils are also found in these two versions. There's a very logical reason for fats existing as either liquid or solid. Certain foods, such as sauces, salad dressings, baked goods, and margarine, require oil in their processing. Hydrogenated oils, unlike regular oils, are thicker

■ *Cheaper ice cream is more healthy than the expensive "creamy" ones. Creamy means more saturated butterfat. Cheaper means more sugar and gums (fiber)—often called bulking agents and thickeners.*

and more creamy. At room temperature they are solid. These oils do not leak out of the product or pool at the top. They keep the product creamy. Margarine and hydrogenated fats help give baked goods texture and palatability. If you use a liquid oil for baking or sauces, it will drip out of the food or pool at the top of the sauce when it returns to room temperature.

The solution is to "hydrogenate" the oil. You should equate the word *hydrogenation* with "limited usage" when you're reading labels. Some experts believe that hydrogenation changes an oil, and its ability to raise blood cholesterol is increased and possibly exposes you to health risks. With new fat substitutes being developed through new genetic engineering science, we believe hydrogenated fats will disappear from foods.

I'd Like Some Toast. Smear It with Fat, Please.

We recommend that you at least reduce your use of margarine and butter. If you can eliminate it altogether, so much the better. Margarine is a hydrogenated fat, and it is best to be on the prudent side of using fats. Several preliminary studies made in Holland suggest vegetable oil margarine can raise your cholesterol and "bad" cholesterol (LDL) levels. When you think of margarine or butter, think of *fat*. You're smearing *fat* on your bread with a *fat* knife. You place your dinner roll on the *fat* plate. You put a pat of *fat* on your pancakes. Instead of buttering your ear of corn, you *fatten* it. Your recipes call for a half cup of *fat* at room temperature. Isn't it amazing how our idea of something delicious changes when you call it by its true name! Be smart and stop fattening your food.

Fats and Blood Cholesterol

STAY OUT OF THE CHOLESTEROL CONTROVERSY!

Our recommendations at BLI are based upon what appears to be a considerable consensus of scientific opinion. You may have heard that a "controversy" about the importance of cholesterol exists. It's true. It is a very complicated area and is one that would take the majority of non-scientific people much too long to completely understand. Whatever the outcome of this complex research tug-of-war, you can bet that recommendations will remain to lower your cholesterol and saturated fat intake. So, we ask you not to wait until the discussion is over. You and your children can get a safe start right now!

Factual evidence and common sense cry out that we support the recommendations of the current scientific consensus. We do agree that research relating the level of blood cholesterol to risk of heart

■ *Only one of three Americans knows that cholesterol is different from fat and is found only in animals or dairy products. If it's a plant, "it ain't got cholesterol!"*

disease is becoming outdated as a new, more precise understanding of the actual factors related to blood vessel disease is developed. Whatever the ultimate conclusions, your level of blood cholesterol is a significant risk factor. You should try to keep it at a safe level.

We don't want to confuse you, but practically speaking, your dietary intake of cholesterol is and will be important regardless of what the new research uncovers. As you reduce your intake of foods high in cholesterol, you will automatically reduce your intake of all fats (including saturated fat) and calories. Simultaneously, you will increase your intake of carbohydrate and fiber. We think this is an intelligent and safe strategy because by adhering to it you can only win.

What Is Safe?

Cholesterol is measured by the number of milligrams found in one deciliter of blood. Milligrams per deciliter, symbolized by mg/dl, is a concentration measure like, for example, ounces per quart. When your blood cholesterol is elevated beyond 200 mg/dl, your risk of cardiovascular disease is above normal. That is because your level of blood cholesterol is related to the probability of having blood vessel disease (blockages) in your coronary arteries. Studies analyzing the composition of artery lesions or blockages indicate that cholesterol is a key ingredient. So, it stands to reason that if you eat less dietary cholesterol, you are less likely to have lesions or blockages in your coronary arteries.

■ *For every 1% you lower your blood cholesterol, you decrease your risk of heart disease by 2%.*

That's a good deal!

Lipid Research Center Study, National Heart, Lung, and Blood Institute

■ *Increasing the family's intake of water soluble fiber—gums, pectins and mucilages—by including oat and rice bran cereal and/or thickeners made with pectin, can help reduce calories, fat, and cholesterol. It may possibly reduce blood cholesterol levels.*

CHOLESTEROL VALUES OF COMMON FOODS

3½-OUNCE SERVING COOKED:	AMOUNT OF CHOLESTEROL
Fruits, grains, vegetables	9 milligrams
Oysters	45 milligrams
Scallops	55 milligrams
Fish, lean	55 milligrams
Clams	65 milligrams
Chicken/Turkey, light meat (without skin)	70 milligrams
Beef, lean	75 milligrams
Chicken/Turkey, dark meat (without skin)	80 milligrams
Lobster	85 milligrams
Dairy (cheese)	95 milligrams
Crab	100 milligrams
Shrimp	130 milligrams
Egg Yolk, one	225 milligrams
Beef Liver	440 milligrams
Beef Kidney	700 milligrams

While there is little research activity in the area of general arterial disease, it appears that your coronary arteries are not the only ones affected by lesions and blockages. Arteries in other areas of your body will also be subject to lesions when exposed to excess fats and cholesterol. Consequently, you improve circulation in many areas of your body when you make the proper diet and exercise changes.

DEFINING CHOLESTEROL ONCE AND FOR ALL

Most people make the mistake of assuming that cholesterol is the same as fat, and they use the two terms interchangeably. Cholesterol and fat are from the same "family" of fats, but they have different functions. Diet affects them independently. Cholesterol is a waxy substance and is essential to life's function in ways that differ from fat. Cholesterol is a key ingredient in each cell membrane wall. It is necessary for proper metabolism and the syntheses of certain hormones—especially sex hormones. It is manufactured in your liver, and you never need to eat additional cholesterol to meet your bodily needs. If you decided to avoid eating anything containing cholesterol for the rest of your life, there would be no shortage because you have your own "cholesterol factory." It is only when we eat foods that are rich in cholesterol that we begin to have problems.

Every person has his or her own sensitivity to a change in diet. Some people experience major changes with a cholesterol-lowering diet while others have only moderate changes. The immediacy of the effect is also a variable—fast, slow, or anything in between. Generally, if you remain on a cholesterol and saturated fat dietary reduction program, there is a very good chance that you will "max out," or finally reach a safe cholesterol level. If you can't, which is unlikely, see your physician.

Check Out the Family

About 5 percent of the population will not react to a change in diet and will require medication to lower their cholesterol if it is in a high-risk range. Some of these people give up on diets too early because they'd rather take a pill than change their diets. Consult your physician for a cholesterol screening and further information on cholesterol-lowering drugs.

We recommend that you check the cholesterol level of all adults in the family. If one or both of the parents have or have had a significantly elevated cholesterol (greater than 250 mg/dl), every member of the family should be checked regardless of age. If anyone's cholesterol is over 200 mg/dl, your first step is to retest and then work on changing your eating habits. If this doesn't work, you will have to get further tests to assess the specifics of your case. Be sure to stay in touch with your physician.

■ *New evidence suggests that oxidized cholesterol and fats play a key role in artery disease. So, reduce your intake of fats and cholesterol regardless of your blood values.*

■ *A recent study in Louisiana revealed that preschoolers eat twice the saturated fat recommended by the American Heart Association. Their cholesterol intake averaged 180 mg per 1,000 calories. The American Heart Association recommends 100 mg per 1,000 calories.*

■ *THE BETTER LIFE INSTITUTE FAMILY HEALTH PLAN*

The Good Guys

Regular aerobic exercise has the indirect effect of lowering your cholesterol level. Later in this chapter, we will explain high density lipoproteins (HDL), but for now, remember that those are the good guys. HDL's tend to increase with exercise, which means there will also be a slight decrease in your blood cholesterol as well as a decrease in the risk of heart disease.

A Word about Eggs (and Not in Your Face)

Many people have the strange notion that eating egg yolks or whole eggs will not have an effect on their cholesterol. Unfortunately for the egg industry, whole eggs have a high cholesterol content, possibly the highest of any common food source of Americans—a fact that has been supported by independent scientific committees, major medical schools, and scientific study groups.

Some people think that if an egg is eaten raw, it will not affect their cholesterol. A raw or cooked whole egg *will* affect your cholesterol. In addition, eating raw egg exposes you to the risk of salmonella. While such risk is low, it is increasing due to the manner in which we feed chickens. So avoid any egg-related risks by eating only cooked eggs, and if possible, just egg whites or Egg Beaters™ or the new lower cholesterol eggs that are now available. Instead of the usual 225 milligrams per yolk they have about 125 milligrams per yolk. They cost more, but for a lot of people they're worth it.

Egg whites are pure high quality protein with no fat or cholesterol in them. Prepare them as omelettes with lots of vegetables.

Polyunsaturated Fats and Blood Cholesterol

All polyunsaturated fats and oils tend to lower blood cholesterol. For this reason, in the past they were recommended as a substitute for other types of saturated and monosaturated fats. However, recent trends in science have de-emphasized the role that corn, safflower, sunflower, and soybean polyunsaturated fats should play in your diet and food preparation. The reason is that some possibly significant health problems have been linked to use of polyunsaturated fats in high amounts. You will see less emphasis upon them and more on plant oils that are high in monounsaturated fats (peanut, olive, canola, avocado, and nut oils).

Fish have an oil that is high in polyunsaturated fats also. But, fish and shellfish poly oils are slightly different in structure from regular polyunsaturated fats. These polys are called "Omega 3," and they tend to improve circulation and lower cholesterol, LDL (which we will explain later), and blood triglycerides. They also have an anti-inflammatory or calming effect on your blood vessel walls. Finally, they tend to reduce the tendency of your blood to clot, which is a problem for those with high risk for circulatory disease. Still, excess fats and oils of any kind are not desirable. For this reason we recommend that you include fish in your weekly diet as many times as possible and substitute fish for meat, dairy products, and even chicken.

Monounsaturated Fats and Blood Cholesterol

Olive, peanut, rapeseed (canola), avocado, nut, and vegetable oils are high in monounsaturated fats. These oils will lower your blood cholesterol, although less than polyunsaturated fats will. However, unlike polys, the safety record for monos is excellent. People have eaten monos for thousands of years, and you will see an increasing reliance upon them when fat is required in a recipe or recommended by health groups. When you see the term "vegetable oil," it is likely to be a high mono oil. In the future, we will engineer new mono oils and devise new plants to grow them. You will soon see them replace polyunsaturated fats in margarine. But remember, margarine is *hydrogenated oil*—a very different type of fat than the original oil. If you wish to use margarine on a limited basis, we suggest you use "lite" tub-type margarine.

Saturated Fats and Blood Cholesterol

Beef, pork, lamb, veal, and dairy products, including butter, are higher in saturated fats than other food groups. Chicken and turkey are higher in monos. As noted earlier, fish and shellfish are higher in a special type of poly (Omega 3). *Dietary intake of saturated fat has almost double the effect on your blood cholesterol as dietary intake of cholesterol.* That's why nutritionists tend to place more emphasis on decreasing the intake of saturated fat rather than just cholesterol itself. Obviously, you should reduce or avoid all saturated fats and the foods in which they're contained naturally or with which they're prepared.

These, then, are the three different families of fats. Remember, the oil (liquid) or fat (solid) you use in food preparation or that you eat contains all three fat families.

What the Better Life Program Does

The Better Life Institute Family Program provides guidelines to reduce your dietary intake of ALL fats and oils to about 20 percent of your total daily caloric intake. We also are very emphatic about eliminating or greatly reducing the amount of oil used in food preparation. Since you are lowering the total amount of ALL oils and fats while you are learning to "make friends with a plant," you are effec-

The little bag of peanuts provided on airplanes has about 100 calories. Seventy percent of those calories are fat.

Butter fat and dairy fat are highly saturated. Whole milk cheese has about 75% percent of its calories from fat.

THE BETTER LIFE INSTITUTE FAMILY HEALTH PLAN

tively lowering your exposure to many health risks. In this way, the BLI program gives you and your family an additional *safety margin for health*.

In summary, you can lower your blood cholesterol by:

1. Reducing the amount of saturated fat you eat every day or at every meal.
2. Reducing your daily intake of foods high in cholesterol.
3. Reducing your total dietary fat intake.
4. Reducing your overall caloric intake. This will usually result in the overall reduction of fat and cholesterol.
5. Do not increase your intake of polyunsaturated or monounsaturated fats to reduce your cholesterol.

Okay, Gang. Summer's over and now it's time to go to FAT SCHOOL!

Fat School

LEARNING MORE ABOUT FAT

The "fat story" gets a little more complicated than what we have already discussed. It is very important that you become familiar with some additional terms and concepts that are on the cutting edge of heart research, treatment, and prevention.

Lipoproteins

You already know that cholesterol is a waxy substance that is different from fat. And if you've ever tried to mix oil or wax with water, you know that a waxy or fatty substance does not mix well with water. Since most of your blood is water, how can cholesterol and fat travel in your bloodstream since neither substance can mix with water? The answer is that they travel through your bloodstream in combination with protein. The combination of protein and fat in one vehicle that can travel through your bloodstream easily is called a *lipoprotein*. (*Lipid* is a scientific term for fat.) There are a number of different types of lipoprotein that travel through your bloodstream. For the sake of simplicity we will identify and discuss the three familiar types of lipoproteins that have made the news: Low Density Lipoprotein (LDL), Very Low Density Lipoprotein (VLDL), and High Density Lipoprotein HDL).

Each of these types is explained as follows:

LDL

LDL, or Low Density Lipoprotein, carries fat and cholesterol to the artery wall and deposits it in the wall of that blood vessel. The higher your level of LDL, the greater your risk of heart disease and other arterial disease. If you are an adult, an LDL rate higher than 125 mg/dl exposes you to increased risk. For children, LDL should be below 90 mg/dl.

VLDL

VLDL, or Very Low Density Lipoprotein, is very fat rich and directly influences your total blood fat, which we call triglycerides. The higher your VLDL, the greater the amount of fat or triglycerides in your bloodstream. The VLDL also indirectly affects the amount of LDL we have in our bloodstreams.

Triglycerides is a fancy term for fat in your bloodstream. It makes your blood thicker and more prone to clotting. If your blood triglycerides exceed 150 mg/dl you are at excess risk.

Sometimes VLDL is used interchangeably with triglycerides. This can also be a risk factor for heart or artery disease. New evidence on VLDL and triglycerides suggests that post menopausal women have a high cardiovascular risk factor if their triglycerides exceed 150 mg/dl. If you are a middle-aged man with a low HDL (below 40 mg/dl) and a triglyceride level above 150 mg/dl, you are considered a high risk for heart disease. BLI recommends a triglycerides level of below 125 mg/dl for everyone. It's obvious that you are healthier if you have a low level of blood fat.

HDL

HDL, High Density Lipoprotein, carries fat and cholesterol AWAY from the artery wall and acts as a cleansing agent. It is well documented that if you have a high level of HDL, you have a lower risk of heart or artery disease. We believe that an HDL of 60 mg/dl or higher is best.

GET YOUR FATS IN ORDER

Scientists and physicians have devised a screening system to determine if you are at excess risk for heart disease from blood cholesterol. National recommendations are that you have a maximum of 200 mg/dl blood cholesterol. If your cholesterol level is higher, it is recommended that you try to lower it with dietary change. If that isn't successful, you'll need to assess your LDL level and other risk factors. BLI recommends a blood cholesterol of 190 mg/dl or lower—and of course, the lower the better!

New evidence suggests that if your cholesterol is below 160 mg/dl or your LDL is below 100 mg/dl, it may be possible to shrink or reverse deposits and lesions on blood vessel walls. Four studies showed reversal. Three of them were conducted with drugs and the fourth used a 10 percent fat calorie diet. Since drugs have side effects, it is best to get your cholesterol and LDL down as low as possible by changing your diet and reducing your fat and cholesterol intake. At BLI, we consider these drugs to be an option only if all other dietary means are ineffective. If you must use the drugs, use the minimum amount that is necessary. All cholesterol lowering drugs have significant long-term side effects. A decision to use a drug is a long-term decision so be extra sure you really need a drug to do the job. Discuss this with your physician.

Food Influences on LDL, VLDL, and HDL

There are several dietary and health-related actions you can take to decrease your heart disease and artery disease risk.

You can decrease your LDL by:

- decreasing your total intake of saturated fat AND cholesterol.
- decreasing your total fat intake.
- eating more fish rather than meat as your entree (not more than once per day).
- decreasing your total calorie intake.

You can decrease your VLDL or triglycerides by:

- decreasing your total fat intake.
- decreasing your intake of foods high in sugar.
- achieving proper weight control on a lower fat and calorie restricted diet and then maintaining proper weight.
- reducing or eliminating alcohol intake.
- engaging in a regular aerobic exercise program (check with your physician regarding a safe, vigorous program).

You can increase your HDL by:

- achieving proper weight control and maintaining it.
- reducing your total fat intake.
- stopping smoking.
- engaging in a regular aerobic exercise program (check with your physician).
- eating more fish as your entree.

The "Magnificent Seven"

For the past decade the ultimate word on dietary guidelines has been rather vague. At a time when we are laboring under the strains of degenerative diseases that are significantly related to the food we eat, we feel you need more than vague dietary guidelines. Moreover, the children of today are the adults of tomorrow. Surely we can provide something more beneficial, nutritionwise, than "eat a little better; good luck and God bless"! For example, the U.S. Department of Agriculture, the U.S. Department of Health and Human Services, and the National Research Council offer us the following advice:

- Eat a variety of foods.
- Maintain a healthy weight.
- Choose a diet low in saturated fat and cholesterol.
- Choose a diet with plenty of vegetables, fruits, and whole grain products.
- Use sugars only in moderation.
- Use salt and sodium only in moderation.
- If you drink alcoholic beverages, do so in moderation.

These dietary guidelines, in our opinion and the opinion of many health professionals, are too vague and too benign. There is not enough "meat" to guide our country into the future.

The Better Life Institute cannot guarantee better health by virtue of our more aggressive dietary recommendations. But if you follow our program, you have much more "insurance" for yourself and your family, for the short- and long-term. And there's little if any sacrifice in taste and ease of preparation. In our opinion, our guidelines, the "Magnificent Seven," are right on the money. The Better Life Institute has built a program around them—not with more "meat," but with more "fiber"!

Consider yourself better informed on fats and cholesterol than 99⅞ people in 100. As you read the next chapters, look for suggestions that will help you and your family achieve your weight and heart health goals. In fact, all of our recipes are designed for these purposes. After tasting these recipes, you'll realize that the foods prepared the "Better Life way" will be enjoyed by everyone.

"YES, I CAN"

- I can learn the difference between *guidance* and *bossiness*.
- I can be more aware of the importance of the example I set for my family.
- I can allow my children to instruct or guide me in areas that they know better than I.

FAMILY CIRCLE
Let your children lead some of the Family Circle meetings. If you do make sure you don't "boss" them from the sidelines. Give them the ball and let them run with it—unless they fumble.

■ *THE BETTER LIFE INSTITUTE FAMILY HEALTH PLAN*

Ask if the family would mind if Grandpa and Grandma attend Family Circle. Let the entire family join in to help and enjoy each other.

Plan to go out for some dessert, or a family treat immediately after Family Circle. It adds a little "zip" to the meeting.

The Better Life Exercise Program

Those Were the Days, My Friend

We all have wonderful memories of the stories our parents told us about their lives in "the good ole days." Time and time again, we listened to magical tales of what life was like "then." Every story would usually start with the old refrain, "When I was your age . . .

- I walked two miles to school."
- It was my job to carry the coal bucket."
- I helped your grandpa with all his chores on the farm."
- I cleaned house with your grandma every day."
- I was a paperboy and gave my money to your grandma every week."

Everyday life was indeed different for our parents as it is and will be for our children. The basics of everyday life required a great deal more activity on their part than is required today. People walked, chopped, carried, scrubbed, washed, sawed, and dug as matter of factly as they breathed the air. Strong arms, legs, and torso were a necessity for both men and women. When Sunday came around they truly looked forward to a day of rest. Since time immemorial, men and women have used the Sabbath day for rest and spiritual reflection—a day to relax and refresh. On the Sabbath they listened, spoke, watched, and sat. It was a wonderful respite. It was sorely needed. They had to labor physically for what they got. Then they restored and refreshed themselves on the Sabbath and started all over again the next day.

FROM MUSCLES TO MINDS IN TWO GENERATIONS
For most people today rigorous physical activity is not a part of daily life. We press buttons, set timers, make restaurant reservations, mi-

crowave food, dial telephones, drive our children everywhere, and pay others to take care of many of the simple physical needs of living that our grandparents did for themselves. We don't need strong arms, torsos, and legs. In today's workplace we need the physical apparatus that our forefathers used yesteryear for leisure: ears, eyes, fingers, mouths, and bottoms to sit on. The rest of us is rarely used. We are the first generation to make what we might call the big switch—from muscles to minds.

The transition to a sit, watch, talk, and button-pushing society has many advantages in terms of productivity, technology, intellectual achievement, and leisure time. But shouldn't someone inform our bodies how wonderful this "high tech, sit and do world" is? Our bodies don't seem to have gotten the message. From the status of our overall health, it appears that our bodies are not agreeing with "new high tech."

Rx: Exercise!

Much of what we call *degenerative disease* is related to our lack of physical activity. So much so that we are now going through a decade where physical exercise is either "prescribed" by physicians or recommended for most Americans as general health "shoulds." In fact if exercise is not recommended, it is because that individual is too ill to exercise.

Today the streets are full of joggers and bikers. Exercise clubs can be found in every neighborhood. Every morning before work and every evening after work, hundreds of thousands of people are dressed in sweats and tights, bouncing up and down to "keep it up," "all together," and "only ten more reps" exhortations of young firm-bodied aerobic instructors. And our homes are full of bikes, treadmills, stair climbers, and an assortment of ropes, rubber bands, springs, and weights. (Unfortunately, many of us have never made the transition from "purchase" to "use.") We are all overexposed to pleas from doctors and health associations to exercise, exercise, exercise.

Many of us have heard the message, but few of us have paid attention to the message. Regular aerobic exercise is important to health! But most of us will use any means possible to avoid getting out of our comfortable chairs and moving our feet and arms. Exercise, just like eating, means the personal change of habits that are known and comfortable, a giving up of the that's-the-way-I've-always-done-it mindset.

OUR KIDS ARE MORE LIKE US THAN WE ARE!

Unfortunately, times have changed also for our children. First of all, beyond age five our children do not dutifully follow us around the

■ *THE BETTER LIFE INSTITUTE FAMILY HEALTH PLAN*

house and garden eager to help or ask to do our menial, routine physical tasks for us. They are busy with their own lives, and too many children are doing mostly sitting, watching, talking, and eating.

The Apple Doesn't Fall Far from the Tree

Gone are the days when little boys rushed home from school eager to go out in all kinds of weather to play the seasonal pick-up game. If little boys play at all, it is in organized midget, mini, teenie-weenie, little, pony, colt, or whatever-the-name leagues. And now, little girls also participate in these leagues. How many times lately have you seen the children of your neighborhood playing hop-scotch or jumping rope?

Recent estimates by national fitness associations are shocking. By age twelve only 12 percent of our children engage in any regular exercise outside of school intramural activities. The President's Council on Physical Fitness points out that by the sixth grade as many as one child in four is at excess risk for heart disease.

It is equally unfortunate that the lion's share of any physical activity our children do have is involved with team sports. These activities do have some virtues. However, building lifelong, enjoyable aerobic exercise habits is not one of them. Team sports rarely consist of activities that children can enjoy as they grow into adulthood or that they can do on an individual basis or at a more convenient time. Race walking, jogging, swimming, biking, hiking, aerobic dance, and cross country skiing are great exercise for people of just about any age if they are in condition. But it is very difficult to get a team of forty-year-old people to leap and run at baseball, football, or basketball, despite the pictures painted by beer and soft drink commercials.

Our children need to learn the value of forming healthy aerobic exercise habits, either at school or at home. They live in a society that does not support these activities. And, as with eating habits, the earlier they learn to practice daily these time-tested virtues, the more vigorous, enjoyable, and probably longer their lives will be. Opportunities for them, and you, abound in family life. You can share many wonderful moments with your children when you exercise together. It's also a great way to show them your support.

OK, GUYS, LET'S DO IT!

We know you know exercise is necessary to improve your family's health. What we're trying to do is help you get going and keep on going. And we need to say a word of caution: Keep your exercise program in perspective. Despite the tales and heroic feats of triathaloners and marathoners, researchers are in agreement that *moderate* exercise on a long-term basis is better for you than short-term "go for

■ *By age twelve only 12% of our children regularly participate in sports or physical activities.*

Dr. Lawrence Wolfe,
National Fitness
Institute

the gold" rigorous exercise. What we don't want to do is make exercise a new vocation or "calling" in your life.

On Your Mark, Get Set, Walk!

Your exercise does not have to be complicated by formulas for maximum oxygen uptake, calorie burn, or the differences between anaerobic and aerobic metabolism. All you have to do is put one foot in front of the other at the right rate and for the right length of time. It's that simple. You don't have to learn any new athletic skills. Everybody knows how to walk! Nor do you need expensive equipment. Just a strong pair of walking shoes and your commitment to *do it!*

What Does Moderate Mean?

Let's put some numbers behind exercise and the term *moderate*. Moderate is:

- regular aerobic exercise four or more times a week.
- exercising for thirty minutes to an hour.
- exercise that includes a five minute warm-up and a five minute cool-down.
- a short muscle-toning session with small five- to ten-pound weights, depending on your strength.

Your Exercise Primer

We apologize ahead of time for this, but we think it's important to provide you with some of the basics relating to exactly why you and your family should exercise. There are three components to a good exercise program:

1. Aerobic, or cardiovascular, fitness
2. Muscle tone
3. Muscle strength

AEROBIC, OR CARDIOVASCULAR, FITNESS

Aerobic simply means "with oxygen." That's exactly what walking, jogging, biking, swimming, and cross-country skiing do. These kinds of exercise activities provide more oxygen to your heart muscle and to all the other cells, tissue, and organs in your body. We all know life cannot exist without oxygen and getting that extra jolt of oxygen is energizing.

> ■ *Your exercise does not have to be complicated. All you have to do is put one foot in front of the other at the right rate and for the right length of time.*

CARDIOVASCULAR RISK TEST
How Likely Are You to Have a Heart Attack?
Circle your score in each category and total.

	SCORE
STRESS	
Hardly ever tense	0
Tense several times a day	1
Constantly on edge	2

	SCORE
WEIGHT[1]	
Average	0
Up to 20% overweight	1
More than 20% overweight	2

BLOOD PRESSURE[2]
(Diastolic)

Under 90	0
90 to 95	1
Over 95	2

BLOOD CHOLESTEROL LEVEL[3]

Age 20–29	Below 150	0
	150 to 200	1
	Over 200	2
Age 30–39	Below 200	0
	200 to 220	1
	Over 220	2
Age 40 & Over	Below 220	0
	220 to 240	1
	Over 240	2

EXERCISE

Aerobic activity 3 or 4 times a week	0
Aerobic activity 1 or 2 times a week	1
No aerobic activity	2

SMOKING

Non-smoker	0
Under 1 pack per day	1
Over 1 pack per day	2

Your Total: _____

HEART ATTACK—REDUCING THE RISK
WHAT YOUR SCORE MEANS

0 to 4: Low Risk   5 to 8: Average Risk   9 to 12: High Risk

The higher your score, the greater your risk of developing heart disease. You can lower your odds by changing your lifestyle.

[1]If you are a man, your ideal weight = 110 lbs. plus 5 lbs. for every inch over 5 feet.
 If you are a woman, your ideal weight = 100 lbs. plus 5 lbs for every inch over 5 feet.
[2]In blood pressure readings, the diastolic is the lower number; the systolic, the top number.
[3]Cholesterol level is measured by a blood test. See your doctor.

Aerobic exercise is rhythmic or repetitive. It's not necessarily a "fun" tennis game. The repetition sometimes makes it tedious or boring, but it doesn't have to be. With the selection of proper activities, it's a form of exercise that you and your family, at every age, can practice on your own or with others.

Toning and Muscle Strength

We place these remaining two features of exercise in the same category for practical reasons. If you engage in any of the above aerobic activities with a stretch and cool-down period, you will tone and strengthen the muscles in your arms, legs, and torso. There is no need to build big muscles unless you lift weights for a living. Most of us never lift anything heavier than a vacuum cleaner.

Whether it's blood vessel disease or its common recognizable consequences—heart disease, high blood pressure, diabetes, stroke, kidney, liver, eye, ear, or skin problems, or weight control—exercise is the key to good health, and it provides the behavioral and motivational "tie that binds."

Exercise, Health, and Degenerative Disease

PRIMING THE PUMP

Proper nutrition helps to provide high quality fuel and oxygen (blood) to all your cells, tissue, and organs. It also helps to keep the walls of your blood vessels clean and open. That's a little more than half the job. Exercise pumps, or forces, blood through your blood vessels and increases the delivery of nutrients and oxygen to all the target parts of your body—cells, tissue, and organs. In addition exercise tends to widen blood vessels. This also increases "fuel delivery." You can see why exercise is very important to enhanced blood circulation and prevents degenerative disease. There's another positive effect of exercise that's a little more complicated to explain. It's called *collateral circulation.*

How Do I Get Collaterals?

When you exercise physical activity increases in many parts of your body. Your heart muscle needs to work harder to deliver fuel, or blood, to your muscles, which work harder as you exercise. The increased activity of your heart and other muscles requires the delivery of additional nutrients and oxygen for food and energy. Your body tries to adapt to your increased nutrition and oxygen needs during exercise. The blood vessels slowly stretch to reach out further and provide your heart and other muscles with what they need to do the job, which is an increased blood supply.

A City Map of Blood Vessels

For the purpose of a graphic example, let's think of our arteries as streets within our bodies. The large arteries could be called boule-

THE BETTER LIFE INSTITUTE FAMILY HEALTH PLAN

COLLATERAL CIRCULATION

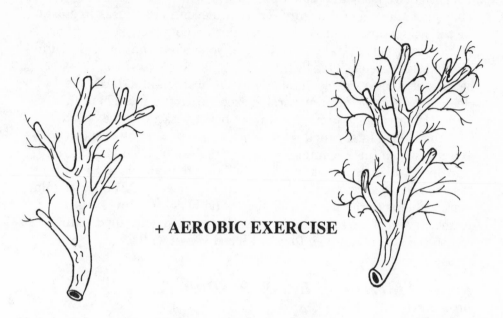

+ **AEROBIC EXERCISE**

vards and the smaller ones side streets. Regular aerobic exercise allows you to build small alleyways and maybe even a few footpaths off the alleys. These alleyways are called *collaterals*. The more you exercise, in terms of intensity and duration, the more collaterals you build.

Think of it this way. A fifty-year-old person who has exercised regularly for ten years has about twenty miles of boulevards, sidestreets, and alleyways or blood vessels of various sizes. A fifty-year-old who has not exercised regularly has only about fifteen miles of these same thoroughfares.

Avoiding Blood Vessel Gridlock

The person with twenty miles of blood vessels has more insurance against poor circulation. It's well documented that collateral circulation simply because the person exercised regularly has saved many lives after a heart attack. They had the good fortune to have enough additional "alleyways" to partially offset the oxygen-choking effect on the heart muscle. It saved their lives. Logic dictates that blood vessels delivering fuel to other areas of your body that are challenged by the need for more oxygen during aerobic exercise are challenged to *stretch* as well. Thus, exercise builds more circulation by increasing the size of blood vessels, or by building a few more "alleyways" through collateral circulation.

THE BETTER LIFE EXERCISE PROGRAM ■

OTHER CIRCULATORY EFFECTS

More Bonuses from Exercise

That's not the end of the story. There are even more pluses in store for the person and family with a regular aerobic exercise program. We've discussed several components of your blood that are related to blood vessel disease. One of them, HDL, is called *good cholesterol* because it removes cholesterol from your artery walls. HDL is a cleansing agent. A regular aerobic exercise program tends to increase your HDL and helps protect you from blood vessel disease.

Your blood fats, called *triglycerides,* also tend to be reduced with exercise which further improves your circulation. With less fat in your blood, it is less thick and is less likely to build clots. Blood that clots too easily increases the risk of arterial deposits. Finally, regular exercise helps to regulate blood sugar and blood insulin levels. Higher levels of sugar and insulin in the bloodstream tend to increase the risk of damage to small blood vessel walls.

RISK TO LIFE OF BEING OVERWEIGHT
(in years)

AGE	MARKEDLY OVERWEIGHT (more than 30%)		MODERATELY OVERWEIGHT (10–30%)	
	MEN	WOMEN	MEN	WOMEN
20	−15.8	−7.2	−13.8	−4.8
25	−10.6	−6.1	−9.6	−4.9
30	−7.9	−5.5	−5.5	−3.6
35	−6.1	−4.9	−4.2	−4.0
40	−5.1	−4.6	−3.3	−3.5
45	−4.3	−5.1	−2.4	−3.8
50	−4.6	−4.1	−2.4	−2.8
55	−5.4	−3.2	−2.0	−2.2

Source: Metropolitan Life Insurance Company

Once you are on a safe yet vigorous exercise routine, your heart starts its own personal "conditioning program." You will remember from earlier chapters that the heart is a muscle. It's large and complex, but nevertheless it is a muscle. If you use your muscles more often, they are in better condition. Several medical studies have documented significant differences in your ability to process and use oxygen in your cells when you exercise regularly. You become a much

THE BETTER LIFE INSTITUTE FAMILY HEALTH PLAN

more efficient oxygen-using machine. That's exactly what is meant
by conditioning.

Getting Better "Mileage" from Your Heart

Every muscle becomes stronger when it is exercised and conditioned.
As you exercise, your leg and arm muscles strengthen, and they experience less fatigue from a workload that would have strained them
earlier. In other words, now they can do the same job with less effort.
Exercise has the same effect on your heart muscle. It becomes
stronger, and along with wider blood vessels supplying more nutrition and oxygen, it pumps fuel through your body with more
strength. You will "huff and puff" less and less until you stop
huffing and puffing! The net result is a decreased pulse rate and
lower blood pressure. Thus, your heart does less work doing the same
job, and your blood vessels experience lower pressure as blood flows
through them. With lower blood pressure, you have a reduced risk of
blood vessel cracking and blockage. In general, you reduce the overall wear and tear on your circulatory system.

Regular exercise does something else that benefits your heart. It
helps control and reduce your weight. Instead of your heart and blood
vessels having to service a Ford Thunderbird, they service a Ford
Escort. By lightening the load, there's less chance for degenerative
disease.

FADS AND FALLACIES

Remember all the hoopla and hype when those passive exercise machines were being introduced? Sorry, folks, but Lulu has always said,
"There ain't no such thing as passive exercise!"

According to marketers of this approach to exercise, you can just
lie on a table and let the machine do the work for you. However, physicians and exercise physiologists know better! The only thing that
gets exercise is the machine. *You* must work your muscles to create
tension from muscle extension and flexion. Electric stimulators,
steam boxes, and other gadgets may tickle your fancy (as well as
your wallet) for easy "no sweat exercise." But you must face a cold,
hard fact of life: There is no lazy way to exercise!

Turning on the Heat

Using a sauna or steam bath will not provide any exercise either. All
that happens is you dehydrate your body. If you have heart disease or
high blood pressure, you should use these treatments only with a
doctor's advice. These heat treatments tend to raise your blood pressure and can put you in a dangerous situation. And children should

■ *Sweating is very
healthy, but you
should replace lost
water. When you are
reducing your
weight, you want to
lose fat, not water.*

■ *Make sure your
kids drink enough
water. Eight glasses
a day for an adult is
a good rule of
thumb.*

never be allowed to use these treatments. They have smaller bodies with smaller cooling systems. They can overheat to a life-threatening point!

Your body strives to maintain a natural water level, and proper water level is essential to your life and health. Any attempt on your part to lose weight by squeezing water out of your body with pills is very unhealthy—unless you have a medical problem. Sweating is very healthy, but you should replace lost water. You want to lose fat, not water. When you lose water you lose key vitamins, electrolytes, and minerals, and the loss adversely affects all bodily functions. Always, always drink water and replenish that which you lost by sweating. Make sure your kids drink enough water. Eight glasses a day for an adult is a good rule of thumb.

Water is an excellent drink. Low sugar or sugar-free drinks are also good. An occasional glass of fruit juice is fine, but remember, fruit juice has lots of sugar in it. That's why it's sweet. Caffeinated beverages defeat the purpose of drinking to replace water because they promote water loss.

It's smart to avoid dehydration, not treat it.

Plastic sweatsuits and herbal wraps also cause you to dehydrate and can be dangerous. They do not "cleanse" you. You just lose plain old water along with essential vitamins and minerals. Wrapping yourself in hot sheets and letting an attendant douse you with herb-flavored liquids is a great idea if you have a sudden urge to become a teabag. Leaping into icewater baths should be called a "leap of death." Such rapid change in body temperature can place your system under tremendous stress, and it can dangerously increase your blood pressure. It's okay for polar bears but not for human beings. If you seriously want to be macho, eat vegetables and run miles, and you can then tear people apart when you celebrate your one hundredth birthday!

START NOW. BETTER YET, START YESTERDAY!

The earlier you start a regular aerobic exercise program, the better the state of your circulatory system will be, and as you get older you will have bigger and wider blood vessel boulevards, sidestreets, and alleyways. As we've said before, you will increase your protection against blood vessel and degenerative diseases.

Children need to develop proper positive attitudes toward exercise. Helping them do that is an important parental responsibility. Both parent and child win. You will be setting a healthy example for your children and improving your own health at the same time. And your children will be forming good habits that will benefit them for the rest of their lives. Just think how different your adult life would have been up until now if you had started proper exercise habits in your youth and maintained them into your adulthood. What a wonderful opportunity for everyone!

Exercise and Weight Loss Control

We've already discussed proper nutrition and calorie reduction as these two factors relate to weight loss and weight control. Exercise is equally important in keeping weight under control. Without a regular exercise program, you can never hope to lose weight healthfully or to keep it off. If you exercise regularly, it is easy to maintain your weight and more difficult to gain weight. Whether you look at exercise as a way to lose weight or a way to maintain weight, exercise is the *key*.

There are many reasons why exercise is important. Some are easy to understand and some require a little imagination on your part. Let's get the easy ones out of the way first.

■ *Whether you look at exercise as a way to lose weight or a way to maintain weight, exercise is the key.*

MAKING WITHDRAWALS FROM YOUR ENERGY BANK

Exercise places increased energy demands on your body. The way you meet the increased demand for energy is by reaching into your "energy bank." Your energy bank is easy to locate on your body. Just reach out and touch all those parts that are well padded. You know the parts we mean. They're the parts you always try to hide. That's your energy bank. When you exercise more, you use up more energy and will lose more fat over a period of time. Think of it as making periodic withdrawals from the bank.

AND THE WINNER IS . . . EXERCISE!

People who change their eating habits and exercise regularly in a lifestyle change program, benefit with faster and more visible results. The extra bonus associated with increased exercise is that it tends to reduce your appetite and relax you. Research and our years of experience have told us that exercise is an effective way to manage stress. You eat less, you feel better, and you burn more calories when you exercise. Now you can understand why exercise is a win, win, win situation.

Let's Go to School!

Think of your body as being composed of two parts. The first part is lean body mass consisting of bone, blood, muscle, and organs. The second part is fat body mass consisting of (ugh!) your fat! When you

THE ENERGY COST OF ACTIVITIES

ACTIVITY	CALORIES PER POUND PER HOUR	ACTIVITY	CALORIES PER POUND PER HOUR
Bedmaking	1.9	Piano playing (Beethoven's "Appassionate")	1.1
Bicycling	4.0	Piano playing (Liszt's "Tarantella")	1.4
Bicycling (moderate speed)	1.6	Reading aloud	0.7
Boxing	5.7	Rowing	5.0
Carpentry (heavy)	1.5	Rowing in race	7.8
Cello playing	1.1	Running	3.7
Cleaning windows	1.7	Sawing wood	3.1
Crocheting	0.7	Sewing, hand	0.7
Dancing, moderate active	2.2	Sewing, foot-driven machine	0.8
Dancing rhumba	2.8	Sewing, electric machine	0.7
Dancing waltz	1.9	Singing in loud voice	0.9
Dishwashing	0.9	Sitting quietly	0.7
Dressing and undressing	0.8	Skating	2.1
Driving car	0.9	Skiing (moderate speed)	5.2
Eating	0.7	Standing at attention	0.8
Exercise		Standing relaxed	0.7
Very light	0.9	Sweeping with broom, bare floor	1.1
Light	1.1	Sweeping with carpet sweeper	1.2
Moderate	1.9	Sweeping with vacuum sweeper	2.2
Heavy	3.0	Swimming (2 mi. per hr.)	4.1
Very heavy	4.0	Tailoring	0.9
Fencing	3.8	Tennis	2.8
Football	3.6	Typing, rapidly	1.0
Gardening, weeding	2.3	Typing, electric typewriter	0.7
Golf	1.2	Violin playing	0.8
Horseback riding, walk	1.1	Walking (3 mi. per hr.)	1.4
Horseback riding, trot	2.5	Walking rapidly (4 mi. per hr.)	2.0
Horseback riding, gallop	3.5	Walking at high speed (5.3 mi. per hr.)	4.3
Ironing (5-lb. iron)	1.0	Walking downstairs, calories per pound per 15 steps	0.011
Knitting sweater	0.8	Walking upstairs, calories per pound per 15 steps	0.034
Laboratory work	1.5	Washing floors	1.0
Laundry, light	0.6	Wiring	0.7
Lying still, awake	0.5		
Office work, standing	0.8		
Organ playing (1/3 handwork)	1.2		
Painting furniture	1.2		
Paring potatoes	0.8		
Playing cards	0.7		
Playing table tennis	2.5		
Piano playing (Mendelssohn's "Song Without Words")	0.9		

THE BETTER LIFE INSTITUTE FAMILY HEALTH PLAN

exercise two things happen. You build muscle or lean body mass, and you expend energy or burn calories to meet your exercise energy needs. Let's stop and think about this for a minute. If you use all the calories you take in through eating, you'll have to tap your energy reserves—your "fat bank" or fatty tissue—for energy.

LOOKING LEAN AND MEAN

Your goal when you try to lose weight is to reduce your fat body mass and increase your lean body mass, your muscle tissue. Essentially you are developing a body with a little bit of fat and a lot of muscle. That is where the "lean look" comes in. It doesn't mean you will look like an iron-pumper. There are many athletes, basketball players, runners, swimmers, and dancers, for example, who have very lean, long muscles and very little body fat who also do not have big, bulky muscles. When you reduce your body fat and increase your lean muscle mass, you are turning yourself into a "lean, mean, fighting machine."

THE EXERCISE/METABOLISM CONNECTION

Muscle tissue actually needs more calories to stay alive than fatty tissue needs. The more muscle you have, the greater your caloric needs, and usually you can eat more without gaining weight. Additionally, a high level of lean body mass raises your metabolism rate.

As an example, let's compare the caloric needs of two men who each weigh 175 pounds. One has 10 percent body fat and the other has 20 percent body fat. The man with 10 percent body fat and 90 percent lean body mass needs more calories to maintain his weight at 175 pounds and keep his lean body mass, or muscle, alive. The reasons are quite simple: Muscle, or protein, needs more calories to maintain life than fatty tissue needs. As the amount of lean body mass increases, the metabolism rate rises. So the 10 percent fat man not only needs more calories to feed his muscle mass and maintain his weight, he also burns his calories faster than the 20 percent fat man. Conversely the HIGHER the percentage of body fat, the LOWER the metabolism rate. The man with 20 percent body fat and less muscle will gain weight on an 1800 calorie diet while the 10 percent body-fat man will lose weight on the same amount of calories! The well-muscled man's exercise program helps to increase his metabolism. He can eat, enjoy life, and not worry or think about food.

The same body composition facts are equally true for women. However, women have more difficulty controlling their weight than men do. They are naturally "blessed" with a greater percentage of body fat and they have smaller body sizes. Therefore, they require fewer calories than men and they need a regular aerobic exercise pro-

■ Cellulite *is nothing more than a name clever marketers created to sell new products. Cellulite is merely fat that collects directly under the skin. It "pouches" because the elastic tissue holding it ages as you age. The only way to get rid of it is to exercise aerobically and lose weight. It takes time, but when you work at it, "cellulite" can disappear.*

gram to increase their metabolism and build muscle to control their weight. A healthy woman age twenty should be about 18 percent body fat. A healthy sixty-year-old woman should be about 25 percent body fat.

As you can see, a scale will not tell the entire story. You can be pudgy and still be at "normal" weight. It's body composition that makes the difference. Invest in a tape measure and watch those inches disappear as you become "lean and mean."

Age becomes a factor in weight control as you pass your thirtieth birthday. There's a tendency for your metabolism to slow down as you get older. In addition, your hormones change with age. Add to that equation more sitting and less exercising, more stress, and more eating, and you wind up not only with an older body, but a bigger one containing more body fat. Yuck!

That's why we said, "Start your exercise program yesterday." It's never too soon to start and it's never too late. Exercise offsets many of the aging and metabolic factors that influence weight gain and body fat gain. Discuss your plans with your physician before you start either a weight loss or exercise program. But don't put it off.

It is both unhealthy and ineffective to consider weight loss or weight control without using the powerful "one-two punch" of both diet and exercise. As with love and marriage, "you can't have one without the other."

Muscle does not turn into fat if you don't use it. "If you don't use it, you lose it" is actually what happens. It shrinks and loses mass. Then since you are not exercising, you replace it with fatty tissue. Thus it appears that fat has replaced muscle. You can rejuvenate those old muscles with a good aerobic exercise program.

A NOTE ABOUT YOUNG CHILDREN

In general children should also exercise aerobically. We are usually overwhelmed by the capacity that our youngsters have for unlimited and spirited activity. It's certainly better than sitting in front of the television and eating a bag of potato chips! Beyond age six there are really no special qualifications or concerns about exercise for your children. We suggest you discuss your child's specific exercise needs with your family physician or pediatrician.

There may be some medical factors that limit their exercise, but there's nothing about being a child that makes exercise dangerous or unhealthy. You must understand, however, that their bodies are smaller than yours. Those little legs can't walk as long or as fast as yours can. They also may not be as well coordinated as you are. Whatever exercise activity you engage in with your children, please make sure that it's fun and not competitive with you or their brothers and sisters. Everybody should win at family exercise.

One special note of caution about children's exercise: Since their bodies are smaller, their cardiovascular systems, blood vessels, and hearts are smaller. If your children are below age sixteen, they should not use hot tubs or jacuzzis unless the temperature is below ninety degrees fahrenheit. Furthermore they should not remain in

THE BETTER LIFE INSTITUTE FAMILY HEALTH PLAN

The Vices and Virtues of Body Composition

10% Body Fat
90% Lean Body Mass

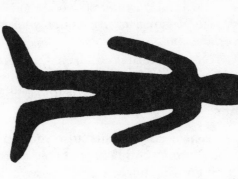

175 pounds
2000 calories to
maintain weight

20% Body Fat
80% Lean Body Mass

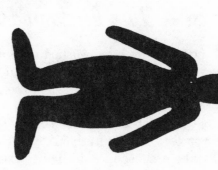

175 pounds
1800 calories to
maintain weight

30% Body Fat
70% Lean Body Mass

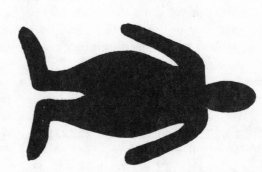

175 pounds
1600 calories to
maintain weight

Fat weighs less than body mass. The greater your percentage of body fat, for the same weight (175 lbs.), the greater your body size.

the water as long as an adult. Their "cooling system and radiator" is their cardiovascular system (blood is mostly water). Because of its smaller size, it is not as efficient as yours, which means that children can overheat more quickly.

We recommend that children six years old and under never be given the same aerobic exercise requirements used by older children or adults. A rule of thumb for younger children and exercise is the following:

1. When considering the distance your child can walk, just divide his age by three. A child six years old can safely walk two miles at a pace SLOWER than an adult. Always use your common sense with your children.
2. A child below age eight should not walk faster than 3 miles an hour or a mile in 20 minutes. Between eight and twelve, use a 3½ mile an hour pace.

Exercise—The Hidden Benefits

Over all the years we have worked with adults and families, we can recall very few people who said they truly enjoyed their exercise program at first. But once they selected the right program and exercised regularly for several months, it became a habit and was actually a pleasurable experience. Exercise is something you know is good for you, and you feel better after you do it. But there is a common tendency to make excuses in order not to exercise. Regular exercise may present a challenge to you and your family. For that reason, we need to look at the excuses for not exercising.

BUILDING IN EXCUSES

If you survey a thousand people like yourself, you will find most of them have thought about doing exercise and know it is important but have not yet done it. About 200 people will flirt with a regular program, but only fifty will actually build a regular exercise habit. Most fitness and exercise clubs, for example, rely upon a 90 percent attrition rate for memberships. That means nine out of ten people who purchase memberships will not use the club more than three times a year after the first month.

We eat to live. Therefore, we can face food and try to make some adjustments in our eating habits. But, we don't *have to* exercise. The additional effort to get up off the couch when one is comfortable has dimmed many of the best laid intentions to exercise. But for those who do, there are many hidden benefits in store. These pluses may in the long term be more important than the very obvious benefits.

■ *THE BETTER LIFE INSTITUTE FAMILY HEALTH PLAN*

"I Don't Get No Respect"

Comedian Rodney Dangerfield always brings down the house with his signature line, "I don't get no respect!" Rodney is saying that other people don't place a high value on what he does. We suspect that the character he plays feels the same way about his own actions and that's the reason he gets no respect. Our personal values, what we personally think is right and wrong or good and bad about and for ourselves, form the basis of our individual self-respect. When our actions are consistent with our values, we think well of ourselves and retain our self-respect—and vice versa. It's that plain and simple.

If, for example, you place a high value on being a "good" parent, and you feel you do a good job at it, you have self-respect. We have many goods, bads, rights, and wrongs in our lives . . . about our health, eating, exercise, work, child (to our parents), spouse, and friends. They are opportunities for you and your family to build self-respect. Self-respect is a precious personal quality, and we could all do better with a good dose of it. How does exercise relate to self-respect?

Getting Your Exercise Act Together and Taking It on the Road

Many people think about getting out there to exercise every day. Yet, as we mentioned, few people actually do it. If you are one of the few who do make the decision to exercise regularly, you are making your actions consistent with your values. You believe exercise is good for you, and you actualize your belief. You feel good about yourself, as we all do when we do something we know is important and good for us, especially if we have had difficulty doing it in the past.

Self-respect goes a long way in life—whether you are a child or an adult. The way you earn it is not complicated or expensive. You just have to do things with yourself that you believe are important. Think of exercise as an opportunity to help you build your own self-respect and an opportunity for the other members of the family to build theirs. What a wonderful quality to begin to nurture in children at the youngest possible age! That's why something as simple as exercise can go a long way for you and others whom you love. So, get some respect—exercise!

Self-discipline

SELF-DISCIPLINE LEADS TO SELF-ESTEEM

Many parents have complained to us that their children need self-discipline. We think that many children feel the same way about their parents! For a child the term *self-discipline* has no meaning in the abstract. But a child does understand that he must pick up his clothes and close closet doors. He must take out the garbage even if he doesn't like doing it. When he does, that's self-discipline.

Exercise activities fall in the same category. Sit down with your child and discuss the importance of exercise. Together you can select the proper exercise program and support. With your help your child can learn the importance of self-discipline and self-respect by doing his or her exercise program. The most valuable lessons in life are simple ones and are usually experienced through practical activities. Exercise is an opportunity to provide your child with the lifelong gift of self-respect and self-esteem. That *can do* attitude is of incalculable value in life. And, by the way, there's an opportunity for you to learn a few things for yourself as well. Remember "do as I do"?

We measure ourselves continuously against others every day of our lives. It is equally important to strive to improve ourselves. When you do compete against others, you can't control how they do. You only have control over what you do. But life presents many opportunities for all of us to try to do better, comparing ourselves to ourselves instead of to others. Exercise presents a very obvious and frequent opportunity to compare past performance with present. It also allows us to try to improve.

Your performance is very obvious and easy to measure. When a child is presented with a tangible experience, such as the exercise to learn, he or she has the opportunity to do better and improve. A practical experience in self-improvement or self-esteem is a natural part of the exercise activity. In addition, improvement is "inevitable" because the effects of continuous practice and conditioning are bound to lead to improvement. Thus exercise is a natural everyday opportunity to increase confidence and self-respect. Remember to leave the competitive edge for competition. Don't compete with the members of your family.

When you think of exercise, think of *opportunities, situations,* and *solutions* to improve health and strengthen family life.

IT'S ALL IN THE FAMILY

Whether yours is a two-parent or single-parent family, exercise activities can be meaningful to family life. For every parent, regardless of family status, a walk with your child can be a very nourishing activity. Exercise provides a natural and enjoyable opportunity to do something constructive and personal together without distractions. Exercise bridges differences between parent and child whether age or culture. It can build understanding and respect between the two of you. If you are a weekend parent, it gives you the opportunity to resume your direct parental responsibilities and allows your child to be parented.

■ *THE BETTER LIFE INSTITUTE FAMILY HEALTH PLAN*

■ *Walking is an exercise activity most children, parents, and grandparents can enjoy together. Think of walking as* health and family medicine.

There are many exercise activities that should not be "medicine" for you and your children to do together. Remember, exercise should be fun for both you and your children. If planned correctly, it gives your child the opportunity to work with you on a mutually important activity. Swimming with your children gives all of you the opportunity to "horse around." This helps kids find an acceptable way to deal with the little frustrations they have with their parents. It also allows parents to be a little childish and get down to their kids' play level. Remember when you were a child and played "Marco Polo"? If you play it with your children, you'll love it all over again.

Don't forget to invite Grandma or Grandpa along for a walk. Perhaps your child can invite them and sort of "chaperone" them if the situation is appropriate. Exercise can bring many generations in a family together, and all are doing something of value together. Sometimes smaller children with smaller legs do quite well with elderly people whose legs are older. Think about it.

Remember, exercise should be fun.

We cannot overemphasize the fact that exercise should be fun and relaxing. It should provide wonderful family memories for all. Try to plan vacations that have natural exercise built in. Trekking, camping, hiking, swimming, and skiing are examples of family vacations that can bring you all closer together.

"It's How You Play the Game"
One final, brief word on exercise activities: There is a time for competition, but family activities or family exercise is not one of them. Whether you realize it or not, you are a bigger-than-life person to your children. Accept it as an indisputable biological fact. You can't get out of it. For this reason, be very careful about competition with your children. In many it brings out confusing feelings. They want to impress their parents and be good at the activity, but they also want their parents to be good at it as well.

Heads, I Win—Tails, You Lose
Your children can experience conflict in either winning or losing. You are older and may not consider it a case of winning or losing. But many children feel it is. Try to keep this important "childish" perception in mind and remember: if you "win," you "lose"; if you "lose," you "lose."

A similar situation exists among brothers and sisters. Teach children not to "go for the jugular" when playing games together. Try to teach them to help their brothers and sisters. Family sports and competition are not the same as competition in the outside world. Family sports is a time to love, support, and help each other and still have fun.

The goal is not winning. The goal is doing. In the words of

Knute Rockne, "It's not whether you win or lose, it's how you play the game." You may or may not agree with this philosophy in the outside world, but it's a fair rule for family life. Family life is truly "how you play the game."

YES, I CAN

- I can go to my children's athletic activities and school games.
- I can *energize* my family when I see they are a little "down in the dumps."
- I can listen to my children and spouse when they make special requests and suggestions for exercise and meal planning.

FAMILY CIRCLE

Discuss the time-honored virtues of *patience, perserverance,* and *tolerance.* Ask each person what these concepts mean. Ask for specific instances when these qualities are present.

Ask the children what "situations and solutions" they face at school lunches.

Tell the rest of the family what you do at meals when you are out with friends eating at a restaurant or in their homes.

Learning Your Exercise ABC's

■ ■

Chapter 8

What Wonder Drug:

- **Increases energy . . .**
- **Reduces stress . . .**
- **Counters depression . . .**
- **Helps sleep . . .**
- **Controls the appetite . . .**
- **Costs little or nothing . . .**

The Answer? *EXERCISE!*

When we went to school, the first thing we learned was the alphabet. We vocalized our "ABC's" with a sing-song repetition until they became a habit. We practiced them daily—writing them, spelling them, and speaking them until they became a part of us. Within a short time, we could sing them to our teachers and parents. And during that time, we also learned to write them, using both capitals and small letters. We progressed from little children who had none of the tools for learning to students "armed to the teeth" for new educational and communication experiences. We practiced and practiced. Within six months, we were ready to join an elite group—people who can read. And, we could begin to experience life in ways that are only possible if you know your ABC's.

The ABC's of Physical Movement

When a baby learns to sit, crawl, stand, or walk, he is learning his "ABC's." As his body gets stronger and his motor skills develop, he can learn more and do more. When he is more active, his muscles grow stronger. As his muscles grow stronger, he is capable of more activity. Each week his body is capable of doing more complex activities that require more strength. With everything we do—walk across the room, drink a cup of coffee, eat a meal—we move muscles. It's something we take for granted and don't give much thought to, but it's really part of our "ABC's" of physical movement.

When we reach our forties, sometimes small acts of movement or exercise become difficult. Suddenly we find we get winded from carrying groceries into the house. We begin to huff and puff while taking a brisk walk around the block. And, we might even have to stop and catch our breath after climbing a flight of stairs.

THE "OVER THE HILL" GANG

How did this happen? How did we change from being "fit as a fiddle" to feeling "over the hill," "asleep at the wheel," and "out to lunch"?

It didn't happen overnight. It was a gradual decline caused by failing to keep our bodies physically fit. Do you remember the immortal words of George Bernard Shaw? He said, "Youth is wasted on the young." It's only when we get older that we begin to appreciate the fitness we took for granted when we were kids. When we are not-so-young we become much more aware of the strength and stamina we used to have.

When we first learned our "exercise ABC's," we practiced them every day. We didn't forget the fundamentals because we used them over and over and over. We leaped, jumped, climbed, and crawled our way through our houses, backyards, and school playgrounds. We used our bodies constantly.

WELCOME TO ADULTHOOD

But, eventually there came a time when our activity levels began to decrease. The native spark in our bodies which crackled when we were young tended to grow dimmer and dimmer with increasing years. Bending, climbing, walking, running, and biking may not be routine parts of our everyday lives anymore. These activities are often done begrudgingly . . . only when necessary . . . usually when we can't get others to do it for us. Age isn't the issue. The issue is our lifestyles. And, as the saying goes, "if you don't use it, you lose it." Physical fitness is no exception. If you don't stay fit, you lose your fitness. Like many adults, perhaps you've lost your grasp on your "exercise ABC's." If you're smart, you realize that these fundamentals are not gone forever. The best way to brush up on them is to practice.

Now is the time to roll up your sleeves and start relearning those "exercise ABC's." Don't forget to include the rest of the family because as you're building good habits, the effects are going to spill over to everyone else. And best of all, by making exercise a part of

Regular aerobic exercise helps prevent loss of bone mass, or density, in later adult years, and reduces your risk of a disease called osteoporosis.

THE BETTER LIFE INSTITUTE FAMILY HEALTH PLAN

family life, you and your kids can keep practicing your physical "exercise ABC's" together.

Back to Exercise Basics

Regular exercise is fundamental and basic to living a long, full life. We hope you understand that. Physical fitness is a way in which we get to know and enjoy those beautiful machines, our bodies. While not as rudimentary as the "ABC's" we learned in kindergarten, the following twelve concepts are the basic fundamentals for bringing regular exercise back into your life:

1. You must have the proper "Yes, I can!" mindset. Many people feel that exercise will always be something they hate or prefer not to do. Don't think of your exercise as optional. You have to get over the hurdle of putting off until tomorrow what you should do today. We are all guilty of procrastinating, so stop looking for excuses. Face the basic reality that exercise will actually improve your health and vitality. When you exercise, you're 50 percent closer to a healthier lifestyle. Make your exercise fun.
2. "Slow and steady wins the race." The goal of exercise is to become physically fit. That's all. You don't have to become a competitive athlete. You need a clear vision of what is required—not a romanticized "take no prisoners" version. Very few of us can come even close to those sterling athletic characters in *Chariots of Fire*. And there aren't many of us who can hold a candle to those unbelievable females who humble us every morning on television's aerobic exercise programs. Exercise is not a "stop-start-stop-start" mechanism. You simply need to develop a regular exercise program. Your body requires it for a healthy life.
3. Because our society is so competitive, many of us truly believe we have to be the best at everything we do. Some people go one step further by completely abandoning an activity if they are not the best. Excellence is awesome to watch in the Olympics, but few of us can get a gold, silver, or bronze medal. We don't have to win anything in our daily routines. The goal of your exercise should be to make it fun and invigorating. Let the Olympians train competitively and go for the gold while you cheer and enjoy your own exercise for life—that's the real "gold."
4. Your body has accumulated some mileage over the years, and it can't be exercised as if it were fresh from the showroom. If you impair your health by injuring one of your body parts, you may avoid exercising ever again. And we don't want to let you off the

hook quite that easily. So, see your physician to get advice about a safe aerobic program. Many a problem has been avoided or prevented by a physical exam and exercise cardiogram.

5. Pay attention to the moans and groans your body makes. A pulled muscle, soreness, cramps, and pain are all signals that the machine is not running correctly. Throw away the old beliefs that say "No pain, no gain" and "Go for the burn." Most important of all, if there is any sign of chest, muscle, or joint pain, STOP your activity *immediately* and see your physician. Let him decide if you have a problem. You're not the doctor.

6. Variety is the spice of life when it comes to exercise. The biggest enemy you have is boredom. There's no rule that you have to do the same thing every day. Use a number of different activities to increase your interest. Technically it's called *circuit training,* but you can call it "having fun by doing a lot of different things."

7. You don't have to look like a fashion plate when you exercise. You're going to perspire, or worse than that, you may even start to "sweat"! And there's nothing like good old sweat to bring you down to earth with the rest of us. After a good exercise class, we all look the same. No one else really cares how fancy or color coordinated your clothes are.

8. Never compromise with your walking or exercise shoes. Sometimes the most fashionable-looking shoes are the least appropriate for exercise. And many people don't pay attention to their feet until they start to hurt. But when your feet hurt, you "hurt all over." Some ankle and leg injuries can be caused by worn out or poor fitting shoes or by shoes that don't have proper supports. Good shoes will make your exercise an enjoyable experience.

9. When you exercise, you always lose water even if you are not sweating. If it's not replenished, it can cause serious health problems. Make sure you do not allow yourself to become dehydrated. Plain drinking water works just fine. If you're a serious athlete, you may want to consider a "sports drink." But, don't forget these beverages contain calories and sugar as well as vitamins and minerals.

10. Remember to warm up and cool down. If you can do that for your car, you can do it for your body. It will prevent many muscle and joint injuries. Don't make the mistake of jumping right in to active exercise or stopping quickly. Too many people have a tendency to skip this very important part of exercising.

11. Everyone, regardless of age and physical condition, can and should have some kind of exercise program. If you have any questions concerning your own capabilities, talk to your physician or an exercise physiologist about a program that's right for you.

12. Watch those competitive tendencies that make you want to outdo your teammates. There's nothing that damages family relationships faster than one person always trying to beat someone else. Remember the goal is your fitness, the family's fitness, and being together. Exercise is not about winning a trophy. It's about being healthy. Good sportsmanship helps to build good character. Save your competitive edge for tournaments.

LEARNING TO EXERCISE INDIVIDUALLY AND AS A FAMILY

Both individual exercise and family activities are essential components of your exercise program. Don't think of one without the other; they have different purposes. Whether you swim by yourself or with your family, for example, you improve your fitness level. You'll probably have lots of fun horsing around in the water when you swim with your entire family. When you swim by yourself, you'll concentrate more on fitness and conditioning. Both are important.

The family that exercises together stays together. We want to emphasize that a family exercise program is for *everyone*—toddlers and grandparents included! And don't forget to bring along the dog! It's a way to build a lasting tradition that provides security, support, and many fond memories of moments shared together. The family exercise program should be at a moderate level, allowing everyone to feel successful, individually as well as a part of the group.

Exercise Togetherness

Walking is an activity preferred by the Better Life Institute because it gives all family members an equal opportunity to do something together. There should always be room for individual programs as well as for fun exercise projects such as a hike or bike ride together. Single parents can use exercise time as an opportunity to assume parenting responsibilities in a mutually enjoyable manner. It also provides quiet and enjoyable moments together with their children.

Another aspect of exercise is the *character* it builds. When people of any age know they've set and are keeping a goal, they feel a sense of pride in what they are able to accomplish. The experience of working hard to improve yourself and *doing it yourself* can forge wonderful personal qualities for both parent and child. Family swimming or walking, for example, are exercise activities that provide the opportunity to challenge oneself at one's own pace and still participate in a family activity. Also these activities aren't school- or education-related and, therefore, don't have a hidden scholastic agenda.

Don't forget that exercise is fun, and the exercise plans for the family should be pleasurable. Think of this family activity as recreation and leisure time and not as learning and educational time. If you or the family don't have fun together while you exercise, you are defeating a major purpose of the activity.

We will suggest several forms of exercise in the following section. They are just examples to show you the various objectives and qualities that your family exercise program should have. The goals of your program should be: (1) family unity, (2) enjoyment and fun together, (3) physical fitness, and (4) character building.

There are countless activities a family can do together. The list is inexhaustible: hiking, biking, swimming, walking, rebounding classes, dancing, aerobics classes, and fitness club activities. All are available in your community. The idea is to do something together while encouraging and supporting your family to participate in their own individual programs. Even vacations can be centered around family exercise time. Exercise can be a moment shared, a gentle touch, a hug and kiss after a walk, a lot of laughs and jokes at your own expense, and a time when you can truly help each other. Exercise is "family."

All Together Now!

The exercise you and the family choose will have an important impact on the success of the program and its long-term maintenance. Some activities should be done on a group basis, and some should be individual. They have different but supportive purposes. An ideal exercise program incorporates both because it helps each family member to accomplish personal and family health goals.

WALKING POWER

The best form of exercise is walking. Almost everyone can walk. It is, by far, the easiest type of exercise, and usually this type of exercise causes very few injuries. In fact a good aerobic walk just about every day is all that is needed for a lifetime of fitness. Many adults walk for exercise because they remember the pleasures of walking as a child. It's familiar and comfortable, and it "clears the head." It's an activity that needs no special skills and no special degree of concentration. Young and old alike can do it. And you don't need any fancy equipment. We will suggest many types of activities, but we strongly recommend that walking be the lynchpin of your family exercise program. If you can't think of what to do for exercise—*walk!*

The Hidden Benefits of Walking
We've all heard the phrase "quality versus quantity." It goes without saying that quality time is what counts—not only at work but also at

play. We believe that family exercise time can provide each family member with a certain level of special quality time that we don't experience in other aspects of our lives. When you go for an outdoor walk, there are no telephones, pots boiling over on the stove, or "emergencies" to distract you from what you are doing. Sometimes going for a walk brings you right back to basics: fresh air, trees, birds, and (usually) Mother Nature at her best. Having a good walk with one or more family members provides the perfect setting for having a good talk. Many parents have gotten to know a child much better when they're away from the distractions of everyday life. It's a great time to share ideas, hopes, dreams, and fears. It's a perfect environment for you and your child to get to know each other better.

Getting to Know New Things about Your Children

We cannot emphasize strongly enough the importance of taking time out *frequently* to get to know the members of your family as individuals. Walking together is the only exercise that allows free flowing conversation to occur. There's a need to build a different relationship with each member of your family. We can think of no better way than by walking together. Choose the day and the time and make a date, weather permitting. If Mother Nature doesn't cooperate, shift gears and go to "plan B," which might be an indoor activity. It's rare in family life that your kids and you do things together that give each person the opportunity to know each other as people instead of just as parent and child, brother and sister, grandparent and grandchild. Walking together can help you become friends.

The walk we have in mind is not to be used for educational purposes, lectures, or discipline. It's what we call a *relationship-building walk*. The goal is to build on your foundation as parents. We've had so many parents tell us that going for a walk with their kids gives them all a chance to tread on "neutral ground." They feel it's okay just to talk about what's going on in their lives. And all kinds of questions and laughs pop up. If your kids see that you think it's all right to "open up," you have the opportunity to show them that it's okay for them to talk about personal things.

In the final analysis, you are "parent" and they are "children." But, sometimes the roles can be reversed, and you can get guidance from your children. Let them get to know you in different ways—as a person with a sense of humor, as someone who has a lot of curiosity, and as an individual who doesn't know all the answers. The concept of "family" is more than parents and children living together under one roof. It is a group of people living together who enjoy each other and are dependent upon each other in addition to their roles as parents and children. This is an opportunity for you to share something

LEARNING YOUR EXERCISE ABC'S ■

that doesn't cost any money. It does cost time, but then, we think you'll agree it's a worthy investment.

Don't forget the "exercise" part of walking. It's a healthful activity, and it doesn't matter at what pace you do it. But it can be even more healthful if you walk at a brisk pace that has those wonderful aerobic effects we've already discussed. If you're walking with a small child or a person who obviously doesn't have the ability that you have, you have no choice but to walk at a slower rate. Do try to keep the pace up whenever possible.

A simple rule of thumb for exercise—something we've nicknamed *Lulu's Formula*—is to walk at a rate that makes it possible for you to continue a conversation without getting out of breath. There are many different calculations for what is termed your *Training Heart Rate*. In a later section we will provide you with the formula that is used by the American Heart Association to calculate it. If you are on prescribed medication, check with your doctor about a safe training heart rate level and exercise program.

GETTING INTO THE SWIM OF IT

Rarely can a family use swimming as a regular aerobic activity. It requires a considerable amount of skill as well as superb conditioning and the luxury of a lap pool. However, the rewards of a family commitment to swimming are great. Lap swimming is perhaps the best form of aerobic exercise available to us. There is no risk of joint damage because the body is buoyant and not weight bearing in the water. Your knees, ankles, and hips are gratefully spared from the bouncing and grinding so characteristic of most exercise activities. Also swimming is the one exercise in which you work a variety of muscles at the same time. You could call it a "prime-time" exercise.

Swimming is an activity that is highly enjoyed by children. There is an excitement about swimming that is often not present in other activities. Whether or not you select swimming as a major individual or family exercise, it is a wonderful activity to use to add some sizzle to your family exercise program. It also happens to be a great way to break the sense of monotony that might occur with your other exercises. Water turns out to be a splendid equalizer since children often swim at a level somewhat equal to adults.

A Special Bonus from Swimming

Swimming offers parent and child a special opportunity for enjoyable guidance and instructive experiences. With encouragement and gentle teaching, you can communicate a great deal of love in the water. The water-related skills you teach your child will form a closer bond between the two of you—one that will be remembered forever. We all fondly remember the skills our parents taught us. It was a special

■ *THE BETTER LIFE INSTITUTE FAMILY HEALTH PLAN*

time just between them and us. Swimming instruction requires you to be physically close to your child even to the point of actually holding him or her up in the water. Because of the underlying insecurity most children feel when in the water, it fosters a sense of trust between you.

HOW ABOUT JOINING A FITNESS CLUB?

Many people think that joining an exercise club costs too much money, particularly if you don't use it every day. Fitness clubs aren't just for jocks or young women in leotards who specialize in high power exercise classes. Many clubs provide programs for all members of the family at different times of the day and at different skill levels. Mom can go to an early morning light aerobics class while the boys can use it for basketball after school. The girls can use the exercise machines on the weekends. And Dad might enjoy a noon-time workout.

A night at the fitness club is a great family outing. Everyone can do what they want and then get together afterward for dessert. There are even classes for pre-schoolers to show them that exercise can be fun. And Grandma and Grandpa can have their own special classes to improve their cardiovascular fitness. The entire family can benefit and enjoy group activities and doing things individually.

The club becomes a subject of conversation, jokes, and experiences of the family giving each other support. It can become an enjoyable family meeting place. Membership costs vary considerably. Often special discounts are offered during membership drives, and be sure to check out special family rates. If used wisely, your exercise club can be a win-win-win solution for family fitness.

A BICYCLE BUILT FOR TWO—OR MORE

Bicycle riding is an excellent family exercise because many family members can do it together. This activity also spares your joints from the pounding associated with jogging. What makes it special is that you can plan an enjoyable destination activity such as a picnic, sports activities at a park, a visit to the zoo or a museum, a family swim at the community pool. For a change of pace, you might even consider renting several bicycles built-for-two. It's a wonderful way for families to work as an interdependent team.

SHALL WE DANCE?

Did you ever watch your little one or teenager gyrate to music? You marvel at their ability to twist their bodies into positions you know would probably break yours in half. There's a sense of pure pleasure on their faces that's impossible to miss. Adults also enjoy dancing, but we seem a bit more inhibited in our movements, or shall we say, "civilized." Some people are just plain embarrassed to get up and dance. Nowadays, you really don't need formal lessons to learn certain steps. You just get out there and "do your thing." Dancing is a place where the two worlds of young and old can meet on pleasurable ground. The joint flexibility and aerobic conditioning that dancing provides is comparable to the best of other exercise programs.

Try some of the dances that your children enjoy. If you survive, you might even enjoy them. Tell your kids you want equal time, which means they should try dancing to your kind of music as well. The relaxation, pleasure, and physical fitness derived from dancing makes it a wonderful family experience. Think of all the laughs you'll provide for your kids when you start getting the "right moves" for their latest dance craze. Most importantly, dancing brings parents and children together at a simple level where they all can enjoy each other's company. It's a great way to communicate with your children. After a while you might get very ambitious and throw a family dance party!

Let's not forget Grandma and Grandpa! They can participate in family dancing too, and we guarantee that you and your kids will get an enormous bang out of seeing them jitterbug. The grandfolks can show you some of the dances they did before discos and MTV!

The "Dancing Grannies" are a group of grandmothers who live in Arizona and who have formed a chorus line dance troupe. Many of them have had heart attacks or other health-related problems and several of them had weight problems. They found that dancing was a way to improve their health, maintain their weight, and have lots of fun doing it. They travel the world entertaining and amazing people of all ages. They're high kickers, maybe not as high as when they were twenty, but, truly, how many grandmas do you know that can even kick? If the spirit moves you, you might form your own Family Chorus Line!

IT'S A STRETCH

Many families using the Better Life Institute program have a regular morning stretch routine before breakfast. It's a wonderful way to begin your day physically and together as a family. Your respective schedules may not accommodate a daily routine, but there are certainly specific days of the week on which you can start the day together. All you have to do is set your alarm ten minutes earlier. Then get up instead of pulling the covers over your head. It will only take a few minutes for the whole family to do some easy stretching exercises. Starting the day stretching together makes a powerful statement about personal and family values. And guess what? It's actually fun!

■ *THE BETTER LIFE INSTITUTE FAMILY HEALTH PLAN*

TAKE A HIKE, KIDDO!

There are several hiking and outdoor clubs that sponsor regular family activities. Consider joining the Sierra Club or some similar outdoor association with regularly scheduled activities. There are a number of other ecologically- and educationally-based outdoor activities that the entire family might enjoy. Fortunately kids today are becoming so aware of the delicate balance of nature and how to save the environment that membership in such a conservation-oriented club might be welcomed. It will also give you a meaningful issue to talk about with your kids.

BE A GROUPIE

Local YMCA's or similar neighborhood organizations have regularly scheduled exercise and family activities year round. Rather than trying to be the family social or activity director, let these associations do the master scheduling for you. Join in and plan to participate regularly. This is a great weekend activity. Encourage your children to use these organizations at other times as well. They'll meet other children who share their common values and interests.

RACEWALKING—THE LATEST RAGE

Known by many names such as speedwalking, pace walking, and aerobic walking, racewalking is an activity that many families can enjoy provided there is an allowance made for individual differences in size, conditioning, and strength. Obviously you don't have to adhere to the Olympic rules. Just develop your own version of this active exercise. It's easier on your joints than jogging and will not cause muscle injuries. If you need a more rigorous workout, combine racewalking with the use of small weights in your hands.

The Better Life Institute doesn't recommend jogging for most people unless you have been doing it for several years. We feel there's too much potential for joint and muscle damage. Jogging requires you to be in excellent physical condition, an important prerequisite for withstanding the continuous body trauma of accelerated pounding of the road.

And Now We Proceed to Plan B

The best exercise plans can be sabotaged by bad weather. Have a few bad weather family exercise activities "up your sleeve." There's always the local community "Y" or fitness center available for a family activity. Many shopping malls open their central areas before shopping hours for exercise. You can always plan something at home

LEARNING YOUR EXERCISE ABC'S ■

followed by a special breakfast or lunch out after exercise. This takes the sting out of a canceled activity to which everyone was looking forward. Remember to have some aerobic exercise video tapes available. Sometimes you can find them on sale or you can rent them at the library. They are handy on a rainy or very cold day.

POINTS TO REMEMBER

Always keep in mind that there are many exercise goals for yourself and your family. In discussing exercise we are not just talking about working up a sweat. We want to reiterate that each member of the family has an individual goal. Before you make your plans, ask yourself these questions:

1. Does the exercise activity provide the family an opportunity to work together and support each other?
2. Does the exercise program provide fun and relaxation for the family?
3. Does the exercise program provide the aerobic experience necessary for you as an individual to improve your fitness?
4. Does the exercise program provide opportunities to develop and strengthen individual character within the family?
5. Is the exercise program realistic and can it be maintained for many months, perhaps even years?

Your Individual Exercise Program

Each day hundreds of thousands of people engage in individual activities to improve their fitness. It is not unusual to see people jogging in the park or street with reflective tape on their jogging suits before dawn breaks. Morning aerobic classes at clubs or on television are routine. Lunch hours are often spent exercising instead of chowin' down on a corned beef sandwich. Evenings again find streets, parks, and clubs filled with people who are jumping, swimming, and riding exercise bicycles. The motivations for this tremendous outpouring of physical activity are many and complex.

Some people exercise to manage stress. Others do it to control their weight. The feeling of vigor and youthfulness resulting from regular exercise is also a strong motivator. Let's not forget that regular exercise improves your physical appearance. And, finally, there are those out there who do it to prove something to themselves, whether the issue is youth or character. In most instances, it is impossible to separate the reasons why we exercise. Nor is it important to do so. The important thing about exercise, the "bottom line," is to exercise regularly and begin as soon as possible.

THE BETTER LIFE INSTITUTE FAMILY HEALTH PLAN

Prior to starting your exercise program, we strongly recommend that you be smart and discuss your program with your family physician, whatever your age or medical status. Your doctor has a good grasp on your overall health and family history and can guide you in selecting an appropriate program that has safe yet vigorous limits.

PICKING OUT YOUR OWN EXERCISE PLAN

There are several points to consider in selecting your personal exercise program. It makes sense to select an individual program that is also compatible with your family exercise objectives. But you may have certain specific interests and needs that require you to do something different from the family program. Don't sacrifice your individual program.

We suggest you consider the following to help other family members to select the best individual exercise program for themselves. Considering and talking about these points is a wonderful activity for Family Circle.

SOME POINTS TO CONSIDER

Convenience Is Everything

The greatest obstacle to a regular exercise program is *convenience*. Many people forget the importance of this factor when selecting their programs. If your program is not convenient for you, you will find every excuse in the book not to do it. You'll suddenly find yourself interested in doing household chores or helping the kids with their homework during the times when you should be exercising.

Next to convenience, your exercise program needs to be easy for you to perform. Don't make the mistake of selecting your program solely on the basis of pure fun and enjoyment. You might choose an activity that you enjoy, but you can't do it on a regular basis. Golf and tennis, for example, are great activities when the weather is good or when you have someone to play with. Racquetball is fine if you have a court and partner available. What if your partner gets sick or is out of town? You still need to exercise despite the weather or the availability of a partner. (We'll go into the specifics of selecting an exercise activity later in this chapter.) Please remember that, above all, *convenience* and *ease of performance* will decide whether you remain in a regular, lifelong exercise program.

Time of Day

Select a time of day that offers the least number of competing activities. For many people that time is early in the morning. You can get up early while the household sleeps and do your exercise before people start to stake a claim on your time. The early morning slot also allows you to shower and dress only once during the day. (And, most of us shower in the morning anyway.)

You may select the lunch hour. If that's your choice, you need to consider that you'd have to get out of your clothes, get into exercise clothes, then get out of them again, shower, and finally get back into your work clothes. This routine may work for you. It does for many, but it is costly in time. For those who can manage it, lunch hour exercise provides a welcome break between the morning and afternoon. It's a "stressbuster" that can invigorate you.

Most people are too tired to exercise after work in the evening. However, some people find it a convenient bridge between work and family life. You may find this is a super way of getting all the anxiety, stress, and muscle kinks out of your body before coming home. Lots of folks find a combination of the morning, noon, and evening strategies suits their needs. The important message is to plan your program with as much care as you would any other very important event in your life.

Homing in on Exercise

For most people, exercising at home is far more convenient than exercising regularly at a club. An at-home program requires very little extra time. If you decide to exercise at a fitness club, you should be prepared to spend time commuting and changing clothes. This extra time may be a good break for you and afford you the versatility of a varied exercise program in a controlled atmosphere.

If you decide to exercise at home, you have the advantage of spending time with your family as you exercise. You can also set an excellent example for others in the family. Make the best decision for yourself and make it in the most objective manner possible.

An Inside Plan

As stated earlier, your exercise program should not be dependent on the weather, temperature, humidity, or whether it will be daylight or dark. That's why we advise you to have an at-home contingency plan. Select a simple piece or two of equipment that allow you to exercise under any conditions and at any time of the day.

There's No Safety in Numbers

Many people want to have fun with others when they exercise. This is perfectly reasonable if it is convenient for you. When your exercise depends on others, they may have other priorities at your scheduled time. That's the problem with using handball or team sports like basketball for your basic exercise program. You may be left with no one "to return your ball." By following our advice and considering exercise as preventive medicine needed for a longer life, you understand that regular exercise is not negotiable. No excuses, please. You can't blame someone else so that you can avoid it.

Monotony Busters

Variety is the spice of life and also of exercise. The greatest enemy of regular exercise is monotony and tedium. It's imperative that you plan a program that has some different activities to avoid feeling bored. You might obtain several pieces of equipment to use at home for circuit training. You can alternate between walking outside on nice days and riding your exer-cycle on rainy and cold days. And how about using a fitness club for some "spice" one or two days a week? By planning more variety in your exercise program, you assure your continued interest and enthusiasm. Be aware of how easily you can fall into the poorest routine if you think it saves time. Many people think only of how much time they're spending and not of whether the exercise is varied or more beneficial.

If the majority of your activities take place outside or away from home you must always have a safe back-up program on which to rely.

Mixing and Matching

Of course, you can alternate some family exercise activities with those in your personal program. First, you have to be honest with yourself and make sure your basic personal exercise needs are being met. If possible, plan ahead and make it special so that everyone can look forward to it. Your children will be overjoyed by the opportunity to exercise occasionally with their parents. There may be times when you won't get the best exercise experience, but the trade-off in terms of family time makes it worthwhile.

Slow and Steady Wins for Life

Proper, safe exercise requires slow, steady conditioning. Most people are tempted to do too much in too short a time. Remember, we Americans are very results oriented, which causes many of us to overdo. Aside from the strong possibility of injury from over-exerting yourself, there is the danger of discouragement because of short-term failure. Remember, this is an investment in LIFELONG exercise, not just a get-in-shape "jag" for the week. Help everyone set goals that are safe and can be reached. This is an opportunity to teach intelligent approaches to exercise. Start by allowing yourself to set the example.

CALCULATING YOUR TRAINING HEART RATE

Your *training heart rate* will give you a sense of how much you are exerting physically for a safe and vigorous aerobic experience. It makes no sense to exercise at a level that does little to improve your fitness. When we ask about their exercise, many people have told us, "I walk around the house," "I shop for groceries," and so forth. This type of activity is fine, but it is not aerobic. It does not improve your cardiovascular fitness.

Training heart rates are not precise calculations. They provide only general ranges for aerobic exercise. Your training heart rate is based upon 60 to 75 percent rather than 100 percent of the calculation. This provides you with a safety margin without sacrificing the aerobic effects of exercise. The following formula is provided by the America Heart Association.

> *To determine your training heart rate, subtract your age from 220. Multiply this number by 60 percent and 75 percent.*
> *For example, if you are 40 years old your training heart rate would be:*

$$220 - 40 = 180$$
$$180 \times 60\% = 108 \text{ beats per minute}$$
$$180 \times 75\% = 135 \text{ beats per minute}$$

> *Your goal, therefore, is to maintain a heart rate between 108 and 135 beats per minute for at least 20 minutes every time you work out. (The Better Life Institute recommends a 30 minute workout.)*

It doesn't make any sense to stop exercising for an entire minute just to take your pulse to see if you are in the correct aerobic range. Instead, there's an accurate method where you can take your pulse in a ten second period. Here's how:

- To monitor your heart rate during exercising, place the tips of your first two fingers lightly on the inside of your wrist just below the thumb. Again, press *lightly!*
- Count your pulse for ten seconds and multiply by six. The result is your current heart rate and that number should fall into your safe training heart rate range.
- If your pulse is below your target range, exercise a little harder. If it is higher, slow down a little.
- Check your target range pulse at least once a week.
- If you feel tired, regardless of your pulse rate, slow down or stop.

NEVER, NEVER exercise if you experience pain of any sort during the activity. Stop immediately. Your body is telling you that what you are doing is not good for you.

THE BETTER LIFE INSTITUTE FAMILY HEALTH PLAN

Check with your physician before starting your aerobic exercise program. Don't forget to tell your physician if you are taking any prescribed medication or other medications from another physician.

HEART RATE TARGET ZONES

To find your target zone, look for the age category closest to your age and read the line across. For example, if you are 30, your target zone is 114 to 142 beats per minute. If you are 43, the closest age on the chart is 45; the target zone is 105 to 131 beats per minute.

AGE	60–75% HEART RATE/MIN.	100% HEART RATE/MIN.
20	120–150	200
25	117–146	195
30	114–142	190
35	111–138	185
40	108–135	180
45	105–131	175
50	102–127	170
55	99–123	165
60	96–120	160
65	93–116	155
70	90–113	150

Your maximum heart rate is usually 220 minus your age. However, the above figures are averages and should be used as general guidelines.

Source: National Heart, Lung, and Blood Institute

Sample Exercise Programs

We have provided you and the family with a lot of practical guidelines for a regular aerobic exercise program. Below is a sample walking and jogging program from the National Heart, Lung, and Blood Institute that *serves only as a guide* for everyone. Bear in mind that you can mix and match activities for total muscle conditioning and interest. Our guidelines are adapted from major medical organizations. Notice how these programs shape or graduate your exercise. Remember "slow and steady wins the race." We want you to be in a *lifelong* exercise program and a very, very *long race.* Check your impulse to do too much too quickly.

A SAMPLE WALKING PROGRAM

	WARM UP	TARGET ZONE EXERCISING	COOL DOWN	TOTAL TIME
Week 1				
Session A	Walk slowly 5 min.	Then walk briskly 5 min.	Then walk slowly 5 min.	15 min.
Session B	Repeat above pattern.			
Session C	Repeat above pattern.			

Continue with at least three exercise sessions during each week of the program.

	WARM UP	TARGET ZONE EXERCISING	COOL DOWN	TOTAL TIME
Week 2	Walk slowly 5 min.	Walk briskly 7 min.	Walk slowly 5 min.	17 min.
Week 3	Walk slowly 5 min.	Walk briskly 9 min.	Walk slowly 5 min.	19 min.
Week 4	Walk slowly 5 min.	Walk briskly 11 min.	Walk slowly 5 min.	21 min.
Week 5	Walk slowly 5 min.	Walk briskly 13 min.	Walk slowly 5 min.	23 min.
Week 6	Walk slowly 5 min.	Walk briskly 15 min.	Walk slowly 5 min.	25 min.
Week 7	Walk slowly 5 min.	Walk briskly 18 min.	Walk slowly 5 min.	28 min.
Week 8	Walk slowly 5 min.	Walk briskly 20 min.	Walk slowly 5 min.	30 min.
Week 9	Walk slowly 5 min.	Walk briskly 23 min.	Walk slowly 5 min.	33 min.
Week 10	Walk slowly 5 min.	Walk briskly 26 min.	Walk slowly 5 min.	36 min.
Week 11	Walk slowly 5 min.	Walk briskly 28 min.	Walk slowly 5 min.	38 min.
Week 12	Walk slowly 5 min.	Walk briskly 30 min.	Walk slowly 5 min.	40 min.

Week 13 on:
Check your pulse periodically to see if you are exercising within your target zone. As you get more in shape, try exercising within the upper range of your target zone.

Source: National Heart, Lung, and Blood Institute

THE BETTER LIFE INSTITUTE FAMILY HEALTH PLAN

A SAMPLE JOGGING PROGRAM

	WARM UP	TARGET ZONE EXERCISING	COOL DOWN	TOTAL TIME
Week 1				
Session A	Stretch and limber up for 5 min.	Then walk 10 min. Try not to stop.	Then walk slowly 3 min. and stretch 2 min.	20 min.
Session B	Repeat above pattern.			
Session C	Repeat above pattern.			

Continue with at least three exercise sessions during each week of the program.

	WARM UP	TARGET ZONE EXERCISING	COOL DOWN	TOTAL TIME
Week 2	Stretch and limber 5 min.	Walk 5 min., jog 1 min., walk 5 min., jog 1 min.	Walk slowly 3 min., stretch 2 min.	22 min.
Week 3	Stretch and limber 5 min.	Walk 5 min., jog 3 min., walk 5 min., jog 3 min.	Walk slowly 3 min., stretch 2 min.	26 min.
Week 4	Stretch and limber 5 min.	Walk 4 min., jog 5 min., walk 4 min., jog 5 min.	Walk slowly 3 min., stretch 2 min.	28 min.
Week 5	Stretch and limber 5 min.	Walk 4 min., jog 5 min., walk 4 min., jog 5 min.	Walk slowly 3 min., stretch 2 min.	28 min.
Week 6	Stretch and limber 5 min.	Walk 4 min., jog 6 min., walk 4 min., jog 6 min.	Walk slowly 3 min., stretch 2 min.	30 min.
Week 7	Stretch and limber 5 min.	Walk 4 min., jog 7 min., walk 4 min., jog 7 min.	Walk slowly 3 min., stretch 2 min.	32 min.
Week 8	Stretch and limber 5 min.	Walk 4 min., jog 8 min., walk 4 min., jog 8 min.	Walk slowly 3 min., stretch 2 min.	34 min.
Week 9	Stretch and limber 5 min.	Walk 4 min., jog 9 min., walk 4 min., jog 9 min.	Walk slowly 3 min., stretch 2 min.	36 min.
Week 10	Stretch and limber 5 min.	Walk 4 min., jog 13 min.	Walk slowly 3 min., stretch 2 min.	27 min.

A SAMPLE JOGGING PROGRAM—Continued

	WARM UP	TARGET ZONE EXERCISING	COOL DOWN	TOTAL TIME
Week 11	Stretch and limber 5 min.	Walk 4 min., jog 15 min.	Walk slowly 3 min., stretch 2 min.	29 min.
Week 12	Stretch and limber 5 min.	Walk 4 min., jog 17 min.	Walk slowly 3 min., stretch 2 min.	31 min.
Week 13	Stretch and limber 5 min.	Walk 2 min., jog slowly 2 min., jog 17 min.	Walk slowly 3 min., stretch 2 min.	31 min.
Week 14	Stretch and limber 5 min.	Walk 1 min., jog slowly 3 min., jog 17 min.	Walk slowly 3 min., stretch 2 min.	31 min.
Week 15	Stretch and limber 5 min.	Jog slowly 3 min., jog 17 min.	Walk slowly 3 min., stretch 2 min.	30 min.

Week 16 on:
Check your pulse periodically to see if you are exercising within your target zone. As you become more fit, try exercising within the upper range of your target zone.

Source: National Heart, Lung, and Blood Institute

CHARTING YOUR PROGRESS

If something is important, its importance is worth evaluating. One way to do this with your family exercise program is to make each person's exercise activity more visible to the individual and to everyone in the family. We recommend using a simple chart to give each person a feeling of accountability and accomplishment when they exercise. Children find it fun and motivating to keep charts of their activities. It is something they do routinely to monitor their progress at school. A chart translates what you are trying to teach into a more visible and measurable experience. Using an exercise chart also provides children with the feeling they are actually making some progress in their lives. It teaches them to accept responsibility for what they actually do and is a form of accountability for what they set out to do.

Finally, a family exercise progress chart says clearly that a family exercise program exists. It is there for all family members to see,

THE BETTER LIFE INSTITUTE FAMILY HEALTH PLAN

HOW ARE WE DOING THIS WEEK, FAMILY?

DAY	ACTIVITY	DID YA DO IT?
Monday		
Tuesday		
Wednesday		
Thursday		
Friday		
Saturday		
Sunday		

TOTAL _____ ×7 = _____

and it tells the children you care. It also states emphatically that you are all on the same family team.

Plan to discuss the progress chart at Family Circle. It's an excellent way to provide objective information about everyone's exercise status without criticism. Furthermore it's an opportunity to compliment everyone on their program and for keeping the chart up to date—even if their progress is not perfect. It's all up there in black and white (or whichever colors you choose). Your chart is a wonderful vehicle for providing additional support and for offering those much needed pats on the back.

We suggest that you use a chart that states what each member of the family is going to do and whether they've accomplished it. Use it in a weekly time frame. The chart on page 145 is a good example of the type to use. Make some copies of it and keep it in a visible place. You can even use little gold stars or some fun stickers which will make the recording of exercise progress more motivating.

A Nag Is a Horse of a Different Color
Nobody likes to be nagged. The person who does the nagging does not know how to motivate people effectively. Motivation is most successful with a carrot instead of a whip, and let's face it, nagging is actually a verbal whip. It's very tempting to use the chart to criticize someone who's not doing well on the program and nag him to do better. Instead, use the chart to build a better sense of responsibility in all family members. During Family Circle, ask if anyone is having difficulty keeping records or doing their exercise. Let the chart and the sense of public accountability speak to the person. In this way no one needs to feel angry at another person for criticizing or nagging them. Each one simply knows it is their responsibility and no one else's. *Encouragement* will get you everywhere!

Comparing one member unfavorably to another is one of the worst things that can be done in a family. Statements like, "Look at the chart. Your brother is doing it; why can't you?" only serve to cause friction within the family. They should be avoided. Instead of comparing family members, let each person stand as an individual. Take into consideration that there will be those days when someone is out of sorts and has not exercised. Don't chastise or nag. Give support and encouragement for the next day.

Exercise Equipment

THE RIGHT STUFF AND THE DUST-GATHERERS
If we could have a dollar for every piece of exercise equipment lying around family basements gathering dust and rust, standing in family

rooms covered with coats and sweaters, or abandoned to garages, we would be millionaires! It's not the exercise equipment that's the problem; it's the commitment to exercise. Some people even feel that buying a piece of exercise equipment will motivate them to use it. That works for about a week, and then that shiny piece of equipment begins to gather dust. It may eventually be used as a rack for drying laundry or old rags.

The primary factors that influence exercise are your family's motivation and commitment—something you cannot buy. However, when you need equipment it does help to buy the right kind. It does not have to be the most expensive or have the most flashing lights and bells on it. It needs only to be something that you and the family will use. Your best rule of thumb should be that the equipment's value will go up according to the number of people who will use it the most number of times. A jump rope, for example, or an elastic stretcher may not be very flashy, but most of the family can use them in their various programs.

There are many alternatives available, and we'll discuss their uses and their advantages. We've had a lot of experience with exercise equipment, both personally and professionally, so we have strong opinions. Let us have our say, but bear in mind that you are the best judge of the equipment's usefulness for your family.

Stationary Bicycles

If someone asks you if you have an *ergonometer*, don't run to your hot water heating system to see if it's one of your dials. That's just a fancy name for an exercise bike with a lot of bells and whistles on it. Bikes are by far the most popular piece of exercise equipment in American homes. They don't use electricity. They're relatively inexpensive. And they don't take up much room. Another big plus is that they don't require learning any special skills.

There are two types of bikes. The most popular bike gives you a workout by primarily working your leg muscles. It looks like a bike on a stand. The second type of bike has handlebars that allow you to combine upper and lower body exercise. This type of bike is far more versatile than one with just pedals and fixed handlebars. It allows you to rotate your program and tone more muscle groups. It is less strenuous also, because you can alternate between upper and lower body during your workout. We suggest you buy the second type of bike.

A recumbent bike is one where you sit very low. It allows you to "push pedal" rather than sit over the pedals. This produces less strain on the back muscles and is worth considering if any member of the family has back problems.

Exercise bikes are safe, and there is little stress on your joints because you are sitting, not standing, while exercising. Try to buy a bike with a timer. If yours doesn't have a timer, keep a clock close at hand. Be sure to get a bike that is sturdy and won't tip over regardless of who is using it. Get one with a large seat. It's safer and more comfortable. You may have to get blocks for the pedals if your children use it. There are many complicated features to bicycles, but remember, the purpose is to move the pedals and handlebars. The rest is extra.

Treadmills

Walking is the simplest and the most practical form of exercise. You already know how to walk, so, for starters, you can save money on lessons. If you want an indoor walking machine, we suggest you consider a motorized treadmill. This is not the one that has rollers with a belt that you must propel yourself. This piece of equipment is relatively expensive, so be sure that you do some comparison shopping before you buy.

There are many variations on treadmills, and each new twist adds many dollars to the price. At minimum, the one you buy should have a timer. Getting a motorized elevation option allows you to walk either fast or slowly up an incline. Make certain the motor is powerful and the treadmill works on your house's electrical current. The treadmill should be sturdy enough to support your weight, and it should have side rails to help you with your balance. Treadmills are not safe for older people or children since they can fall off. One last thought: you can get some upper body exercise while walking on your treadmill if you hold some light weights.

Rebounders

It sounds like the name of a character from a science fiction film, but a rebounder is simply a mini-trampoline. Children love to bounce on them. If you buy one, it needs to be wide with strong legs and no space between the frame and netting. Both kids and adults can fall through the springs. Rebounders give you a quite varied workout. You can use all your muscles together or in any combination you choose. Using a set of light weights will give you more upper body exercise and additional toning.

Because rebounders are cushioned, there is little stress on your joints. However, you need some skill in order to use a rebounder properly. It is important to learn how to use it safely. Video tapes are available to guide you and make using a rebounder a more enjoyable activity. This device can be easily stored and is light enough to be moved around. You can place it in front of the television to use it while watching an exercise program and then remove it for the rest of the day. And they're not expensive.

Cross-country Ski Machines

This machine provides a vigorous workout and requires a very high level of coordination, skill, and conditioning. They are not useful for children because to use the system correctly the user must be at least a certain height, and they can be dangerous if not used properly. Many people have acquired or aggravated back and hip problems because they used a ski machine incorrectly. We don't recommend this type of machine. It requires too much conscious effort to operate it without injury.

Stair-climbing Machines

Stair climbers come in many forms. We suggest you get either the motorized step or pedal models. We do not suggest purchasing a self-propelled step machine. As with treadmills, there are many expensive variations. The machine should be heavy and sturdy and have a timer. Children can safely use this type of machine. The energy expenditure required to operate a stair climber is greater than with any other machine. It can be a problem for people with high blood pressure. Studies indicate that blood pressure tends to rise more quickly on stair climbers than on other exercise equipment.

Rowing Machines

"Row, row, row your machine gently down the family room." People like the idea of rowing for exercise. In general, it is not an effective repetitive conditioning activity. Many people tire very quickly on a rowing machine and get little aerobic effect from the exercise. A rowing machine must be used correctly, or it can cause back injuries. Primarily for this reason we don't recommend them for children. In addition, children tend to be too small to fit into the machine's dimensions properly.

Weight-lifting Equipment

Muscle building is not part of the Better Life Program; muscle toning is. We believe you can build and tone your muscles easily and safely without the use of weights or heavy resistance equipment. We also feel that a weight lifting orientation is not healthy since it rarely involves aerobic and cardiovascular conditioning. Proponents of weight lifting will argue its aerobic effects, but there is little in research or in actual practice to substantiate this claim.

Children should not lift weights until they are older than sixteen years of age because it can be harmful to their structural development. Weight lifting encourages large body mass, and many body builders become obsessed with enlarging their musculature. Recently a large number of teenage weight lifters have been taking illegal anabolic steroids to increase their bulk. Unfortunately some high school coaches have encouraged this practice to "beef up" their football squads. New studies reveal that these steroids can cause cancer as well as sexual and glandular dysfunction. Also, if a weight lifter stops training for any length of time, he may very quickly become fat because he still has his appetite and often a sluggish metabolism.

A word to the wise: Don't tell a weight lifter what we said "face to face." It could be disastrous. If you're in good condition, though, you can shout it to him at a distance of at least fifty yards without any worry. He'll never catch you!

Gadgets, Rubber Bands, and Other Gizmos

There are hundreds of small gizmos, gadgets, widgets, and rubber bands touted as "fitness systems." They come with little booklets describing with imagination how the little thing can actually be used. Surprisingly most of them will, in fact, work if you use them correctly, and they are relatively inexpensive. We ask you to consider these gadgets because some of them can be used when traveling. They may be fun for the family and are not likely to be harmful for children. Some of these little gadgets may be perfect for your small children who can't use exercise equipment. It helps them have a sense of belonging in the family program.

SOME FINAL ADVICE ON EQUIPMENT

The purpose of buying exercise equipment is to make exercise more convenient and enjoyable. The machinery is always there in your home no matter what the weather may be, and you can use it for a few minutes any time of the day or night. The greatest obstacle to its regular use is boredom. Exercise equipment provides repetitive exercise, and to many the minutes on the machine seem like hours. That's why you should be careful when selecting equipment. A more expensive digital program can provide you with variety in the program and more interest. Some equipment varies resistance and speed automatically. Select your equipment with an eye toward keeping your interest level high.

Since all exercise equipment provides repetitive activity, it is worthwhile to consider an activity that allows you to read or watch television to pass the time. Bikes, treadmills, and stair climbers require activity that is automatic. You don't have to pay much attention to the actual exercise. Time certainly passes faster on a treadmill while watching "Good Morning, Wherever You Are." However, rowing machines and cross-country ski machines require concentration on the activity. Since monotony is your greatest enemy during exercise, it may be better to get two less expensive pieces of equipment that everybody can use to provide variety rather than one expensive machine and give yourself some enjoyable distractions to help pass the time. Listening to music or a book on tape can help alleviate boredom. Many people place their exercise equipment by the phone so they can occupy themselves. Video movies provide a lot of entertainment and also help pass the time. Watch the right horror movie and it will increase your heart rate without you moving the pedals on your bike!

An Important Word of Advice

Changing your personal health habits will be a great challenge. There are differences between nutrition and exercise that are worth emphasizing. You cannot avoid eating, and therefore, your efforts to change eating habits are merely an improvement of an existing and necessary set of actions. However, exercise is an "extra" in the equation. You don't *have* to exercise. It is entirely voluntary. For this reason, it is more difficult to maintain a regular exercise program. You have to face this reality. It will require discipline and effort beyond what you anticipate. That's why it is important for you to get the "mechanics" out of the way. Be very, very smart about designing your program. You want it to be as convenient and interesting as possible, but in the final analysis, it will be your commitment that makes the difference.

Please bend over backward to avoid criticizing or getting upset with yourself or any other family member. That accomplishes nothing and discourages everyone from continuing on the programs or working to do better. Regular exercise is a difficult habit to develop. It requires patience and support. Use the development of proper exercise habits as a *bootstrap* to develop positive and supportive family attitudes. Teach everyone to help and support each other and to provide an occasional compliment and an encouraging word. The goals are health, family unity, and happiness. Don't lose sight of these goals by using exercise as a *whipping boy* or a situation to teach critical lessons. There are many children who shy away from exercise activities and sports simply because of their experiences with their parents. These parents jumped all over their children when they didn't perform well or stick to their activity. Exercise is an opportunity for you and your children to build solid, enjoyable, positive relationships for a lifetime. Show some caring and love. Encourage your children. Help them by giving them all of your support. Enjoy the precious moments of your children during their childhood. The time will be gone before you know it.

The Gift That Keeps on Giving

There's an advertisement on television once in a while that says, "Give a gift that lasts. . . . Give her a diamond." Think of exercise in the same way. It truly is a "gift that lasts." It doesn't cost as much as a diamond, but we would be willing to bet that a gift of exercise will increase in value to you more than any precious stone. That's something you can bank on!

YES, I CAN

- I can say "I choose to," rather than "I have to." I can teach this to the rest of my family.
- I can start today to nibble on heart-healthy, lower calorie snacks. I can make sure that they are placed where the family can see them and eat them.
- I can have dessert a few hours *after* dinner, rather than with dinner.

FAMILY CIRCLE

Review the weekly exercise chart and ask each person how they feel about their exercise program. Ask if anyone needs any help, encouragement, skills, or a change in the activity.

Use the weekly exercise review to compliment people. Never allow any family member to criticize another. Always ask everyone to speak in a positive, supportive manner.

Ask one of the kids to demonstrate some stretching or toning activities that he or she uses. Try it yourself and see if you can do it. Don't be afraid to let your family see that the kids can do something you can't.

Step into the Kitchen

■ ■

A Personal Message

Welcome to the Better Life Program. You'll notice that we don't call it the "Best Life Program." The reason is simply because I've been able to live on "better" for fourteen years and so has my family. That reason in itself is what makes it the "best."

I decided to make necessary changes in my life way back in 1977. Back then, we did not have the public information or the knowledge of nutrition that we have today. Diet, exercise, lifestyle, disease were considered and discussed, but not in a synergistic way. We didn't know or truly understand how one affects the other. But I had gotten to the point of being sick and tired of being sick and tired, and fat! I decided to take some action!

I got rid of all the fattening foods in my diet, and I started to walk every day. I learned quickly and succeeded very well. But my challenge to meet the needs of my family was the catalyst for me to learn more and more. I realized that I wanted and needed a lifestyle program that was easy, practical, enjoyable, effective, and as painless as possible! Everyone wants good results, and I was no different. We all have a difficult time in the struggle of getting to where we want to go, and I was no exception.

My challenge in those days was the same one I have today: take the basic principles for a healthy lifestyle and incorporate them into a busy world for busy people. This can be done by using the best of what modern technology has to offer in time-saving foods, techniques, and programs.

In this food section of *The Better Life Institute Family Health Plan,* I will lay out the basics, and you and the family will know how to make the changes you need in your eating. All these ideas and recipes have been tested on my nine children and an ever-growing

STEP INTO THE KITCHEN ■

number of grandchildren. The food plans have all "passed muster." And *muster* in my family probably means the same thing as it does in yours: tasty, quick, and easy to prepare.

Cooking for your family will not be like asking you to step into the cockpit of a Boeing 747 on the assumption that you know how to pilot that bird into the wild, blue yonder. This will be easy. You already know your way around your kitchen. You've spent years shopping for groceries, entertaining friends, cooking wonderful holiday meals. I suspect that you've eaten in most every type of restaurant and coffee shop as well.

You don't have to throw everything out and start from scratch. You already have all the experience and skills you'll need. In fact, you're probably overqualified.

I've divided this part of the book into four sections. I suggest you read them in order because there's a natural flow to learning the Better Life Institute way to cook. I've organized the material in the way that makes sense to me and that I think will make sense to you. The final section contains lots of recipes that I've used over the years. The more you read, the more you'll realize how much you already know. That's the beauty of Better Life cooking.

I'm going to show you how to take the *unhealthy* out of your family's food and keep in the *healthy* part. We'll walk through the supermarket and read labels. We'll plan menus and cook recipes together. We'll even eat at fast food places as well as in up-scale restaurants. We'll discuss parties, brown bag lunches, holidays, and other events that might present a situation for family discussion. Trust me in that I'm a very practical and basic person.

With love and best wishes,

Pat

Pat

■■■■■■■■■■■■
A Tour of the Kitchen

■ *An Overview of What's Ahead*

Section 1

WHAT CAN WE EAT?

In Section 1, you'll see the "big picture." We'll go over the types of foods that you and your family can eat for a healthy lifestyle: soups, salads, poultry . . . you'll get a general "fix" on how we can use all types of foods. I've also listed some specific suggestions for each meal at the end of this section.

Section 2

WHAT DO WE BUY?

We all have our talents. Shopping is one of the things I do best, and shopping for food is no exception. Take a sprint through the supermarket with me. You'll learn what products to buy for meals, snacks, and school lunches. You'll also learn how to really read a label. A food label may look like Greek to you, but it's really very easy to understand. I think your family should also know how to read and understand a label so I've included a label reading exercise for Family Circle.

Section 3

LET'S PUT IT ALL TOGETHER!

It's time now to build meals, snacks, and school lunches, and you'll need some help to do the planning and develop the menus. In this section, I've provided you with a week's worth of menu plans. There is a 1200 calorie menu plan for the weight conscious female and a 1500 calorie menu plan for the weight conscious male. Also included is an 1800 calorie menu plan for those who just want to maintain weight. These plans are merely general guidelines to give you a sense of direction. If you have teenagers with bottomless stomachs that you just can't seem to fill up take my 1800 calorie plan and add more food to it. You can provide larger servings or add some additional foods. Just be sure the food is healthy. Remember, we all want to grow healthy kids.

Families eat many of their meals away from home, so it's important for everyone to know how to eat healthfully everywhere they go, which includes restaurants, fast food shops, parties, and being on the road. "Surviving and thriving" away from home is easy once you

STEP INTO THE KITCHEN ■

know how. We have tips for the whole family everyone can use away from home.

Section 4

IT'S EATIN' TIME!
This is the fun part. Better Life family foods add enjoyment to family life. Every recipe I've included knocked the socks off someone in my family. Since most of my family are professional eaters, however, this was not an enormous feat. However, I'll confess that I've concocted some dishes in my lifetime that no one wanted to try. But I tried again, just like you do.

The nice part about all my cooking is that it's easy. My husband is so proud of how simple and tasty my foods are that he labeled my ability in the kitchen as "dum-dum cookin'." Don't laugh. That's a compliment! There's nothing that makes me happier than turning out a great dish in no time flat and practically in my sleep. That's what this section is all about.

I do so look forward to holiday meals and entertaining at home. No one has ever come to my home for a party or at holiday time and admitted the next morning that they went hungry or didn't have all their favorite holiday treats. I'll share some of my winners with you.

Once you try my recipes, you'll quickly see how you can "tweek" them and make them better to suit your own taste. They'll also give you ideas for adapting some of your recipes. I'm helping you more by showing you how to adapt your own cooking style to the Better Life program than by teaching you new recipes.

You'll find a quick reference to calorie counting at the end of this section.

THE BETTER LIFE INSTITUTE FAMILY HEALTH PLAN

What Can We Eat?

- *Better Life Cooking: Practical Guidelines*
- *Food Groups*
- *Meal Suggestions*

Section 1

Better Life Cooking: Practical Guidelines

"EASY AS PIE!"

Since you've read the preceding chapters, you know the basic do's and don'ts of more healthy eating and exercise. What we're going into now is the practical guidelines you can follow to make your life practical, livable, and enjoyable. Contrary to other programs, you won't need a scale or a computer or a math degree from M.I.T. to follow this one. We've purposely made it easy as pie, just for you.

- Enjoy eating chicken, turkey, fish, other seafood, and very lean meats. Your average size portion should be about *4 cooked ounces per meal.* For those of you who are used to eating Moby Dick on a plate, this might be a little difficult to get used to. But now that you know cholesterol is found only in animal foods, you'll understand why we limit the portion sizes.
- Beans, vegetables, fruits, and grains are the mainstay for a better life. We call these foods carbohydrates, and they are your body's favorite fuel. This category also includes pasta, rice, and whole grains.
- Use only skim and nonfat dairy products. Whole dairy products are very high in saturated fats, and saturated fats help to push up your cholesterol. Besides fats are very high in calories, which is why they should be limited in a healthy diet.
- Go easy on sugar, sweet foods, and sweetened foods. Americans eat too many sweets, 142 pounds of sugar per person, per year! That's a fact. We suggest you use Nutrasweet™ along with sugar, honey, molasses, and fructose, and that you do it in moderation. You'll reduce your overall exposure to sugar. (See Nutrasweet™ information.)
- Use the white of the egg. An average egg yolk contains about 225 mg. of cholesterol, more than an average suggested day's diet intake should be. There are products on the market and we will discuss recipes that will help you avoid the yolk.
- Caffeine is a stimulating drug and should be limited. Decaffeinated coffee, tea, and soft drinks are available and taste just like the real thing.
- Watch your alcohol consumption since alcohol is a drug. A glass of wine, a lite beer, or an occasional mixed drink is perfectly acceptable if you so choose. Just watch your frequency and consumption.
- Stop spreading *fat* on your bread! That's what butter and margarine are: *fat!* Go easy on the 100 calories per tablespoon that

both butter and margarine contain. Use diet margarines when desired.

- Take a brisk walk frequently. It will clear your mind, help you deal with stress, and get the metabolism going.
- Stop to give thanks to your Creator. Say your prayers. Learn to relax and smell the roses. Being alive is a wonderful state in which to be.

It's as easy as all that. Easy as pie.

Food Groups

LET'S TALK ABOUT THE BASIC FOODS

Okay, now that you've gotten the basics, let's talk food. These are the foods that we eat and enjoy daily, the foods we always take for granted and never think about. Before you and your family plan your menu and the grocery shopping list, you should know about the healthy foods, the ones you can eat.

We suggest you have a discussion during Family Circle about what each food is, what it does for the body, which foods each member of the family enjoys, and which foods you'll incorporate into your family menu plan. This discussion will get all family members involved in choices and compromises and will not only act as a learning session about foods, but also a learning session on how to give a little to win a lot!

Cereals

Both hot and cold cereals are the breakfast choice of most Americans. They are easy and convenient and there's little clean up. Cereals that are good for you (some are very high in sugar!) give you lots of nutritional "cluck" for the buck you spend on them. Normally children will eat cereal without a fight. When shopping make sure you purchase the healthiest cereal that is good tasting when you add skim milk, sweetener, and fruit. An abundance of good ones is in the grocery stores.

If you purchase it, you'll eat it. If you don't buy it, it won't be around to tempt you.

Be careful when you buy cereals that are loaded with sugar and some of the granolas that are very high in fat. We'll discuss how to read a label so that you'll be able to make the correct choices for both you and your family. Be on alert also for the cereals that are advertised on television and aimed at kids. Because they contain so much sugar some of them are more like candy than cereal.

Speaking of advertising, just because a product has a catchy ad doesn't mean it's good for you and yours. Use Family Circle to talk about the way advertising affects us and sometimes causes us to want to buy foods and other items that we really don't want and often are unhealthy. Discuss this topic with your family. Our friend Lulu says, *"What you eat today, you will wear tomorrow."* Experiment with the different new cereals the industry keeps putting out. They seem to appear with amazing speed. I've listed a variety of cereals in the grocery shopping section, and I encourage you to add your choices to the list.

Some hot cereals cook very quickly in the microwave or in a

bowl with boiling water added. I learned a quick trick a long time ago that is a boon for busy people who don't have time in the morning to cook hot cereal. The night before I put the hot cereal ingredients in a crock-pot. Just mix water and whole grains in the pot and set it on the lowest setting. While you sleep, the cereal is cooking, and all you have to do in the morning is dish it up, doctor it up, and eat it up! And don't forget the microwave oven for fast, clean cooking in minutes.

Fruit

Fruit is good food to enjoy any time—for dessert, for a snack, in a fruit plate for lunch. Fruit contains natural sweetness, relatively few calories, fiber, vitamins, and minerals, and it tastes good. Those of you watching your sugar may have to limit your fruit intake to 3 to 4 pieces a day. A medium orange has only 65 calories. When choosing canned fruits select the juice or water packed kind and stay away from the syrup packed.

Here's the word on dried fruits: Enjoy them but not to excess. These foods pack lots of calories. A half cup of raisins has about 275 calories! Compare that to a French roll that has 75 calories and an apple that has 80 calories. When you compare you can see a big difference. Raisins seem so tiny we think they can't possibly contain many calories, but they do. Now, if you add raisins to muffins or sprinkle a few raisins on cereals, that's okay. And raisins are an excellent snack and source of energy for little bodies. Just know where to set your limits. There's one more thing about raisins: (I don't want my favorite dentist to get after me) be sure you and your kids brush your teeth after eating sweet, sticky foods.

Fruit Juices

Fruit juices are very pleasant tasting and give you a quick shot of fruit sugar with very little fiber. Juice goes right into your bloodstream, whereas whole fruit takes a longer time to digest since it has lots of fiber to be processed. A small glass of fruit juice is perfectly okay. Just be careful that you don't substitute juices for water as a frequent beverage. An 8-ounce glass of orange juice has 110 calories but little or no fiber.

Tomato juice and V-8™ juice do not have the sugar content that other juices have, and therefore, they do not have the quick sugar impact or the calories ounce per ounce as sweet juices. Tomato and V-8™ juices do contain sodium, however, so if you're on a sodium-restricted diet, purchase the low or nonsodium type. A zip-lock can of tomato juice, a few crackers, and a piece of fruit can save you from a hot pastrami sandwich when you're in a hurry.

■ **THE BETTER LIFE INSTITUTE FAMILY HEALTH PLAN**

Pancakes, Waffles, and French Toast

These foods are good eating, any time! Elsewhere in this book you'll find recipes for "The Big Breakfast Three" that can be made at home, quick and easy, as well as suggestions for the frozen kind that even a chimpanzee can make with its feet. (That's one of Lulu's favorite expressions for "simple.") Be very careful of the globs of butter that you put on your plate because many times the butter or margarine has more calories than the pancakes, waffles, or French toast! Use a light syrup available in the grocery store and enjoy!

Eggs and Omelettes

As mentioned previously, egg yolk is high in cholesterol. At the Better Life Institute we advise about 200 mg. of cholesterol in the diet per day and one yolk alone is more than that. Now, if you eat an egg yolk or a food prepared with an egg yolk once in a while, your eyeballs won't fall out! But Americans have been gorging on whole eggs for too long. The average American breakfast has to be changed! Just think about the cholesterol in a three-egg ham and cheese omelette! We like to use Egg Beaters,™ both plain and vegetable, as well as plain ol' egg whites. Sounds strange to a lot of you, I know, but try these suggestions:

1. Beat up the egg whites with a drop of vegetable food coloring. Throw the yolks out, put them down the drain, or better still, give them to the dog. He'll have a lovely, shiny coat and you won't feel like you have been wasteful.
2. If your cholesterol is below 180, beat up 1 whole egg with 6 egg whites. This will give you a yellow color and about 75 mg. of cholesterol per serving if you serve three people.
3. Use Egg Beaters.™ They are quick, easy, and convenient, and there's no guilt. And no, I do not have stock in the company! It's just a product I like very much.
4. Try the new lower cholesterol whole eggs available in the egg section of your grocery store.

Jams, Jellies, Syrups

There is a very nice variety on the market of no-sugar, low sugar, calorie-controlled foods that will make your eating quite enjoyable. Most major food companies that make these products also make a variety that suits the Better Life Program. And I've included some make-at-home recipes for you to try.

Breads, Muffins, Coffeecakes, and Other Hot Baked Goodies

Breads are mainly made with flour, water, yeast, salt, sometimes sugar, and a little fat. There are many good breads to enjoy: French,

Italian, sourdough, and whole grain breads, bagels, pita bread, and the new lite calorie-controlled breads, to name a few. A French roll has only about 75 calories. One tablespoon of butter or margarine has 100 calories. An avocado has 300 calories. A large apple has about 80 calories. Big difference, huh? Bread is good food. But be careful about pigging out on good foods! And forget the fatty spread! Please, just once try toast or an English muffin without butter. Use a dab of jelly instead. Smearing fat on these filling, relatively low calorie foods is a habit we continue without thinking.

Muffins are not created equal. It depends on who did the baking and the mixing. Try to stay with muffins that are made with whole grains (bran, etc.) or those that have berries, grated apple, etc. in them. Muffins don't need the butter to be enjoyed either. It's amazing how good a muffin tastes all by itself.

CALORIES IN YOUR FAVORITE PIE

Pecan	431	Sweet Potato	243
Pumpkin	241	Cherry	308
Apple	302	Raisin	319
Coconut Custard	268	A ½-cup portion of nonfat	
An Apple or Orange	80	fruit yogurt or no fat	
Mincemeat	320	ice cream	90

YOU DECIDE!

WHEN TEMPTATION STRIKES REMEMBER:

2 oatmeal cookies =
- 1 slice of bread
- 1 teaspoon fat
- 1 teaspoon sugar

1 slice of layer cake with chocolate icing =
- 1 slice of bread
- 3 teaspoons fat
- 6 teaspoons sugar

1 slice of apple pie =
- 2 slices of bread
- 4 teaspoons fat
- 6 teaspoons sugar
- ¼ apple

Coffeecakes and Other Goodies: Take a bread recipe, add fat (you still call it butter, shortening, margarine) and lots of sugar, put icing, nuts, and other good stuff on it, and you have coffeecake. And you don't even have to eat it. Just stuff it down your pantyhose because that's exactly where it goes. If someone puts a gun to your head and

THE BETTER LIFE INSTITUTE FAMILY HEALTH PLAN

forces you to eat that coffeecake, allow him or her to do so only on a special occasion. Then walk an extra mile that day!

There is a new line of once-forbidden goodies made by Entenmann's Bakery that are no fat, no cholesterol. They do contain lots of sugar, so when you do the goodie thing once-in-a-while, these products might fit your need. I am including some recipes in this book that those of you who would like to try your hand at quick and easy goodies can do at home. There's also some interesting information that can help you put sweets into the proper perspective.

Turkey and Other Poultry

Let's talk turkey. We're all learning about the benefits of eating animal products that have less fat and less saturated fats. That's turkey, chicken, and seafood.

Poultry is good food so enjoy it in 4 oz. cooked portions, but let me offer a word of caution. Some processed turkey and chicken products have a lot of fat in them because they've been processed with the skin of the animal (all fat), not to mention lots of additives, preservatives, and fillers. When choosing a product *always read the label*. Another thing, not all manufacturers make their products the same way. In other words, not all ground raw turkey or chicken is the same! Read the label and ask questions of the butcher. I've recently found a superior grade of turkey ham, bacon, sausage, and ground meat in my local grocery store. I'm sure that you have it in your town also. But you'll have to search it out because it's not going to look for you!

Children like hot dogs. It's amazing to me. Our children did not come out of the delivery room knowing about hot dogs, yet at three years of age, the average child knows everything there is to know about hot dogs and hamburgers! It's all part of the *All-American Syndrome*. All I can say to the concerned parent is this: "Choose wisely and eat prudently, and you'll do just fine."

Turkey ham is made from the thigh of the animal and is smoked and processed just like the pork product. Turkey bacon is the dark and the white meats of the turkey pressed together to give the appearance of bacon. It cooks up with little shrinkage and has very little fat in it. As is true of other foods, not all turkey sausage is created equal. Check with your butcher for the very leanest product available. I've found that these turkey products—ham, bacon, and sausage—make a healthy diet very easy and much more palatable than the one I started thirteen years ago!

Lamb, Pork, Veal, Beef, Game

Most red meats are very high in fat, and more importantly, saturated fats, the kind we all want to avoid. Therefore, we suggest that whenever you do choose to eat these foods, that you pick the leanest of the lean, and also trim all the fat off of that. In the marketplace today there is a selection of very lean beef and pork products that will meet the Better Life guidelines. The animals that this meat comes from were specially fed so that the flesh of the animal is lower in saturated fat and cholesterol. Look for these products when the spirit moves you to have red meat.

Wild game is, by and large, okay to eat. Don't forget that wild game was grown in the wilds, not in a corn-crib, fed with hormones, etc. Some wild game runs a bit higher in fat, but venison, quail, pheasant, rabbit, etc. are perfectly okay. Duck is high in fat. Just make sure that you don't eat more than 4 ounces cooked at any meal.

Fish and Seafood

Remember when fish was known as "brain food"? It is good food for smart people! We suggest that people on a heart-healthy diet eat fish or seafood 3 times per week. Fish is low in calories and fat, and the fat that is in fish is a good-for-the-body fat that health professionals are suggesting that people eat.

Up until a few years ago, it was believed that shellfish was too high in cholesterol for the heart-healthy person to eat, but with new up-to-date calculations, we can now enjoy shellfish in moderation. Again this does not mean a platter of deep-fried shrimp at the all-you-can-eat-buffet. I've included recipes that you may enjoy preparing which use different fish in different ways.

Butter, Margarine, Oils, Shortenings, and Other Fats

When you must use a butter or margarine, use the soft-tub type diet margarine if possible. Whenever you use an oil, make it canola oil, olive oil, one of the nut oils such as walnut or peanut, or avocado oil. These are the monounsaturates we've spoken about. There are fat substitutes on the market, or soon to be on the market, that will make all your cooking a lot easier. Again always read the labels before you make a purchase. Then watch how you use them. A tablespoon of butter or margarine has 100 calories, a tablespoon of diet margarine has about 50 calories, a tablespoon of oil has about 120 calories.

Dairy Products

Whole milk—the All-American food to grow strong bodies, or so we once thought. But our thinking is changing since we've become aware that dairy products can be very high in saturated fats. The solution to this situation is to use skim and nonfat dairy products whenever possible, then everyone wins! For a product to be considered

THE BETTER LIFE INSTITUTE FAMILY HEALTH PLAN

skim or nonfat, the label must state the product has 1 percent or less milkfat. (I can find ½ percent milk in my local market.) You'll get all the vitamins and minerals that milk offers without the fat whenever you "go skim."

Don't let the label on a package of cheese mislead you. Always read the label, as I will show you, and then make a decision as to (1) what to purchase and (2) how to use a given product. Remember you're the boss of you. Don't be swayed by the ads or the labels until you take the time to calculate the percentage of fat by total calories. Purchase 1 percent milkfat cottage cheese and nonfat plain and flavored yogurts. For the many people who have a lactose intolerance, we suggest a dairy substitute such as Lactaid.™ This product and others like it are available in the dairy section. Parmesan cheese is acceptable when used as a condiment. Reduced calorie Laughing Cow™ wedges, Weight Watchers,™ Alpine Lace,™ Lifetime,™ and Lite Line™ products are also acceptable.

Vegetable Food Sprays

There are several varieties of vegetable oil food sprays on the market that are excellent to use in a heart-healthy diet plan. Some are flavored. There are butter-flavored sprays, and now you can even get olive oil in a spray can. Whenever possible use a food spray instead of oil, butter, more margarine when you cook or sauté. You'll save lots of fat calories and still have good tasting food. You'll find in most of my recipes that I spray or spritz a pan instead of using oil by the spoonful.

Salad Dressings, Spreads, Mayo, and the Like

Use the lightest products possible. There are some very good no fat, no cholesterol salad dressings available, and now that we have fat substitutes, more healthy foods in this line are available. Salad dressing and mayonnaise can be found in reduced calorie form. Use them sparingly when a recipe calls for them. There are 100 calories in 1 tablespoon of regular mayonnaise; diet mayos have about 45 calories per tablespoon. You save 55 fat calories when you use diet or lite products. Mustards and vinegars of all types are acceptable and low in calories, so enjoy them.

Soups, Sauces, Spices—The "S's"

Again I will tell you to read the label. I'm giving you several soup recipes to make at home. In the grocery stores there are all kinds of healthy soups and some not so healthy soups. Pick and choose. Watch the sodium content, especially if you are on a sodium-restricted diet or if you're sodium sensitive. The biggest problem with soups is the fat that might be in them.

STEP INTO THE KITCHEN ■

Here's a handy tip that will help you get the fat out of the soup. If your soup is homemade place the soup, after straining, in the refrigerator for several hours. The fat will rise to the top and then all you have to do is scrape off the fat and throw it away. The richest and best broth soups turn to jelly when chilled. Don't be upset if your broth turns to jelly! When it's heated, it will return to liquid form again.

If you're using a canned soup and you want to make sure that extra fat is removed, just place the can in the freezer for about 15 minutes before opening and cooking. In the freezer the fat will quickly rise to the top and start to congeal. When you open the can, just scrape off the excess fat and discard. Whenever you make homemade soups, you'll find that the flavors improve if the soup is chilled for several hours before re-heating and serving. The same goes for stews and gravies. My father, who was a professional chef, used to say that the flavors "marry" in the refrigerator. That is, they have an opportunity to compliment one another after they have the opportunity to become acquainted. Maybe the same could be true of people.

Rice, Pasta, Whole Grains

There are good foods for high energy people. Try eating different types and shapes of pasta. Some of the latest shapes and forms have been designed especially for kids, dinosaurs and space ships for example. Grains such as rice, barley, coucous, and kasha are delicious and provide variety and nutrients. Pasta and rice have about 110 calories per ½ cup serving cooked. Compare the 100 calories in 1 tablespoon of butter and the same calories in a half cup of pasta. The pasta will fill you up, not out, like the fats will. Add barley, rice, or pasta to your casseroles and soups. Kids like pasta. Feed it to them with pleasure.

Soft Drinks, Kool-Aid,™ Crystal Light,™ Etc.

As I've said, Americans love the taste of sweet things. We've gotten away from plain water as a beverage or thirst quencher. Try to stay away from sweet beverages and drink water. Then if you want something sweet, do try the many dry mixes and soft drinks that are available. Remember: *There are 11 teaspoons of sugar in one can of a regular soft drink.* That's a lot of sugar. So mix up your liquid intake to include plenty of water, some fruit juices, some calorie-controlled drinks, and on occasion, go for the regular stuff if you so wish!

Ice Cream and Frozen Desserts

There are so many choices out there, you shouldn't have any problem in this department. Just read the labels and choose the flavor and type that suits you and your family best. Some yogurt desserts are delicious. Real ice cream can have 270 calories per ½ cup serving (vanilla flavor). Compare that to the new fat free, cholesterol free variety at 90 calories per serving. Don't forget, "What you eat today, you wear tomorrow." Fruit juice popsicles are great for the kids.

Crackers, Cookies, Chips: The 3 "C's"

I'll repeat what I've said before. *Read the label!* Not all C's are created equal! But there's an excellent selection of crackers and cookies on the grocers' shelves. I've listed several brands that I've found locally on the shopping list. All are about 30 percent total fat calories but can be considered okay as long as you don't pig-out on them. Chips are a different story. Most chips, at this time, are fried. Those that say they're baked invariably contain lots of fat, no matter how they were cooked. Read the label carefully. Try bagel chips or the new Dorito™ light chips as an occasional treat, but not as a snack or a part of your meal.

Candy

Sweet and good to the taste buds, candy is bad for the teeth and the caloric content is very high. Pick and choose what you're going to allow yourself and your family to eat, and don't buy the big economy pack that always seems to be on sale. "A moment on the lips, forever on the hips," or so I've been told many times by the experts! (Lulu definitely qualifies as an expert.) I love to splurge on gummy bears and licorice once in a while, but I stay away from the fatty-chocolate-gooey-nutty stuff I love! Somehow one piece is too much and, at the same time, never enough! Grab a piece of fruit instead. And for those of you who call yourselves "chocoholics": remember that chocolate candy is very high in *fat*. For instance a Baby Ruth™ candy bar has 12.0 grams of fat, 36.0 grams of carbohydrate, 4.0 grams of protein, and *260 calories!*

Canned, Frozen, and Packaged Foods

Most of us dream of living in an ideal world where foods are picked fresh daily and go from the garden to the table the same day. That's a dream for most of us. We live in a busy, practical world, and we should stop fighting it and use the very best of what modern technology and industry has to offer. Choose the canned food items that will help you in your busy lifestyle, such as canned tomatoes and tomato products, canned beans, and beets for salads. Drain and rinse the salty liquid off before cooking or using. Frozen foods, when chosen properly, are delicious and easy to prepare.

When was the last time you shelled peas or had the time to shell peas? Frozen peas can fill the bill very nicely! We use frozen vegetables in soups and stews, as side dishes at dinner, and in salads. Almost every kid I know will eat macaroni and cheese without a battle. So feed it to them. Just make it with skim milk and add a powdered butter flavor for the buttery taste instead of fatty butter or margarine. Try skim evaporated milk for a richer taste.

I keep a package of dry scalloped potatoes in my cupboard and make them using skim evaporated milk and butter flavored powder, and I add sliced onion before baking them in the oven. This makes a great dish to serve with baked turkey ham and vegetarian baked beans. Read the labels on all packaged foods and see what's best for you. Remember that 60 percent of something is better than 100 percent of nothing. A healthier lifestyle doesn't have to mean sprouts, dry oatmeal, and deprivation. Those days are gone forever, I hope.

Gelatins, Puddings, Etc.
Go for the no sugar products that taste very good and are quite versatile. You'll see that I use these products frequently, and I would encourage you to do so also.

Spices, Flavoring, and Dairy Powders
Spices make your foods come alive. Experiment with different spices until you achieve just the right taste. Many new spice blends are excellent since the blends are just right for a recipe without one particular spice overpowering a special dish.

Flavorings are a great substitute. For instance, coconut is high in fat, yet the taste is very pleasant. So substitute coconut flavoring in a recipe. The same goes for rum or brandy or banana flavorings.

Something new called "dairy flavored powders" has recently come on the spice shelf and they're very good. The powders come in cheese, butter and sour cream, and onion flavors and have no fat or cholesterol. They can be used to spice up foods with the familiar flavors so many of us are used to. Try them.

Organic Foods
For those of you who are confused about how to purchase the healthiest fresh products, the term *organic* can be misleading.

Laws on organic foods vary widely from state to state. In one state, for example, for a food to be labeled organic, it must be grown on land where no chemicals have been applied for at least three years. In yet another state, farmers can label their produce organic after just one year of chemical-free growing. Know your state laws before assuming that what you purchase is what you think you're purchasing!

And *always*, as a safety precaution, wash all fresh produce well before eating.

Make your life practical, livable, and enjoyable. Use your plain good common sense. And you'll also see that you save money when you shop and eat healthy. Junk foods cost lots of money. Compare grocery bills after one month on the program and see if I'm right!

Meal Suggestions

THE BETTER LIFE SAMPLE MENU

Step number one in planning a menu for your family is to sit down and review the list of suggested foods in a healthy eating plan, an excellent topic of conversation for Family Circle.

Discuss the suggested foods with family members and get their ideas on what foods to eat on what day. Every family has a different schedule, so plan for your lifestyle, not the neighbors'. Choose foods that the majority likes. When the family sees that a healthy eating plan includes pancakes and bacon and spaghetti and hamburgers and even macaroni and cheese, they'll be willing to give it a try. There are recipes in this chapter that will compliment the menu plan. Recipes for the starred (*) items are included.

During the discussion make a list of the foods each family member suggests. Then when the meal is prepared, give some credit to the person who suggested the menu as well as the person or persons who prepared it.

WHAT YOU CAN EAT HEALTHY FOR BREAKFAST

BREAKFAST

Hot Cereals
Cold Cereals
Whole Grain Muffins*
Fruit Muffins*
Pancakes*
Waffles*
French Toast*
Fruit

Fruit Juice
Breads, Toast
Scrambled Eggs*
Omelettes to Order*
Turkey Ham, Turkey Bacon,
    Turkey Sausage
Jams, Jelly, Syrup*
Skim Dairy Products

*Recipes included.

WHAT YOU CAN EAT HEALTHY FOR LUNCH AND DINNER

LUNCH

Sandwiches
    Bacon, Lettuce, Tomato*
    Grilled Cheese*
    Tuna Salad*
    Sliced Turkey or Turkey Ham*

Soups
    Chicken Rice*
    Chicken Noodle*
    Vegetable Soup*
    Bean Soup*

LUNCH—Continued

Sandwiches—*Continued*
    Ham and Cheese*
    Bar-B-Que Ham*
    Sloppy "Toms"*
    Chicken Salad*
    "The Burger"*

Soups—*Continued*
    Lentil Soup*
    Barley-Mushroom Soup*
    Cream of Something Soup*
Chili*

*Recipes included.

DINNER

Old-fashioned Meatloaf and
    Variations*
Tacos and Enchiladas*
Swedish Meatballs and
    Variations*
Lasagna*
Manicotti*
Pizza and Variations*

Broiled Fish and Chicken . . . the
    Basics*
Chicken in Wine*
Basic Italian Tomato Sauce*
Bar-B-Que Chicken*
Creole Fish Stew*

*Recipes included.

■ ■ ■ ■ ■ ■ ■ ■ ■ ■ ■ ■ ■

What Do We Buy?

■ *A Sprint Through the Supermarket*
■ *Read Those Labels!*
■ *Ideas . . . and How To's . . . and What Do I Need? . . . Etc.*

Section 2

A Sprint Through the Supermarket

Before you shop, you need to make a grocery list. You've had a discussion about food with your family, and you've made decisions about the foods you'll make at home. Think about what you'll need to pack lunches. What will you need to take to the office for emergencies? How about snacks?

Here is a sample shopping list to use as a guideline.

SAMPLE GROCERY SHOPPING LIST

Whole Wheat and No Fat
    Saltines
Harvest Crisps, 5 Grain and Oat
Triscuits™ and Triscuit Bits™
Pretzels and Bread Sticks
Ry-Krisp™
Melba Toast, Melba Snacks
Rice Cakes, Corn Cakes
Oyster Crackers

Fig Newtons™ and other Fruit
    Newtons™
Golden Fruit Raisin Biscuits™
Graham Crackers
Vanilla Wafers
Gingersnaps
Animal Crackers
Soft Batch™ Oatmeal Raisin
    Cookies
Any crisp "dunkin" cookie

Check out the no fat, no cholesterol cookies.

Fruit Snacks and Roll-ups
Suckers and Lollipops
Raisins and Dry Fruit

Watch hard candies with little kids so that they don't choke.

Oatmeal
Cream of Wheat
Grits
Instant Cereals
Whole Grain Mixed Cereals 7-,
    4-, and 10-Grain Blends

For those of you who never make a list to use as a shopping guide: how can you carry out a plan without a plan? Make a list!

Raisin Bran
Cheerios™
Nutri-Grain™ Cereals
Shredded Wheat
Grape Nuts™
Kix™
Fiber One™
All-Bran™
Wheaties™

Read the labels on all cereals and evaluate them not only for fat content, but also for sugar and fiber content.

Cup-of-Soup:
    Chicken and Noodle
    Tomato
    Hearty Chicken
Bouillon Cubes
Onion Soup (dry mix) and
    variations
Soup Starter

Watch the sodium in all package soups.

Canned Vegetarian Baked Beans
Hot Chili Beans, Beans in Chili
    Gravy (neither is too spicy
    hot)
Canned Beans: Kidney,
    Garbanzo, Black Beans,
    Black Eyed Peas
Dry Beans, all varieties; Dry
    Bean Soup Mix
    with Smokey Ham Spice
Jar Beans, Cooked Great
    Northern Beans
    in 24 and 48 oz. jars

Scalloped Potatoes (omit added
    fat in preparation)
Hamburger Helper™ (use lean
    meat or poultry)
Macaroni and Cheese
Rice Mixes

Oriental Choices:
    Rice Crackers
    Fortune Cookies
    Lite Soy and Terriyaki
        Sauces

Always read the label on all products. Refer to the Label Reading Section for "how to's."

THE BETTER LIFE INSTITUTE FAMILY HEALTH PLAN

Water Chestnuts
Bamboo Shoots
Sweet and Sour Sauce
Hoisin and Oyster Sauces
Brown Sauce
Sesame Oil

Vinegars (all types)
Tabasco 7 Spice Chili Recipe™
    Sauce
Sloppy Joe Sauce
Manwich™ Sauce
Bar-B-Que Sauce
A-1™ Sauce
Lea & Perrins™ Sauce
Catsup
Mustard (all types)
Pickles (all types)
Lite Salad Dressings
No Oil or Fat Salad Dressings
Lite Mayonnaise

Good Seasons™ and Modern Magic Meals™ make very good no oil salad dressing mixes.

New products that fit perfectly into a heart-healthy, calorie-controlled lifestyle are being marketed every day. Take time to check out the new products on your grocer's shelves, and don't forget to read the labels.

Mexican Choices:
    Vegetarian Re-fried Beans
        (no lard)
    Taco and Tostada Shells (dry
        baked)
    Taco Sauces
    Salsas, plain and chunky
    Enchilada Sauce (no lard)
    Green Chiles
    Chili spice mixes (you add
        ground turkey, tomato,
        and beans)

Tuna (water pac)
Salmon (water pac)
Chunky Chicken (water pac)
Canned Clams, Shrimp, Crab
    (water pac; great for salads
    and soups)
Sardines in Tomato Sauce or
    Mustard

Sauces and Gravy Dry Mixes:
  Sweet and Sour Sauce Mix
  Turkey and Chicken Gravy
    Mix
  Brown Gravy Mix
  Mushroom Gravy Mix (good
    for soups and sauces)

Italian Choices:
  Spaghetti Sauce, meatless
  Lasagna Noodles
  Manicotti Noodles
  Pasta Shells (large and
    small)
  Spaghetti Noodles, Elbow
    Macaroni
  No Egg, No Oil Noodles
  "Kids" Pasta
  Parmesan Cheese

Jams and Jellies made with low
  sugar or all fruit
Lite and Fruit Pancake-Waffle
  Syrups
Canned and Frozen Fruit Juices
Tomato Juice (watch sodium)
V-8™ Juice (watch sodium)

Canned Vegetables:
  Tomato Paste
  Tomato Sauce
  Crushed Tomatoes with
    added puree
  Just for Chili diced and
    spiced tomatoes
  Stewed Tomatoes: Original,
    Cajun, Italian
    and Chunky Style
  Beets
  Green Beans
  Asparagus
  Artichoke Hearts
  Hearts of Palm
  Carrots
  Peas

THE BETTER LIFE INSTITUTE FAMILY HEALTH PLAN

Corn
Sweet Potatoes (water, juice,
     or vacuum pac)

No Sugar Gelatin Mixes
No Sugar Pudding Mixes
San Sucre™ Chocolate Mousse
     and Cheesecake Mixes

Frozen Foods:
     Nutri-Grain Waffles™
     Aunt Jemima™ Lite
          Pancakes
     Egg Beaters™ (plain and
          vegetable)
     Low Calorie Whipped
          Toppings
     TV Dinners
     Pizza Crust
     Ravioli and Pastas
     Vegetables and Fruits (watch
          for sodium and sugar)
     Bread Dough and Bagels
     Phyllo (Greek pastry dough)
     Dinner Rolls
     Fruit Juice Bars
     Weight Watchers™ Frozen
          Desserts
     Yogurt Popsicles™
     Yogurt Desserts
     Lite Desserts

**Read the label before buying
frozen entrées. Some are okay;
some are deadly!**

Meat, Fish, Poultry:
     Turkey Breast Roast
     Turkey Ham Roast
     Sliced Turkey Breast
     Sliced Turkey Ham
     Turkey Bacon and Sausage
          (read the label)
     Chicken Breasts
     Fish Fillets and other
          Seafood and Shellfish
     Lean Beef and Veal
     Ground Turkey or Chicken
          (read the label)

**The lunch meats available in the
deli section may be better for
you than the packaged products.**

Hot Dogs (read the label)
Lunch Meats (read the label)

Bakery Items:
     Whole Grain Bread and
          Rolls
     Muffins (read the label)
     Sourdough, Italian, French
          Breads

Canola Oil
Olive Oil
Nut Oils, walnut, peanut, etc.
Avocado Oil
NutraSweet™ or EQUAL™
Fructose (liquid and powdered)
Sugar
Salt Substitutes, Lite Salt, or
     Salt Sense™
Assorted Spices and Flavorings
Onion and Garlic Powder
Liquid Smoke™
Butter, Cheese, and Sour Cream
     Flavored Powders
Lite Coffee-Mate™ creamer
Lite Pancake Mix
Flour
Corn Meal
Nonfat Dry Milk
Skim Evaporated Milk
Assorted Teas and Coffees
De-Caf Coffee
No Sugar Tea Mixes
No Sugar Hot Cocoa Mix
Dry Stuffing (dressing) Mixes
     (prepare without fat)
Bread Crumbs

Canned Fruit:
     No Sugar Applesauce
     Individual Cans, Packs
          Fruits Packed in Juice
     Lite Fruit Pie Fillings
     Cran-Fruit Relishes

Water and Juice Packed
     Fruits
Bottled Waters, plain and
     flavored
Diet Soft Drinks
Crystal Light™ type beverage
     mixes
Spiced apple cider mix, no sugar

Cracker Jacks™ (read the label)
Popcorn
Peanuts
Doritos™ Lite Chips

Watch those peanuts and some microwave popcorn mixes. They can be high in fat and calories!

■ *Look for the new NO FAT, LOW CHOLESTEROL American and cheddar cheeses recently added to your grocer's shelves.*

Dairy:
     Skim (nonfat) Milk
     Buttermilk
     Cottage Cheese and Yogurts
          (1 percent or less
          milkfat)
     Lite Sour Cream
     Eggs
     Tub Margarine, Soft
     Lite Cheeses, made from
          skim milk (*always* read
          the label)

Laughing Cow™ Reduced Calorie Cheese and Neufchatel Cheese are acceptable as condiments or in cooking. Weight Watchers,™ Lite-Line,™ and Alpine Lace™ are also good.

DRUTHERS—INSTEAD OF'S

Druthers. What is this word? It's a Lulu-ism that stands for "What would you rather do?" You'd druther do this or druther do that. You see here a list of *druthers* I've thought of regarding food. I've given you space to think of your own *druthers,* not only for food but also for exercise, family activities, and other things. Have fun making this list.

NO	YES
Egg Noodles	Spaghetti, Macaroni
Ice Cream	Sherbet, Nonfat Yogurt, No Fat Ice Creams
Sour Cream	Lite or No Fat Sour Cream
Bacon from Pork	Turkey Bacon
Beef or Pork Hot Dog	Turkey or Chicken Hot Dog
Mayonnaise	Lite or No Fat Mayo
Layer Cake	Angel Food Cake
Chips	Pretzels
Peanuts	Roasted Chestnuts

STEP INTO THE KITCHEN ■

Common sense will get you everywhere!

Make your own Druther list:

NO	YES
_____	_____
_____	_____
_____	_____
_____	_____
_____	_____
_____	_____
_____	_____
_____	_____
_____	_____
_____	_____
_____	_____
_____	_____
_____	_____
_____	_____
_____	_____
_____	_____
_____	_____
_____	_____
_____	_____
_____	_____
_____	_____
_____	_____
_____	_____
_____	_____
_____	_____

Read Those Labels!

Learning how to read a food label is the *key* to healthy eating. In this section we'll show you step-by-step how this is done *healthfully*. This is an excellent activity for Family Circle, also. You'll see that I've given you step-by-step instructions for the entire family to get involved. Be patient, follow along carefully, and have fun doing and learning it all!

READY, SET? LET'S GO!

1. Choose a package product from your grocery cupboard. Pick up your package and look at the ingredients list. Read it and give it an over-all rating for you in your new healthy lifestyle. We like to rate on a scale of 1 to 10 with 1 being really bad and 10 extra good.

2. The ingredients are listed in the order of predominance by weight, not by calories. Therefore the first ingredient listed is the predominant ingredient in the package with all other ingredients included in decreasing amounts.

3. After looking at the ingredients, rate the product. If the main ingredient is wheat and you have an allergy to wheat, the product will automatically be a "0"! Someone without the wheat allergy may rate the product a 5 or 6 or 7 depending on their specific goals and needs.

4. Look for ingredients in the product that might be considered not so healthy, such as sugar, fat, sodium. Lots of cereals have sugar as the first ingredient listed. Decide how this cereal is to be eaten, by itself or mixed with other whole grain cereals and *who* is going to eat it. A little sugar in a little body packs a bigger wallop than a little sugar in a big body! Think about it!

5. Discuss the ingredients list and the specific ingredients in the product. Use the glossary for words or phrases you may not know the specific meaning of, lite and reduced calories, for example.

6. Involve the entire family group in this project at Family Circle and make it a fun learning process. Get the kids involved in the rating process. Don't be surprised if you get lots of *ugh* and *barf-barf* comments or "How do you pronounce this word?" questions!

Once you've gone over the list of ingredients, then comes the fun part. Please be patient and don't throw in the towel. This is the basis for label reading.

Ready, set? Let's go to the next step!

Look at your label and check out the

NUTRITIONAL ANALYSIS
or
NUTRITION INFORMATION

This is what you'll find:

serving size	protein in grams
servings per package	carbohydrates in grams
calories per serving	sodium in milligrams
fat in grams	cholesterol in milligrams

vitamins and minerals and USRDA recommended allowances

USRDA means the United States Recommended Daily Allowances

Okay now, don't panic. I'm with you all the way! Before you check out the package you're holding, go over the following lesson step by step.

In the Better Life Institute Program, we focus on *fats* in foods because fat is a big culprit in health-related problems. Therefore it behooves everyone to know how to determine whether a packaged product is healthy or unhealthy depending on the amount of fat a specific ingredient contains. Fat is also very high in calories. There are 9 calories in every gram of fat compared to 4 calories in every gram of protein or carbohydrate. You see that fat has over twice as many calories as proteins or carbohydrates have. The sooner you learn how to read a label for fat content, the better off you'll be. It's not difficult, but you do have to learn an easy formula:

*Grams of fat multiplied by 9, divided by total calories,
equals percentage of fat in a product.*

Now don't get excited! It's not as difficult as it first appears! Let me explain.

1. Check and note the amount of fat in grams a product contains.
2. Multiply that number by 9 because each gram of fat has 9 calories.
3. The answer you get is the amount of fat calories in that product.
4. Take the answer you got in Step 2 and divide that number by the total calorie count. This gives you the percentage of fat in the product—the number you want to determine to see if the product falls into the BLI dietary guideline of: **20% fat, 15% protein, 65% complex carbohydrates.**

Here's a sample package to study: Chicken and Vegetables with Vermicelli, Frozen Dinner Entree, Single Serving Twin Pouch.

INFORMATION PANEL

Chicken Pouch Ingredients: WATER, TOMATOES, CHICKEN, BROCCOLI, ONIONS, MUSHROOMS, CAULIFLOWER, ZUCCHINI, MODIFIED CORNSTARCH, CARROTS, PEAS, WHITE WINE, SALT, BUTTER, MONOSODIUM GLUTAMATE, CHICKEN FAT, SUGAR, SPICES, DEHYDRATED GARLIC, DEHYDRATED ONIONS, CHICKEN BROTH, TURMERIC, NATURAL FLAVORINGS.

Vermicelli Pouch: COOKED VERMICELLI, PARMESAN CHEESE, CORN OIL, SALT.

NUTRITIONAL INFORMATION	**PER SERVING**
SERVING SIZE	12¾ oz.
SERVINGS PER CONTAINER	1
CALORIES	270
PROTEIN	22 gm.
CARBOHYDRATE	32 gm.
FAT	6 gm.

PERCENTAGE OF U.S. RECOMMENDED DAILY ALLOWANCES (USRDA)

PROTEIN	35	RIBOFLAVIN	15
VITAMIN A	15	NIACIN	20
VITAMIN C	30	CALCIUM	10
THIAMINE	6	IRON	15

DIET EXCHANGE INFORMATION AVAILABLE UPON REQUEST.

This product will serve 1 person. It is a main-dish TV meal.

If you look at the label on this frozen entrée package, you might be taken aback to note that a product advertised as diet food and having under 300 calories contains chicken fat, corn oil, parmesan cheese, etc. What you have to determine, as a conscientious consumer, is the *amount* of fat, oil, and cheese in this product. Does it have a shovel-full or a thimble-full of fat?

Let's try our exercise and check out the fat content:

1. There are 6 grams of fat in this product.
2. Multiply 6×9 (6 grams of fat in the product times 9 calories per gram) to get 54 calories.
3. Now, divide the 54 fat calories by the number of total calories (54 divided by 270) and you get .20, or 20 percent.
4. This product with chicken fat, corn oil, and parmesan cheese, is 20 percent fat.
5. Does this product fall within the BLI dietary guidelines? How do you rate it? Would you use it? Could you use it?

STEP INTO THE KITCHEN ■

You decide what's best for you!

For practice, let's compare two labels: 2 cans of tuna—1 water pack, 1 oil pack. Read the list of ingredients first.

<table>
<tr><td>

CHUNK LIGHT TUNA IN WATER

NUTRITIONAL INFORMA-
TION PER SERVING
(including liquid)

SERVING SIZE . . . . 2 oz.
SERVINGS PER
    CONTAINER 3.3
CALORIES 60
PROTEIN . . . . 15 gm
FAT . . . . less than 1 gm
SODIUM . . . . 310 mg
CARBOHYDRATES . . . . . less
                  than 1 gm

PERCENTAGE OF U.S. REC-
OMMENDED DAILY ALLOW-
ANCE (USRDA) PER
SERVING

PROTEIN 25
VITAMIN A . . . . *
VITAMIN C . . . . *
THIAMIN (B_1) . . . . *
RIBOFLAVIN (B_2) 2
NIACIN 35
CALCIUM . . . . *
IRON 4
VITAMIN E 2
VITAMIN B_6 10
VITAMIN B_{12} 25

*CONTAINS LESS THAN 2% OF
    THE USRDA OF THESE NU-
    TRIENTS.

INGREDIENTS: Light Tuna,
Water, Vegetable Broth, Salt.
    Fat content less than 1 gram;
60 calories per serving

</td><td>

CHUNK LIGHT TUNA IN OIL

NUTRITIONAL INFORMA-
TION PER SERVING
(including liquid)

SERVING SIZE . . . . 2 oz.
SERVINGS PER
    CONTAINER 3.3
CALORIES 150
PROTEIN . . . . 13 gm
FAT . . . . 13 gm
SODIUM . . . . 310 mg
CARBOHYDRATES . . . . . less
                  than 1 gm

PERCENTAGE OF U.S. REC-
OMMENDED DAILY ALLOW-
ANCE (USRDA) PER
SERVING

PROTEIN 25
VITAMIN A . . . . *
VITAMIN C . . . . *
THIAMIN (B_1) . . . . *
RIBOFLAVIN (B_2) 2
NIACIN 35
CALCIUM . . . . *
IRON 4
VITAMIN E 6
VITAMIN B_6 15
VITAMIN B_{12} 25

*CONTAINS LESS THAN 2% OF
    THE USRDA OF THESE NU-
    TRIENTS.

INGREDIENTS: Light Tuna,
Soybean Oil, Vegetable Broth,
Salt.
    Fat content 13 grams; 150
calories per serving

</td></tr>
</table>

Now do your analysis:

$$1 \text{ gram fat}$$
$$\times\ 9 \text{ calories per gram of fat}$$
$$9 \text{ fat calories}$$

$$13 \text{ grams fat}$$
$$\times\ 9 \text{ calories per gram of fat}$$
$$117 \text{ fat calories}$$

$$\frac{9 \text{ fat calories}}{150 \text{ total calories}} = 15\% \text{ fat}$$

$$\frac{117 \text{ fat calories}}{150 \text{ total calories}} = 78\% \text{ fat}$$

These two cans of tuna, made by the same company, made of the same light chunk tuna, in the same size cans (6½ oz. each), are very different fat-wise, calorie-wise, and health-wise. Even if you pour off the oil in the oil-pack tuna, some of the oil will remain. Besides the oil permeates the tuna while in the can, adding calories and an unhealthy food item to your diet.

Obviously the water-pack tuna is the one to purchase and eat for all the good reasons. The reason we show you both labels is to make you aware that tuna in cans is not always the same. Nor are all packaged products that say: **NO SALT, NATURAL, LIGHT, HEALTHY, LESS, LEAN** healthy and good for you to eat. Read the label. Evaluate the product.

Remember if you purchase a product, take it home, and put it in your refrigerator or your grocery cupboard, you'll eat it! It's in the cards. So the best thing to do is be a conscientious consumer *before* you buy. Make it fun and make it a challenge. You'll see and feel the results.

Food labels are designed to be attractive and informative, yet sometimes the information can be confusing. Be sure to keep that in mind and take your time. You'll catch on in no time at all.

The Food and Drug Administration (FDA) requires a food label to state the name and address of the manufacturer and to list the ingredients in descending order of weight. That means the ingredients that contribute the most weight to the product are listed first. Any nutritional claims must be backed up with nutrient information. At this very moment, the FDA is acting to improve labeling laws. Watch for these new regulations and labels.

Calorie information is optional. If included, the label must give the serving size; the per serving amounts of calories, protein, fat, carbohydrate; and the percentage of the U.S. Recommended Daily Allowances of five vitamins (A, B_1, B_2, B_3, C), two minerals (calcium and iron), and protein. This information must also be provided if the label makes any claim about a particular nutrient in a food or if the product is enriched or fortified. This federal regulation is the consumer's best basis for comparison shopping.

Terms such as *lite, light, natural,* or *organic* have no standard definitions and are often misleading to unsuspecting consumers.

Lite can refer to color, taste, texture, calories, or weight. Lite olive oil, for instance, is milder in flavor and lighter in color than regular olive oil, but the fat and calories are the same. A careful look at the ingredient list or the nutrient chart is needed to determine why a product is *lite*.

Any product can be labeled *natural* by any manufacturer which, of course, does not make it more healthful. The term *natural* may only be used on meat or poultry if no artificial flavors, colors, preservatives, or synthetic ingredients have been used. Sometimes *100% natural* is confused with *100% pure* which means the product consists of a single ingredient (and maybe water). Juices and applesauce are common examples of 100% pure.

Organic usually implies that no synthetic fertilizers or pesticides were used when growing, processing, or packaging the food, but this definition is not backed by federal law. In other words, there is no guarantee that organic foods are completely free from pesticides, fungicides, or fertilizers.

The following list of legal definitions will help you make informed food choices by making you a more confident label reader.

Lean: No more than 10% fat by weight, not by calories.

Extra Lean: No more than 5% fat by weight, not by calories.

Leaner: At least 25% less fat (by weight) than the original product.

Dietetic: One or more ingredients (usually sodium or sugar) has been changed, substituted, or restricted. Not necessarily low in calories.

Sugar-free/Sugarless: Contains no sucrose (table sugar), but might contain corn syrup, fructose, honey, sorbitol, or other sweeteners. Not necessarily low in calories.

Very Low Sodium: No more than 35 mg. sodium per serving.

Low Sodium: No more than 140 mg. sodium per serving.

Reduced Sodium: At least 25% less sodium than the original product.

No Salt Added and Salt-free: No salt added in processing. However, the food could have significant amounts of natural sodium or sodium from other sources, such as soy sauce or preservatives.

Low in Calories: No more than 40 calories per serving and no more than 0.4 calories per gram.

Reduced Calories: One-third fewer calories than the product it most resembles, except meat and poultry, which must contain 25% fewer calories than similar products.

No Cholesterol: Currently, no legal definition. Remember, though, that a product labeled *no* or *low cholesterol* may still contain saturated fats that raise blood cholesterol. This label does not mean *no fat*.

THE BETTER LIFE INSTITUTE FAMILY HEALTH PLAN

Enriched: The replacement of nutrients lost in the manufacturing process. Most common is the addition of vitamins B_1, B_2, B_3, and iron to refined grain.

Fortified: The addition of nutrients to foods that did not originally contain them. The additions of vitamins A and D to milk, iodine to salt, and vitamins or minerals to cereals are examples.

If you want to determine how much protein or carbohydrate are in a package, use the same formula I showed you to calculate fat, except this time you'll multiply by 4. There are 4 calories in every gram of protein or carbohydrate. A note to the very conscientious consumer: Remember that when you compute percentage of calories, you must take into consideration that these are TOTAL CALORIES of fat, carbohydrates, and protein. In other words, you might find a product that is 30% fat. In the Better Life Institute Program, we suggest about 20% total fat calories. Does that make the product that is 30% off limits? Not necessarily.

To make your decision ask yourself these questions: What will this food be eaten with? Will you add vegetables, grains, salad, fruit, skim milk to the meal? Just try to make sure that your total fat calories for the day stay around 20% and you'll do just fine! For instance, chicken may be 33% fat added to 2 slices whole wheat bread, 10% fat; lettuce, tomato, onion, 10% fat; mustard 10% fat. Make a chicken sandwich with all of the above and what do you have? Good eating and about 20% total fat calories when you take into consideration the *entire* sandwich!

Did you get all this? We don't want to confuse you, but if you are to become a truly conscientious consumer, you should know all the important information necessary to make a decision before you purchase a product. Not everyone in the household needs to know the entire package of information, but everyone should have an overview of label reading.

Let's encapsulate everything:

grams of fat
$\times$ 9 (calories in gram of fat)

$$\frac{\text{fat calories}}{\text{total calories}} = \% \text{ of calories from fat}$$

grams of protein or carbohydrate
$\times$ 4 (calories in gram of protein or carbohydrate)

$$\frac{\text{protein or carbohydrate calories}}{\text{total calories}} = \% \text{ of calories from protein or carbohydrates}$$

FAT WATCHER INSTRUCTIONS: Find the Total Calories and Grams of Fat per serving on your food label (or calorie counter). On the chart below find the same calorie number (down) and grams of fat (across). The point where the numbers intersect is the percentage of FAT CALORIES in your serving. Remember, try to limit your fat calories to about 20% of *your total calories each day.*

GRAMS OF FAT (per serving)

TOTAL CALORIES (per serving)	1	2	3	4	5	6	7	8	9	10	11	12	13	14
10														
20	45													
30	30	60												
40	23	45	68											
50	18	36	54	72										
60	15	30	45	60	75									
70	13	26	39	51	64	77								
80	11	23	34	45	56	68	79							
90	10	20	30	40	50	60	70	80						
100	9	18	27	36	45	54	63	72	81					
110	8	16	25	33	41	49	57	65	74	82				
120	8	15	23	30	38	45	53	60	68	75	83			
130	7	14	21	28	35	42	48	55	62	69	76	83		
140	6	13	9	26	32	39	45	51	58	64	71	77	84	
150	6	12	18	24	30	36	42	48	54	60	66	72	78	84
160	6	11	17	23	28	34	39	45	51	56	62	68	73	79
170	5	11	16	21	26	32	37	42	48	53	58	64	69	74
180	5	10	15	20	25	30	35	40	45	50	55	60	65	70
190	5	9	14	19	24	28	33	38	41	47	52	57	62	66
200	5	9	14	18	23	27	32	36	41	45	50	54	59	63
210	4	9	13	17	21	26	30	34	39	42	47	51	56	60
220	4	8	12	16	20	25	29	33	37	41	45	49	53	57
230	4	8	12	16	20	23	28	31	35	39	43	47	51	55
240	4	8	11	15	19	23	26	30	33	38	41	45	49	53
250	4	7	11	15	18	22	25	29	32	36	40	43	47	50
260	3	7	10	14	17	21	24	28	31	35	38	42	45	48
270	3	7	10	13	17	20	23	27	30	33	37	40	43	47
280	3	6	10	13	16	19	23	26	29	32	35	39	42	45
290	3	6	9	12	16	19	22	25	28	31	34	37	40	43
300	3	6	9	12	15	18	21	24	27	30	33	36	39	42
310	3	6	9	12	15	17	20	23	26	29	32	35	38	41
320	3	6	8	11	14	17	20	23	25	28	31	34	37	39
330	3	5	8	11	14	16	19	22	25	27	30	33	35	38
340	3	5	8	11	14	16	19	21	24	26	29	32	34	37
350	3	5	8	10	13	15	18	21	23	26	28	31	33	36
360	3	5	8	10	13	15	18	20	23	25	28	30	33	35
370	2	5	7	10	12	15	17	19	22	24	27	29	32	34
380	2	5	7	9	12	14	17	19	22	24	26	28	31	33
390	2	5	7	9	12	14	16	18	21	23	25	28	30	32

FAT CALORIES (per serving)

THE BETTER LIFE INSTITUTE FAMILY HEALTH PLAN

Ideas . . . and How To's . . . and What Do I Need? . . . Etc.

This section will deal with just that. The "tie up" of questions that most people have in this practical world. Questions like:

What do I put in a brown bag for lunch?

What can I keep in the refrigerator or in the office for munching?

What kinds of pots and pans and appliances will I require?

What can I do with left-overs?

Can I change a recipe around to make it healthier? If so, how can I do it?

How can I get more information about food?

Here are Better Life tips and ideas.

■ *To receive a Consumer Information Catalog, a handy catalog of brochures and information on foods available from the U.S. Government, write to:*

U.S. Government Printing Office Superintendent of Documents Public Documents Distribution Center Pueblo, Colorado 81009

"BROWN BAG" LUNCH IDEAS

Brown bag lunches need not be boring once you can think past bologna on bread. These are some healthy ideas for lunches that kids of all ages will enjoy. Check with your family to see how they feel about these suggestions, and encourage them to make their own changes. Allow for an occasional peanut butter and jelly sandwich!

■

#1
Thermos of Chili Combo
Crackers
Celery and Carrot Sticks
Apple Granola Bar
Whole Fruit
Milk

■

#2
Turkey Breast Sandwich with Relishes
Container of Applesauce
Celery and Carrot Sticks and Dill Pickle
Cookies
Beverage

■

#3
Pizza on Pita Bread
Container of Fruit Yogurt
Carrots, Celery, Cherry Tomatoes
Beverage

■

#4
Turkey Ham Sandwich with Relishes
Celery, Carrots, Tomatoes, Dill Pickles
Whole Fruit
Cookie
Beverage

■

#5
Thermos of Dum-Dum Vegetable Soup
Pita Chips and Raw Veggie Snacks
Brownie
Whole Fruit
Beverage

■ *Nature Valley® and Snack Sense® Fiber Bars are excellent choices for snacks or lunches.*

STUFF TO KEEP IN THE OFFICE THAT REQUIRES LITTLE OR NO REFRIGERATION

Emergencies will always come up when you least expect them. "He who is prepared . . . survives best." (Lulu may have said that.) Keep some of these suggested foods in your office for those days when stress-pressures-schedules try to take over and ruin your day.

Tuna and chicken in water pack, 3½ oz. cans
Crackers
Tomato or V-8™ Juice, small cans
Aseptic containers of Fruit Juice
Applesauce
Tea, De-caf Coffee; no-sugar Hot Cocoa mix
Dry Cereal for munching
Fiber-Fruit Bars
Fruit Newton™ Cookies

■ *In a survey of elementary and junior high students 75 percent said they eat the fruit packed in their lunches. Fruit is not traded away like other foods!*

Tufts Newsletter 12/90

SNACKS FOR THE REFRIGERATOR AND CUPBOARD

Munching, munching, someone's always munching around the house. Keep those munchies healthy and available at all times. Here are some suggestions:

Munching-type Cereals (eat right out of the box)
Raw Veggies cut into finger-sized pieces
Fresh Fruit of all kinds
Raisins and other dry Fruits
Sliced Apples sprinkled with cinnamon and EQUAL,™ sugar, or fructose
Air-popped Popcorn*
Pita Chips*
Shredded Wheat Nibbles*
Healthy Crackers and Skim Cheese
Cinnamon Toast*

*Recipes included.

Fruit Yogurts (nonfat)
Frozen Ice Desserts, calorie and fat controlled
Fruit Juice Popsicles
Fruit Juice
Diet Pop and flavored Bottled Waters
No sugar Crystal Light,™ Kool Aid,™ etc.
Pretzels and Bagel Chips

POTS, PANS, AND THINGS

The question always comes up, "Do I need a lot of special equipment to cook healthy?" The answer is, "No, except for a few inexpensive items."

Just as a carpenter needs special tools to do his job, and a surgeon requires special equipment to do his very special work, so do you if you're going to cook, eat, and live a healthy lifestyle. Just what do you need?

- Non-stick omelette, egg pans are a must. A non-stick Dutch oven is great for cooking without burning.
- Invest in a stock pot if you cook for a crowd, or if you enjoy cooking and freezing. Most kitchens already have a large pot collecting dust.
- Non-stick cookie sheets and baking pans are nice to have around. Just spray and bake.
- Zip-lock plastic bags are a must. They're great for storing and freezing, for lunches, and to help keep bugs out and flavor in.
- Plastic containers with good tight lids are great for lunches, storage, etc. Also thermos bottles for food "to go."
- Plastic spoons to pack in lunches will keep the silverware in the family and not in the trash can.
- I love a blender and a food processor.
- Plastic and wooden cooking utensils are necessary.
- A wok is nice to have if you enjoy stir frying.
- When the children were home and I was trying to be all things to all people, I used disposable paper products on busy days to avoid the arguments about who was going to do the dishes. Use the biodegradable kind and help protect the environment while helping yourself!

Let's Put It All Together!

- *Seven-Day Meal Planner*
- *Surviving and Thriving in Restaurants*
- *Eating Fast Food on the Run*

Section 3

Seven-Day Meal Planner

This Seven-Day Meal Planner has been designed with the family in mind. You'll see that the entire family eats the same foods, except in different amounts. No Mom's diet, and kids' food, and Dad's dinner. At the Better Life Institute we encourage everyone to make their meals as easy and simple as possible.

A FEW WORDS OF CAUTION

1. Never start a calorie-restricted diet before talking to your physician. We suggest a healthy adult female eat 1200 calories if she wishes to lose weight and a healthy adult male eat 1500 calories if he wishes to lose weight.
2. Never put your children on a diet before talking with your pediatrician or physician.
3. Remember to eat a healthy snack between meals.
   - A glass of milk
   - A graham cracker and a cup of tea
   - A piece of fruit
   - A glass of tomato or V-8™ juice
4. Remember to take a vitamin and mineral supplement whenever you or any member of your family is on a calorie-restricted program.
5. Use this Seven-Day Meal Planner as a guide. Move meals and recipes around to meet the needs of your family.

DAY 1

BREAKFAST	1200 CAL	1500 CAL	1800 CAL
Hot Cereal	½ cup	1 cup	1 cup
Cantaloupe	½ melon	½ melon	½ melon
Skim Milk	1 cup	1 cup	1 cup
Whole Wheat Toast	1 slice	2 slices	2 slices
Lo-Cal Jam	1 Tbs.	2 Tbs.	2 Tbs.
Egg Beaters™ (egg whites)	3 egg whites	3 egg whites	3 egg whites
Salsa or Catsup	2 Tbs.	3 Tbs.	3 Tbs.
Nonfat Yogurt OR		½ cup	1 cup
1% Cottage Cheese		½ cup	1 cup
Coffee, Tea de-caffeinated			

DAY 1—Continued

LUNCH	1200 CAL	1500 CAL	1800 CAL
Green Salad	Unlimited	Unlimited	Unlimited
Italian Dressing	3 Tbs.	5 Tbs.	5 Tbs.
Turkey Breast	3½ oz.	3½ oz.	3½ oz.
French Roll	1 small	2 small	2 small
Vegetable Soup	1 bowl	1 bowl	1 bowl
Apple or Orange	1 each	2 each	2 each
Skim Milk	½ cup	1 cup	1 cup
Coffee, Tea de-caffeinated			

DINNER	1200 CAL	1500 CAL	1800 CAL
Tomato Salad	1 average tomato, sliced with capers		
Ranch Dressing	2 Tbs.	3 Tbs.	3 Tbs.
Lasagna	8 oz.	10 oz.	12 oz.
Tomato Sauce	½ cup	¾ cup	¾ cup
Garlic Toast	—	1 slice	2 slices
Lo-Cal Pudding	½ cup	½ cup	½ cup
Coffee, Tea de-caffeinated			

DAY 2

BREAKFAST	1200 CAL	1500 CAL	1800 CAL
Cold Cereal (dry)	1 oz.	2 oz.	2 oz.
Skim Milk	1 cup	1 cup	1 cup
Banana (medium)	1 each	1 each	1 each
Bran Muffin	1 each	1 each	2 each
Lo-Cal Jam	1 Tbs.	2 Tbs.	2 Tbs.
Egg Beaters™ (egg whites)	3 egg whites	3 egg whites	3 egg whites
Salsa	3 Tbs.	3 Tbs.	3 Tbs.
Nonfat Yogurt OR	—	½ cup	1 cup
1% Cottage Cheese	—	½ cup	1 cup
Coffee, Tea de-caffeinated			

LUNCH	1200 CAL	1500 CAL	1800 CAL
Tossed Salad	Unlimited	Unlimited	Unlimited
Italian Dressing	3 Tbs.	5 Tbs.	5 Tbs.
Turkey Chili and Chopped Onions	¾ cup	1 cup	1½ cups
Pita Bread, toasted	½ each	1 each	1 each

LUNCH—*Continued*	1200 CAL	1500 CAL	1800 CAL
Lo-Cal Gelatin Dessert	1 cup	1 cup	1 cup
Skim Milk	½ cup	1 cup	1 cup
Coffee, Tea de-caffeinated			

DINNER	1200 CAL	1500 CAL	1800 CAL
Pickled Beets and Onions	½ cup	1 cup	1 cup
Breaded Fish Fillets with Lemon	3½ oz.	3½ oz.	3½ oz.
Baked Potato (medium)	1 each	1 each	1½ each
Whipped Sour Cream and Scallions	3 Tbs.	4 Tbs.	6 Tbs.
Steamed Broccoli	Unlimited	Unlimited	Unlimited
Cheesecake Dessert	4 oz.	4 oz.	6 oz.
Coffee, Tea de-caffeinated			

DAY 3

BREAKFAST	1200 CAL	1500 CAL	1800 CAL
Muesli	½ cup	1 cup	1 cup
Spanish Omelettes	3 egg whites	3 egg whites	3 egg whites
Rye Toast	1 slice	2 slices	2 slices
Lo-Cal Jam	1 Tbs.	2 Tbs.	2 Tbs.
Grapefruit	½ each	½ each	½ each
Skim Milk	½ cup	1 cup	1 cup
Nonfat Yogurt OR	—	½ cup	1 cup
1% Cottage Cheese	—	½ cup	1 cup
Coffee, Tea de-caffeinated			

LUNCH	1200 CAL	1500 CAL	1800 CAL
Green Salad	Unlimited	Unlimited	Unlimited
Italian Dressing	3 Tbs.	5 Tbs.	5 Tbs.
Turkey Burgers	3½ oz.	3½ oz.	3½ oz.
Lettuce, Tomato, Onions, Mustard	Unlimited	Unlimited	Unlimited
Sourdough Roll	1 small	2 small	2 small
Skim Milk	½ cup	1 cup	1 cup
Fresh Fruit Cup	1 cup	1 cup	1 cup
Coffee, Tea de-caffeinated			

DAY 3—Continued

DINNER	1200 CAL	1500 CAL	1800 CAL
Cole Slaw Tomato Shells	1 Tomato	1 Tomato	1 Tomato
Oriental Stir-Fry Veggies and Scallops	1½ cups	1½ cups	2 cups
Steamed Rice	½ cup	1 cup	1 cup
Skim Milk	½ cup	1 cup	1 cup
Apple Crisp	4 oz.	4 oz.	6 oz.
Coffee, Tea de-caffeinated			

DAY 4

BREAKFAST	1200 CAL	1500 CAL	1800 CAL
Whole Wheat Pancakes	1 medium	2 medium	2 medium
Lo-Cal Syrup	1 Tbs.	2 Tbs.	3 Tbs.
Strawberries, fresh	1 cup	1 cup	1 cup
Nonfat Yogurt OR	½ cup	1 cup	1 cup
1% Cottage Cheese	¼ cup	¾ cup	1 cup
Skim Milk	½ cup	1 cup	1 cup
Coffee, Tea de-caffeinated			

LUNCH	1200 CAL	1500 CAL	1800 CAL
Sliced Cucumber Salad	Unlimited	Unlimited	Unlimited
Chicken Cacciatore	4 oz.	8 oz.	8 oz.
Pasta (noodles)	½ cup	1 cup	1 cup
Vegetable Medley	Unlimited	Unlimited	Unlimited
Italian Bread	—	1 slice	2 slices
Lo-Cal Pudding	½ cup	½ cup	¾ cup
Skim Milk	—	½ cup	1 cup
Coffee, Tea de-caffeinated			

DINNER	1200 CAL	1500 CAL	1800 CAL
Tossed Salad	Unlimited	Unlimited	Unlimited
Yogurt Mustard Dressing	2 Tbs.	3 Tbs.	3 Tbs.
Lentil Rice Soup OR	½ cup	¾ cup	1 cup

DINNER—*Continued*	1200 CAL	1500 CAL	1800 CAL
Mushroom Barley			
Soup	½ cup	¾ cup	1 cup
Whole Wheat Roll	—	1 each	1 each
Yogurt Fruit Dessert			
OR	½ cup	¾ cup	¾ cup
Banana Ice Cream	½ cup	¾ cup	¾ cup
Skim Milk	—	½ cup	1 cup
Coffee, Tea			
de-caffeinated			

DAY 5

BREAKFAST	1200 CAL	1500 CAL	1800 CAL
Hot Cereal	½ cup	1 cup	1 cup
Cantaloupe	½ melon	½ melon	½ melon
Skim Milk	1 cup	1 cup	1 cup
Scrambled Egg			
Beaters™	3 egg whites	3 egg whites	3 egg whites
Salsa or Catsup	2 Tbs.	3 Tbs.	3 Tbs.
Whole Wheat Toast	1 slice	2 slices	2 slices
Lo-Cal Jam	1 Tbs.	2 Tbs.	2 Tbs.
Nonfat Yogurt	—	½ cup	1 cup
Coffee, Tea			
de-caffeinated			

LUNCH	1200 CAL	1500 CAL	1800 CAL
Tossed Salad	Unlimited	Unlimited	Unlimited
Ranch Dressing	2 Tbs.	3 Tbs.	3 Tbs.
Minestrone	1 cup	1½ cups	2 cups
Parmesan Cheese	1 tsp.	1 Tbs.	1 Tbs.
Garlic Toast	1 piece	2 pieces	2 pieces
Fruit Salad	1 cup	1 cup	1 cup
Zucchini-Apple Muffin	—	1 each	1 each
Skim Milk	—	½ cup	1 cup
Coffee, Tea			
de-caffeinated			

DINNER	1200 CAL	1500 CAL	1800 CAL
Gelatin Fruit Mold	½ cup	1 cup	1 cup
Herb Chicken Breast	½ breast	½ breast	½ breast
Wine Sauce	1 Tbs.	2 Tbs.	3 Tbs.
Herb Noodles	½ cup	1 cup	1 cup

DAY 5—Continued

DINNER—*Continued*

	1200 CAL	1500 CAL	1800 CAL
Glazed Carrots	½ cup	1 cup	1 cup
Bread Sticks or Roll	—	1 each	2 each
Baked Apple	½ each	1 each	1 each
Skim Milk	—	½ cup	1 cup
Coffee, Tea de-caffeinated			

DAY 6

BREAKFAST

	1200 CAL	1500 CAL	1800 CAL
French Toast	1 piece	2 pieces	2 pieces
Syrup-Fruit	1 Tbs.	2 Tbs.	3 Tbs.
Pineapple Wedges (⅛)	1 each	2 each	2 each
1% Cottage Cheese	¼ cup	¾ cup	1 cup
Cold Cereal	—	1 oz.	2 oz.
Skim Milk	½ cup	1 cup	1 cup
Coffee, Tea de-caffeinated			

LUNCH

	1200 CAL	1500 CAL	1800 CAL
Tuna Salad	4 oz.	6 oz.	6 oz.
Pita Bread	½ each	1 each	1 each
Alfalfa Sprouts	Unlimited	Unlimited	Unlimited
Cherry Tomatoes	Unlimited	Unlimited	Unlimited
Potato Salad	¾ cup	¾ cup	1 cup
Skim Milk	—	½ cup	1 cup
Orange	1 each	1 each	1 each
Coffee, Tea de-caffeinated			

DINNER

	1200 CAL	1500 CAL	1800 CAL
Green Salad	Unlimited	Unlimited	Unlimited
Ranch Dressing	1 Tbs.	2 Tbs.	3 Tbs.
Manicotti	1 each	2 each	3 each
Sauce	¾ cup	¾ cup	1 cup
Parmesan Cheese	1 tsp.	1 Tbs.	1 Tbs.
Yogurt-Gelatin Dessert	½ cup	¾ cup	1 cup
Skim Milk	—	½ cup	1 cup
Coffee, Tea de-caffeinated			

DAY 7

BREAKFAST	1200 CAL	1500 CAL	1800 CAL
Waffles	½ large	¾ large	1 large
Applesauce	½ cup	¾ cup	1 cup
Syrup	1 Tbs.	2 Tbs.	3 Tbs.
1% Cottage Cheese	—	½ cup	½ cup
Skim Milk	½ cup	1 cup	1 cup
Scrambled Egg Beaters™	—	2 egg whites	3 egg whites
Salsa or Catsup	—	1 Tbs.	2 Tbs.
Coffee, Tea de-caffeinated			

LUNCH	1200 CAL	1500 CAL	1800 CAL
Cucumbers on Lettuce with Tomato	Unlimited	Unlimited	Unlimited
Veal and Mushrooms	4 oz.	4 oz.	4 oz.
Rice Pilaf	½ cup	1 cup	1 cup
Vegetable Medley	Unlimited	Unlimited	Unlimited
French Bread	—	1 slice	2 slices
Skim Milk	—	½ cup	1 cup
Fresh Berries	1 cup	1 cup	1 cup
Coffee, Tea de-caffeinated			

DINNER	1200 CAL	1500 CAL	1800 CAL
Tostadas	1 each	2 each	3 each
Sour Cream	1 Tbs.	2 Tbs.	3 Tbs.
Salsa	1 Tbs.	2 Tbs.	3 Tbs.
Cantaloupe Wedges	¼ melon	½ melon	½ melon
Skim Milk	—	½ cup	1 cup
Coffee, Tea de-caffeinated			

Surviving and Thriving in Restaurants

This is the next step in healthy living. Again, we'll emphasize watching your fat intake, since many foods eaten on the run are fried and really loaded with unhealthy calories. In this section are some tips and ideas for when you eat out and some sample menus for ethnic restaurants.

1. Choose restaurants wisely. Don't fall into the all-you-can-eat-buffet trap. Foods in buffet lines can be very heavy in cream, fatty sauces, and gravies and salads loaded with mayo and oil. Choose foods that are lighter or foods that allow you to control the sauces and gravies. That's where the fat calories are.
2. Eat a roll or drink a cup of de-caf coffee, tea, or a diet soft drink before ordering if you're feeling very hungry or stressed. It will help to take the edge off.
3. Order and eat your salad, dressing on the side, and a bowl of non-creamy soup *before* you order your entrée! This will also take the edge off your hunger. Here's a great idea to use to control salad dressing calories:

   > Order your salad with the dressing on the side. Dip your fork into the dressing *before* you put the fork into the salad. Put the fork in your mouth and you'll be surprised. You'll use very little dressing and enjoy your salad and a taste of dressing at the same time. Never pour the salad dressing all over your salad. Every tablespoon of dressing put on top of your salad can have 65–100 calories, whereas the green salad is almost calorie free! This is one way to have your cake and eat it too!

4. Order wisely. Never assume. Ask, "How is this dish prepared?" "Can I have it prepared with the sauce on the side?" (You control.) "May I have my toast dry?" (You control the butter or margarine.) "May I have my baked potato dry with a side of salsa and green onions?" *Keep the fat under control.*
5. Make sure you get what you order. Sometimes you'll order very specifically and the cook or waitress will make a mistake. Be nice and let your waitress know that you wanted your food without the sauce or gravy. Be specific but nice. You can catch more flies with honey than with vinegar. (Lulu again.) Order properly and control *your* behavior and be nice to the waiter or waitress. You'll be surprised how well you'll do. Mistakes happen. Be prepared for them and don't get stressed out when they do happen.

■ *THE BETTER LIFE INSTITUTE FAMILY HEALTH PLAN*

Eating Fast Foods on the Run

This is the next step in healthy living. Learning how to eat in restaurants, fast food shops, and even the food truck that comes around at 10:00 A.M. every day is a key to a healthy lifestyle.

Again we'll emphasize watching your *fat* intake. Here are some tips and ideas for "fast" food and some sample menus for ethnic restaurants.

1. Choose the fast food emporium wisely.
2. Choose a muffin, pancake, Egg Beaters,™ cereal, and dry toast and jam for breakfast. Ask for skim milk and fruit with your cereal.
3. For lunch choose a fast food place that grills chicken breast, no skin. Then ask them to "hold the sauce" on your bun and use mustard and catsup instead. The sauce can be very high in fat calories. Top off your meal with a nonfat yogurt dessert and a diet soft drink or fruit juice.
4. Pizza is good food, if you hold the sausage, pepperoni, and fatty cheese! Ask for pizza made with extra sauce and veggies and skim cheese and parmesan.
5. Find a fast food place that offers a salad bar and baked potato. Some also offer a soup bar. You can load up on health food items.
6. Watch out for deep-fat fried foods even if they say "no cholesterol." They're still fried in fat and high in calories.

The biggest problem in fast food places is *fat*. Many of the foods are fried or sauced with heavy, fatty sauces. If you stay away from these foods, you'll do okay. Check out the "Surviving and Thriving in Restaurants" section for more advice.

LET'S EAT OUT ETHNIC!

Let's take a look at what you can order in an ethnic restaurant. We think you'll be surprised by the large variety of wonderful foods you'll be able to enjoy.

■ *Several fast food emporiums are testing* Lite *burgers, burgers that have less fat and cholesterol than the usual burgers. Check out your favorite place and see.*

■

CAJUN STYLE

Shellfish, Steamed or Boiled with
Lemon, Horseradish, or Cocktail Sauce
Green Salad with Dressing on the Side
(dip your fork)
Blackened Fish (your choice)
Rice and Beans
Sherbet or Sorbet

■

ORIENTAL STYLE

Mao Schu Chicken (no egg)
Won Ton Soup
Hot and Sour Soup
Moo Goo Gai Pan
(Chicken and Vegetables)
Vegetable Lo Mein
Broccoli in Brown Sauce
Fortune Cookie

Note: Hold the MSG and go easy on the oil.

■

GREEK STYLE

Hummas-Tahini with Pita Bread
Greek Salad
(hold the feta cheese and olives)
Cucumber Salad with Dill and Yogurt
Lentil Soup with Vegetables and Spices
Greek Coffee (De-caf of course)

Note: Find specific dishes that do not include fatty lamb or beef and those that
include vegetables and rice.

■

INDIAN STYLE

Breads: Papadum, Chapati, Naan
Soups made with DAHL (Lentils)
Tandoori Chicken
Rice and Vegetables in Curry (if desired)
Bean Dishes cooked with Vegetables and Spices

■

ITALIAN STYLE
Seafood Antipasto
Soup
Pasta Fagioli (Beans and Macaroni)
Minestrone
Pasta al Brodo (Pasta in Chicken Broth)
Salads: Green and Seafood
Pasta Primavera
Pasta Marinara
Lobster Diavolo
Chicken Cacciatore
Italian Ice

■

JAPANESE STYLE
Yakitori
(Chicken broiled in Terriyaki Sauce)
Clear Soups; Noodle Soups
Seafood and Cucumber Salad in Rice Vinegar
Sukiyaki Chicken
Steamed Rice
Noodle and Vegetable Dishes

Note: Watch your sodium intake.

■

MEXICAN STYLE
Plain, warm Tortillas and Salsa
(Hold the deep fried chips!)
Gazpacho
Chicken Tostado
(Hold the sour cream and guacamole sauce)
Fajitas—Chicken and Shrimp (roll your own)
Seafood or Chicken Vera Cruz
Spanish Rice

Note: Watch the high calorie guacamole and sour cream and fried chips.

It's Eatin' Time!

- *Healthfully Ever After:*
  The Better Life Institute Way
- *Breakfast*
- *Lunch*
- *Main Dishes*
- *Vegetables*
- *Desserts*
- *Holidays and Snacks*
- *Menu Ideas for the Single Non-Cooking*
  Person
- *How to Adapt a Recipe*
- *Quick Calorie-Counting Guide*
- *Family Circle Suggestions*

Section 4

Healthfully Ever After:
The Better Life Institute Way

The following recipe section contains a collection of recipes with family in mind. Since we're all heavily involved in family and children of our own in addition to running programs for kids of all ages, we believe that we have a good inkling of what people like to eat. At the Better Life Institute we make everything as easy and as simple as possible. We encourage you to experiment with your own twists and spices and have fun doing so. We include these recipes with lots of love and best wishes!

PAT AND STEVE

Breakfast

EGGS AND OMELETTES THE BLI WAY

They are: high protein. Little or no fat or cholesterol. Low in calories if you're interested in weight loss. Quick and easy to prepare. What more can we say?

1. Use Egg Beaters™ or egg whites with a drop of yellow vegetable food color. Throw the yolk away! The yolk has about 225 mg. of cholesterol in it. More than a day's supply! See practical guidelines on page 165 for a discussion on eggs.
2. Follow the measurements on the container of Egg Beaters™; two egg whites equal 1 whole egg. Four egg whites is an excellent portion for a person, and has only 80 calories.
3. Always use a nonstick pan to cook in.
4. Use a vegetable food spray, olive oil, regular, or butter flavored to season the pan instead of butter or margarine.
5. Try sauces, i.e. Mexican salsa, spaghetti sauce, Creole or Cajun sauces, chili, or just plain ole catsup on top of your eggs or omelettes.
6. Sauté onions, green peppers, mushrooms, diced turkey ham, etc. in the pan before adding the egg mixture.
7. Don't just think of eggs for breakfast. An omelette along with a salad and a roll can make a great lunch or an easy light dinner. Lots of cluck for your buck!

Make a Ham and Cheese Omelette using Modern Magic Meals™ Smokey Ham Spice and Cheese Dust while cooking.

To make scrambled eggs, just beat the egg whites or the Egg Beaters™ with a little salt and pepper. Pour into a heated, food sprayed non-stick skillet. Mix and cook until cooked through.

To make an omelette, follow directions for scrambling eggs, just don't mix them after you pour the mix into the pan. Allow the eggs to set. Lift the edge of the omelette and tip the pan to allow the uncooked egg to flow to the edge of the pan and cook. If you're an expert you might try flipping the omelette, but only if you're an expert.

French "Lite" Toast

Everyone's favorite, regardless of age!

½ cup Egg Beaters™
¼ cup skim evaporated milk
½ teaspoon cinnamon
⅓ teaspoon vanilla
4 slices bread

Mix all ingredients except bread in blender. Pour into a bowl and dip the bread in the egg batter. Spray a non-stick pan or griddle with vegetable food spray. Cook the battered bread on the griddle until brown, turning once. Serve with a low calorie pancake syrup. Enjoy!

Pancakes the Easy Way

Purchase a package of LIGHT pancake mix from the store. Follow directions using skim milk and egg white, instead of whole eggs (2 egg whites equal 1 whole egg). Cook and enjoy.

Waffles

Follow directions for Pancakes adding 1 tablespoon canola oil to the batter.

■ *Use Modern Magic Meals™ Cinnamon Spice*

■ *Spray a waffle iron with vegetable food spray to prevent the waffle from sticking.*

■ *Try a butter-flavored food spray instead of butter or margarine on your foods and save many, many fat calories! Remember there are 100 calories in every tablespoon of butter or margarine.*

■ *Don't forget there's a selection of frozen pancakes and waffles in the freezer section of your grocery store. Read the labels and choose the healthiest available. Always use a Lite maple or fruit syrup and forget about the fat (butter) on top!*

■ *Modern Magic Meals™ Buttery DeLite food spray and Maple Syrup make pancakes and waffles taste delicious and healthy.*

Pumpkin Muffins

I make up a batch of muffins, bake, cool, and store in a zip-lock bag in the refrigerator for "hungry moments."

1½ cups flour
½ cup sugar or ⅓ cup fruc- tose
2 teaspoons baking powder
¼ tablespoon salt
1 teaspoon pumpkin pie spice

½ cup skim evaporated milk
½ cup pumpkin
¼ cup canola oil
2 egg whites
½ cup raisins (optional)

Place all dry ingredients and raisins in a large mixing bowl and make a well in the center. Add wet ingredients in the well and mix. Do not beat. Spray a muffin tin with food spray. Spoon mixture into the tin. Bake in 350° oven 20 minutes. Makes 8 large muffins.

Old Fashioned Buttermilk Biscuits

Biscuits are good for what ails you and are great any time. Serve a low sugar jam or maple syrup on a hot biscuit and enjoy! (Trust me when I tell you that hot biscuits don't need butter or margarine. Try one once with just jam or syrup. Is that a deal?)

2 cups flour
2 teaspoons sugar
2 teaspoons baking powder
½ teaspoon soda

½ teaspoon salt
⅓ cup canola oil
⅔ cup buttermilk

Heat oven to 450°. Mix all dry ingredients in a large bowl. Cut in (kids love to do this) the oil until mixture is mealy. Stir in buttermilk. Dough should be soft and puffy. Place dough on floured board and knead 20 times (get the kids involved). Roll out to ½-inch thick. Cut into rounds and place on a non-stick baking pan. Bake 10–12 minutes.

Easy Muffins

This is a quick and easy muffin that you can make up, cool, package, and freeze. I always suggest that you put a serving for you or your family in a zip-lock bag and freeze. Then all you have to do is pull out your muffin bag, defrost or drop in a lunch bag, and eat when hungry. Make a big batch for a rainy day.

2 cups lite pancake mix
1 teaspoon cinnamon
1/3 cup powdered fructose
   (or sugar)

1/2 cup applesauce
2 egg whites
3/4 cup skim milk
2 tablespoons canola oil

Use Modern Magic Meals™ Rice Bran Muffin mix.

Place dry ingredients in a bowl and mix. Add wet ingredients and mix. Do not beat the batter. Spoon into muffin tin that has been sprayed with vegetable food spray. Bake in a 350° oven 25 minutes or until browned on top. Makes 12 large muffins.

Bran Muffins the Easy Way

Another quick and easy, make-ahead recipe. This one has bran in it.

1¼ cups lite pancake mix
1 teaspoon baking powder
2 cups All Bran™ cereal
1/3 cup powdered fructose or
   sugar

1/2 cup mincemeat
1 cup skim milk
2 egg whites
1/4 cup canola oil

Modern Magic Meals™ Muesli cereal is excellent in this recipe.

Place all dry ingredients in a large mixing bowl. Add wet ingredients and mix well. Do not beat. Spoon into a muffin tin that has been sprayed with vegetable food spray. Bake in a 350° oven 25–30 minutes or until muffins are browned on top. Makes 12 large muffins.

Corn Bread

Corn bread is great any time and with just about anything from jam and fruit to chili and beans. Make a batch, freeze, and enjoy!

1 cup cornmeal	1/2 teaspoon salt
1 cup flour	1 cup skim evaporated milk
2 tablespoons sugar	1/4 cup canola oil
4 teaspoons baking powder	2 egg whites

Place dry ingredients in a large mixing bowl. Mix and make a well in the center of the flours. Add wet ingredients and mix well. Do not beat. Pour or spoon batter into non-stick muffin tins or baking pan that has been sprayed with vegetable food spray. Bake in a 350° oven until browned on top.

Steamed "Coffee Can" Bread

This recipe takes a little more time to set up and cook. It's a fun project for a rainy day or a special occasion. You'll need 4 empty 1 lb. size coffee cans and a large canning type pot with a rack in it to make this recipe. Our ancestors used to make bread this way in the winter when the wooden stove was going all the time to keep the house warm. No energy was wasted and the smell of bread on the stove was heart-warming!

1 cup flour	1/2 teaspoon salt
1 cup cornmeal	2 cups buttermilk
1 cup whole wheat flour	1 cup molasses
2 teaspoons baking soda	1 cup raisins

Spray the 4 coffee cans with vegetable food spray. Mix the dry ingredients in a bowl. Make a well in the center. Add the wet ingredients. Mix, but do not beat. Spoon batter into coffee cans. Place coffee can on the rack in the large pot. Pour water in the pot up to the top of the rack. Cover the pot and steam the bread about 3 hours or until tests done with a toothpick. Serve warm with "Buttery Spread."

Buttery Spread

Surprisingly good!

1 pint cottage cheese (1% milkfat)
¼ cup water
4 tablespoons dry nonfat milk
3 tablespoons dry butter-flavored powder
sweetener to taste

Process all ingredients in a food processor until light and creamy. Sweeten to taste and use as a spread on muffins, pancakes, etc.

Modern Magic Meals™ Butter Dust is an excellent ingredient for homemade dishes.

Easy Jam

Jams and syrups made with less sugar are available in your grocery store. Look for them and keep them on the shelf or try these simple yet delicious recipes. These also make very nice gifts at holiday time or for a special person who needs cheering up.

1 pkg. (20 oz.) frozen berries
1 small pkg. berry flavor no sugar gelatin

Place berries in a medium saucepan. Bring to a boil. Add the dry gelatin mix. Stir. Remove from heat. Cover and allow to sit for 15 minutes. In a blender jar, blend a few minutes until well mixed and smooth. Spoon into a glass or plastic container with a tight lid. Store in the refrigerator.

Easy Syrup

1 pkg. (20 oz.) frozen berries
1 large (12 oz.) can apple juice concentrate
1 small pkg. Knox™ unflavored gelatin

Place the berries in a large saucepan. Add the juice and bring to a boil. Simmer 5 minutes. Add the gelatin. Mix. Take off the heat and allow to cool. Blend in a blender jar and pour into jars or bottles with tight lids. Store in the refrigerator.

Modern Magic Meals™ Maple Syrup is unique since it comes dry and you mix it with water and has only 8 calories per tablespoon.

Bircher Muesli

One of the tricks to get the children involved in a healthy eating program is to do exactly that . . . get them involved. Here is a recipe that children of all ages enjoy fixing and eating.

Bircher Muesli is the granddaddy of some of the new dry, cold cereals available today. It was originated in Switzerland, I've been told, by health-conscious exercisers who were looking for long-lasting carbohydrate calories to sustain them while climbing the Alps.

It is messy stuff for breakfast that kids of all ages like to mix and eat!

In a food processor chop:

1 apple, peeled and cored
1 orange, peeled and sectioned

Pour the apple-orange mixture over:

1 cup nonfat yogurt
1 cup quick cooking oats, uncooked
1 teaspoon coconut flavoring
1/2 cup crushed pineapple packed in juice

Mix all ingredients well. Moisten to desired consistency with nonfat milk. Sweeten with sweetener of choice. Eat!

Quick and Easy Muesli

I've taken the old recipe for Bircher Muesli and adapted it to a quick and easy recipe that will take only minutes to prepare. The enjoyment will last much longer.

In a large mixing bowl mix:

1 cup yogurt
1 cup quick cooking oats, uncooked
1 teaspoon coconut flavoring
1/2 cup crushed pineapple in juice
2 tablespoons each apple juice and orange juice concentrate

■ *THE BETTER LIFE INSTITUTE FAMILY HEALTH PLAN*

Moisten to desired consistency with nonfat milk. Sweeten to taste with sweetener of choice. Enjoy!

Amy's Mess

Just to show you how children can get involved, Amy is my daughter, my seventh child, who was born with a wooden spoon in her right hand and talking a blue-streak! I'll bet you have an Amy in your family, too! Anyway, Amy started making this "Mess" during high school days when she was always "on the run," "on a diet," "too busy to eat," etc. Since that time, I've encouraged children of all ages to try this recipe. See how you like it.

¹/₄ cup Grape Nuts™
¹/₄ cup nonfat yogurt
¹/₄ cup apple butter

Mix all ingredients and serve immediately to 2 people.

Kiddo's Milkshake

Great for those "on the run" or those just wanting an extra bit of love and attention!

1 cup skim milk
1 banana
1 cup berries

1 carton (6 oz.) yogurt (flavor of choice)
1 tablespoon oat bran

Blend all ingredients in a blender, adding ice as desired. Sweeten to taste. Makes 4 servings.

■ *Positrim*™ *drink mix is an excellent meal replacement with vitamins and minerals included.*

Lunch

LUNCHTIME AND SNACKS, DRESSINGS, AND DIPS

Let's Make a Sandwich

I wonder if the Earl of Sandwich really knew what he was creating when he placed some watercress between 2 slices of buttered bread, smacked his lips, and said, "Now that's a sandwich!" The sandwich is the original convenience snack, invented by this English nobleman because he was too busy playing cards to go into the dining room for a meal.

Sandwiches are real food for real people! Here are some quick and simple ways to create your own specialties as well as enjoy some of your favorite standbys, like grilled cheese and hamburgers. Always have the healthy ingredients in the cupboard and the refrigerator and you're all set to go.

Bacon, Lettuce, and Tomato

4 strips turkey bacon
2 slices bread
lettuce, tomato
lite or no fat mayo

Cook turkey bacon until browned. Drain on a paper towel. Toast bread of choice. Layer bacon, lettuce leaves, sliced tomatoes on 1 slice of bread. Spread lite mayo *lightly* on the other slice of bread. Put sandwich together and cut in half. Serve with a slice of onion, if desired, and a wedge of dill pickle.

Grilled Cheese the BLI Way

2 slices bread, whole grain or Lite
2 slices skim cheese slices, such as Lite Line™ or Weight Watchers™
vegetable food spray, butter flavored

Spray a non-stick pan or griddle with butter flavored vegetable food spray. Assemble the sandwich and place on the griddle. Cook until browned on the bottom side. Turn and brown on the other side. Cut and serve with mustard and a pickle or salsa.

■ *THE BETTER LIFE INSTITUTE FAMILY HEALTH PLAN*

Sliced Turkey Breast or Turkey Ham

2 oz. turkey breast or turkey ham, sliced or shaved
2 slices bread, whole grain or lite
lettuce, tomato
mustard, lite or no fat mayo

Make sandwiches with bread of choice. Spread bread lightly with *lite* mayo if desired and mustard. Add lettuce, tomato, alfalfa sprouts, onions, pickles, etc. as desired.

■ *Purchase a "chub" of turkey ham and ask the butcher to slice or shave the ham for you. Divide the meat into 2-ounce portions. Place each portion in a plastic lunch bag and refrigerate or freeze for future use.*

Ham and Cheese

2 oz. turkey ham
2 slices skim cheese
bread, whole grain or lite
mustard
relishes (if desired)

Take the ham from the ham sandwich and the cheese from the cheese sandwich. Put them together and do your thing the healthy way.

Light Tuna Salad

Great in Pita bread! Very low calorie!

In a large mixing bowl, place:

1 6½ oz. can water pack tuna, drained
½ cup each chopped onion, celery, water chestnuts, apple, radishes
Lite Italian salad dressing or no fat mayo or salad dressing

Gently mix tuna, vegetables and apple in bowl. Toss with lite dressing. Chill. Serves 4. Approximately 50 calories per serving.

"American" Tuna or Chicken Salad

1 6½ oz. can water pack tuna or chicken, drained
1 stalk celery, chopped
½ onion, chopped
lite or no fat mayonnaise to mix

Place drained tuna or chicken, celery and onion in a bowl. Add just enough mayo or salad dressing to moisten. Serve with pickles, tomatoes, green onion, etc. if you wish.

Chicken or Turkey Salads #1

For the more adult tastes. Wonderful for a luncheon or light supper.

Use left-over chicken or turkey, or purchase cooked chicken breast from your local deli. Let someone else help with the work.

3 cups cooked and cubed turkey or chicken breast
1 medium apple, cubed
1 medium pear, cubed
1 cup seedless grapes, halved
½ cup chopped celery
1 cup shredded cabbage
1 teaspoon orange rind
lite or no fat Miracle Whip™

Place all ingredients in a large mixing bowl. Add just enough Lite Miracle Whip™ to moisten. Chill well before serving. Makes 6 servings.

Chicken or Turkey Salads #2

2 cups cooked, diced turkey or chicken
1 small (4 oz.) jar diced red pimento
½ cup green onion, chopped
1 stalk celery, chopped
1 cup seedless grapes, halved
¼ teaspoon each onion and garlic powder
1 teaspoon curry powder
½ cup lite or no fat mayonnaise

Mix all ingredients in a large mixing bowl. Chill well. Serves 4.

Bar-B-Que Ham

turkey ham
bread or roll
Bar-B-Que sauce (from the grocers)
vegetable food spray

Fry sliced turkey ham on a vegetable food sprayed, non-stick griddle or skillet. Cook until browned on one side. Turn. Place 1 teaspoon of bottled Bar-B-Que sauce on top of the ham. Continue to heat for about 2 minutes, turning once. Place the Bar-B-Que ham on bread or roll. Serve.

Sloppy "Toms"—The Easy Way

ground turkey, uncooked
whole wheat buns or bread
vegetable food spray
jar of Sloppy Joe mix (from the grocers)

Spray non-stick skillet with vegetable food spray. Cook ground turkey until lightly browned. Add a jar of Sloppy Joe Sauce mix. (Readily available at your grocery store.) Heat and simmer 10 minutes. Serve spooned over a toasted whole wheat bun. Good!

■ *Modern Magic Meals™ Beef Flavored Spice Mix for Poultry is wonderful when making burgers, meatloaf, stews, and soups. It gives you the* taste of *roast beef without the fat and calories of roast beef.*

Burgers

Real American food for real Americans:

4 oz. per person ground turkey, chicken, or very lean beef
seasonings*
buns or rolls, whole grain or lite
lettuce, tomato, onion, sliced pickles
lite or no fat mayonnaise, mustard

Mix seasonings into ground meat. Shape into individual patties.
Spray skillet, griddle, or grill with vegetable food spray. Cook patties and enjoy!

*Seasoning ideas:
- 1 teaspoon beef bouillon granules and pepper to taste.
- Smoke flavoring spice. (Tastes like burgers cooked over the coals.)
- 1/4 cup oat bran and 2 tablespoons Bar-B-Que Sauce.
- 1 tablespoon low sodium soy sauce and 1/4 teaspoon Oriental spices.
- Mexican or Italian spices.

"Stevie" Burger

Stevie is, of course, my husband who loves vegetables and is always challenging me to do something different with the same old stuff! So for the "kid" who loves to eat tasty, healthy food, here's one for Steven!

■ *Some "Burger No-No's": 1) Do not over-handle the meat; 2) Never press down on the burger when cooking.*

1 carrot
1 stalk celery
1 green pepper
1 small onion
1/4 head broccoli
1 pkg. frozen chopped spinach, defrosted and squeezed dry
1 large zucchini

1/2 cup walnuts
1 1/4 cup egg substitute or 10 egg whites
1 clove garlic, minced
1 tablespoon Worcestershire sauce
3 cups Bran Flakes™ cereal
1/2 teaspoon pepper
Salt to taste

■ *THE BETTER LIFE INSTITUTE FAMILY HEALTH PLAN*

Chop the vegetables, walnuts, and cereal in a food processor into small pieces. Transfer to a large mixing bowl. Add remaining ingredients and mix well. Cover and refrigerate for 20 minutes. Mix again and form mixture into burgers about 3 inches round and 1 inch thick. Spritz a non-stick griddle or pan with vegetable food spray. Place burgers on the griddle and cook until browned on both sides, turning only once. Serve like burgers on a bun with catsup, mustard, lettuce, tomato, onion, etc. Makes about 12 burgers. These freeze very well. And this mixture is also a great stuffing for green peppers and eggplant.

Mexican Bean Patties

These burgers are delicious cold also!

1 15 oz. can Mexican-style beans in sauce
1/2 onion, chopped
1 4 oz. can mild green chiles
1/2 teaspoon chili powder
1/2 cup oat bran
2 egg whites
1/2 cup shredded skim or no fat cheddar cheese

Modern Magic Meals™ Mexican Spices add a not so spicy hot taste. Children can enjoy Mexican foods without the fire.

Drain the beans. Place all ingredients in a food processor and process into a thick mixture. Remove mixture to a bowl, cover, and chill at least 1 hour. Wet your hands and divide mixture into 4 large patties. (Wetting your hands will prevent the mixture from sticking.) Spray a baking sheet with vegetable food spray. Place the patties on the sheet and spray the tops with food spray. Bake in a 350° oven about 30 minutes or until browned. Serve on a bun or in a pita bread pocket with salsa, shredded lettuce, and chopped tomatoes.

Munching Time!
Snack chips are great to have around for when you get "the munchies." These chips are easy to make and when you serve them with a dip and salsa, they're healthy snacks for munching. Before baking all of them all can be sprayed with vegetable food spray and then seasoned with spices of your choice or Parmesan cheese. Allow to cool before storing in a dry container or a zip-lock bag.

Tortilla Chips

Cut soft tortillas into chip-size wedges and bake in a 250° oven on baking pan until "snap" crisp. Approximately 10 calories per chip.

Bagel Chips

Chill bagels until very cold. Slice very thin. Bake on a cookie sheet at 250° until very crisp. Approximately 15 calories per chip.

Pita Chips

Cut pita bread into wedges. Spray wedges with vegetable food spray and sprinkle with Parmesan cheese. Bake in a 250° oven until browned on top.

Salad Dressings

Bottled salad dressings that are low or no fat and calorie-controlled are very good. Try some and find your favorites. Always read the label before you buy a dressing and then choose a variety that suits your fancy.

Try mixing an Italian dressing with either French or Russian dressing, or mix Thousand Island and Ranch dressings. Make your own mystery dressing and see what happens! Or try these.

Ranch Dip

Modern Magic Meals™ Ranch Dressing Mix is great in dip recipes.

1 pkg. (1 oz.) reduced calorie Ranch Dressing Mix
1/2 cup lite mayonnaise
1/2 cup cottage cheese (1% milkfat)
1 cup buttermilk

Blend all ingredients in a blender jar or in food processor until very creamy and smooth. Serve as a dip for chips and vegetables, as a topping for baked potato, or on a taco or tostada.

THE BETTER LIFE INSTITUTE FAMILY HEALTH PLAN

Very Quick Dip for Veggies

1 carton (16 oz.) lite sour cream
1 pkg. dry onion soup mix

Blend. Chill well before serving.

Another Very Quick Dip for Veggies

1 carton (16 oz.) lite sour cream
1 pkg. Mrs. Grass Vegetable Soup Mix™

Blend. Chill well before serving.

■ *Substitute Modern Magic Meals™ Minestrone Soup Mix for Mrs. Grass Vegetable Soup Mix.™*

Mustard Dressing

1 cup nonfat yogurt
3 tablespoons Dijon mustard
Sweetener of choice

Mix the yogurt and mustard. Sweeten to taste. Chill. Serve as a dressing, a dip, or a sauce for fish or chicken.

Soups

Soup is wonderful food! All you have to do is pour some liquid into a pot, add stuff, mix, cook until flavors and smells are just right, season to taste, and eat! Easy, huh? I don't quite understand why so many people are afraid to make soup. For centuries soup was peasant food. It was made in a pot over a fire with anything around thrown into it. I encourage all of you to try your hand at filling your own soup pot. In the meantime, here are some basic, quick, and easy recipes you might like to try.

These broths are very rich and can be used as is or diluted in soups, gravies, sauces, etc. Remember that these recipes are basic recipes. On clean-the-refrigerator day, anything that is not spoiled goes into the soup pot. One day I made the mistake of putting a fresh peach in the bean soup. Much to my surprise, the soup was very good and when it was blended into a puree, the children could not tell what the mystery taste was. Of course, I never told them, until now. I've used chicken and beef bouillon cubes and granules as well as packaged onion and onion-mushroom soups as a basis for a good broth-stock. I've found that using packaged soup starter is a great way to start something wonderful in a pot. Soup freezes well and is great to take to the office or school in a thermos. I always use more water than directed on the package since some of these foods have more sodium than I need or want in my diet. You do your thing your way and have fun!

Basic Chicken Stock

1 frying chicken, cut up (approx. 2 lbs.)
1½ quarts water
1 onion, chopped
1 carrot, peeled and cut in chunks
1 stalk celery, chopped
1 bay leaf
½ teaspoon pepper
½ teaspoon each onion and garlic powder
½ teaspoon mixed Italian spices

Mix all ingredients in a stockpot and bring to a boil. Cover and simmer 2½ hours or until chicken is cooked and tender. Strain and save chicken for use in other dishes. Always discard skin. Correct seasonings in broth to taste. Chill. Skim off fat before using. Broth should yield 4 cups.

Basic Vegetable Broth

8 cups water
4 each large carrots and onions
2 each leeks, celery stalks, parsnips, and scallions
1 16 oz. can tomatoes
2 cloves garlic
2 sprigs parsley
1 bay leaf
10 whole peppercorns

THE BETTER LIFE INSTITUTE FAMILY HEALTH PLAN

Bring water to a boil. Add all ingredients except the bay leaf and peppercorns. Bring to a second boil and add bay leaf and peppercorns. Reduce heat and simmer covered 2 hours, skimming occasionally. Strain soup; discard vegetables. There should be approximately 4 cups remaining. Add salt and pepper to taste.

Mushroom-Barley Soup

(My dear husband's favorite!)

2 quarts de-fatted beef stock
1 onion, chopped fine
1 clove garlic, minced
1/2 teaspoon mixed Italian seasonings
1 tablespoon parsley flakes
1 cup quick-cooking barley
1 lb. fresh mushrooms, sliced

■ *Use bouillon cubes to save time!*

Place all ingredients, except mushrooms and barley, in a large stockpot and bring to a boil. Add barley and mushrooms. Cover and simmer until barley is tender, approximately 20 minutes. If soup is too thick, add more stock. Serve with a sprinkle of Parmesan cheese if desired, and season to taste.

The quick way to make this soup is with an onion-mushroom dry soup mix. Make according to package directions. Bring to a boil and add barley and extra mushrooms if desired.

Lentil Rice Soup

This soup is great for a crock pot. Put everything in the pot in the morning. Set it on low and let it cook all day while you're busy doing something else.

2 quarts de-fatted chicken stock
1 cup dry lentils, washed
1 cup rice
1 25 oz. can crushed tomatoes
1 onion, chopped
1 potato, chopped
2 stalks celery, chopped
2 cloves garlic, minced
2 teaspoons mixed Italian seasonings
2 tablespoons dried parsley flakes
1/4 teaspoon pepper

Combine all ingredients in a large stockpot and bring to a boil. Cover the pan and reduce heat to a simmer. Cook until rice and lentils are tender, approximately 45 minutes. This makes a thick soup, which can be thinned, if desired, with additional de-fatted chicken stock. Season to taste.

Cream of "Something" Soup Base

4 cups skim milk
1 tablespoon chicken flavored bouillon granules
2 tablespoons cornstarch

Place ingredients in a medium non-stick saucepan. Mix ingredients with a wire whisk. Heat, stirring to prevent scorching. Makes 4 cups soup base.

Variations:
- Sauté 1/2 cup finely chopped celery in butter-flavored vegetable food spray. Add to soup base.
- Add 1 10 oz. package frozen chopped broccoli to the soup base and heat to a simmer. Blend the soup and add cheese-flavored powder for Broccoli-Cheese Soup.

- Add 1 6 oz. can minced clams for a white clam chowder.
- Sauté 1 cup sliced mushrooms in butter flavored vegetable food spray. Add to soup base and heat.
- Sauté 1 lb. uncooked, ground turkey sausage. Add 1 tablespoon cornstarch to the cooked sausage and mix. Add soup base and heat to a simmer. Serve over rice, grits, or toast.

Dum-Dum* Chili–Corn Combo

1 15 oz. can chili with beans
1 15 oz. can chili beans in chili gravy
1 10 oz. pkg. frozen corn

Place can of chili with beans in the freezer 15 minutes before opening. When you open the can, scrape off all the fat that has risen to the top. Discard the fat. Place chili and beans, chili beans, and corn in a saucepan. Heat, stirring to prevent sticking. Add extra Mexican spices and hot sauce if desired. Skim any fat off top. Makes 4 generous servings. Great over rice, pasta, etc.

Modern Magic Meals™ Mexican Spices adds flavor but no "heat."

Dum-Dum Soup

Makes a *big* pot. Great for freezing or to feed a crowd.

1 large can (48 oz.) tomato juice
2 tomato juice cans of de-fatted broth or stock
2 1 lb. pkgs. frozen veggies for stew
1½ cups uncooked macaroni
1 16 oz. can beans, rinsed
1 teaspoon mixed Italian seasonings

Place tomato juice and stock in a large stockpot. Bring to a boil. Add remaining ingredients, stir, and bring to a boil. Simmer until macaroni is tender. Correct seasonings. Serve with Parmesan cheese, if desired.

*Any Dum-Dum can do it.

Split Pea Soup

■ *Season with Modern Magic Meals™ Smokey Ham Spice.*

■ *Stock can be made using Modern Magic Meals™ Beef Flavored Spice. Mix with water. Season to taste.*

1 cup dried split peas, washed
2 quarts de-fatted chicken stock
1 each carrot and potato, cut into chunks
2 stalks celery, chopped
1 clove garlic, minced
1 tablespoon dried parsley flakes
2 slices turkey bacon, diced
Salt and pepper to taste

Sauté turkey bacon in a food sprayed Dutch oven until lightly browned. Add remaining ingredients and bring to a boil. Cover and simmer 1 1/2 hours or until soup is thick and peas are tender. Put through a blender or processor until smooth. Season to taste. If too thick, add a little water or skim milk.

Chicken Rice Soup

4 cups chicken stock,* de-fatted
3/4 cup cooked rice

Place stock in a pot and bring to a boil. Add rice and mix. Cover and heat to a simmer. Add diced, cooked vegetables for added nutrition, flavor, and color.

Chicken Noodle Soup

4 cups chicken stock,* de-fatted
1 1/2 cups cooked noodles

Place stock in a pot and bring to a boil. Add cooked noodles and mix. Cover and heat to a simmer. Add diced cooked vegetables for added nutrition, flavor, and color.

*Stock can be homemade, made from bouillon, or canned.

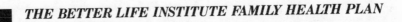 **THE BETTER LIFE INSTITUTE FAMILY HEALTH PLAN**

Bean Soup

½ lb. turkey ham, diced
1 large onion, chopped
1 16 oz. package white beans
1½ quarts water

■ *Add Modern Magic Meals*™ *Smokey Ham Spice for a great taste.*

Prepare beans according to package directions. Sauté diced turkey ham and onion in a soup pot that has been sprayed with vegetable food spray. Do not brown onion. Add 1½ quarts water and the prepared beans to the pot. Cook until beans are tender, adding salt and pepper to taste. You may like to add chopped stewed tomatoes after the beans are cooked.

Dum-Dum* Chicken Vegetable Soup

This recipe is not only quick and easy, it's great for thermos bottles and quick lunches. Serve with crisp rolls and a salad. Top it off with a yogurt dessert and you have a great meal!

1 cup chicken stock
1 small onion, chopped
1 10 oz. package frozen peas and carrots
1 14½ oz. can stewed tomatoes
1 teaspoon mixed Italian Spices
1 6½ oz. can cooked chicken

Mix all ingredients except chicken in a stockpot and bring to a boil. Lower heat and simmer 15 minutes. Add chicken. Cover and turn off heat. Allow to "set" for 5 minutes, then serve.

Quick Meals for People on the Run
When you're in a hurry and you're "stressed out" because there's no time to cook, and your family, spouse, or stomach is growling, here are some quick and easy ideas to solve this situation.

*Any Dum-Dum can do it.

TAKE OUT FOOD

- Call the local pizza man and order a vegetarian pizza with extra sauce and a sprinkle of Parmesan cheese on top.
- Drive into a fast food restaurant and order a charbroiled chicken breast on a bun (hold the mayo) and iced tea or fruit juice.
- Drop by the local Chinese Quick Wok and order dishes stir-fried (not deep-fat fried). That includes chicken, seafood, lots of veggies, a side of steamed rice or chicken, and vegetable fried rice. Ask them to use little oil and *no MSG*. Fortune cookies are okay.
- Drive into a Mexican take out and order a soft chicken taco and a side of Spanish rice. Hold the guacamole and sour cream, and enjoy as much salsa as you choose.

DELI FOODS

- Sliced turkey and smoked turkey are great for sandwiches or casseroles. Purchase a package of dry gravy mix and make a hot turkey sandwich.
- Breads and muffins! Great stuff!
- Mixed fruit and gelatin salads are excellent side dishes.
- Salads without the heavy mayo and oil are good.
- Call in advance and ask the deli to bake or broil several chicken breasts. When you get home, pop a scrubbed potato in the microwave and bake (takes about 6 minutes). Make a salad and set the table. Voilà! Instant dinner!
- Thinly sliced smoked salmon tastes great with a slice of onion on a bagel!

FROM THE GROCERY STORE

- Look for the new Lean and Free (no fat, low cholesterol) cheeses or skim milk cheeses in the refrigerator–cheese section of your store. Purchase a box of whole wheat saltine crackers and a can of vegetable soup. Top off with a large, crisp apple and you're all set.
- Read the label on the new shelf stable entrées as well as the frozen entrées in the grocery store. Some are very healthy and tasty.
- Purchase a "chub" of turkey ham and turkey breast in the meat section. Ask the butcher to slice them for you and keep the sliced meats in the refrigerator or freezer for handy, healthy eating.

THE BETTER LIFE INSTITUTE FAMILY HEALTH PLAN

SOME DUM-DUM IDEAS:

- Mix in a large saucepan:

    1 28 oz. can chopped tomatoes
    1 10 oz. pkg. frozen succotash (corn and lima beans)
    1 pkg. instant rice mix (chicken flavor)
    1½ cups water

    Heat to boiling. Cover and simmer until rice has absorbed all the liquid and serve. Add chopped, cooked turkey, ham, or chicken from the deli. Spice to taste.
- Prepare 1 pkg. macaroni and cheese according to directions, using skim milk and omitting butter. When cooked, add 1 cup frozen green peas and 1 cup chopped, cooked turkey, chicken, or ham from the deli. Serve with a green salad and French bread.
- Prepare 1 pkg. onion-mushroom soup mix according to directions. Add 1 cup quick-cook barley. Cover and simmer until barley is cooked. Add 1 cup sliced mushrooms. Mix and serve as a side dish or a main dish with a salad.
- Make an omelette using Egg Beaters™ with vegetables.* Sprinkle cheese flavored powder on top. Salt and pepper lightly. Makes a great meal or sandwich!
- Water-pack tuna in pita pockets is great. Top with alfalfa sprouts from the produce section and lite Ranch dressing. Quick and easy and no cooking. Little clean up also!

Mystery Foods

"What do I do with left-overs when there's a little of this and a little of that?" Make *Mystery Food of the Day,* that's what! Try something different!

I'm a master at making mystery food. I hate to throw food away, so I just "marry" foods and sometimes I even surprise myself! Try your own mystery foods and see what happens!

1. Mix left-over pasta, vegetables, beans, etc. Add salsa or Italian spaghetti sauce. Place in a vegetable food-sprayed casserole. Sprinkle Parmesan cheese on top and bake until hot. Serve with a salad.
2. Mix all the "little-bits" of hot cereals together before cooking. Cook by using 1 cup cereal to 2 cups water. I've mixed oatmeal, cornmeal, bulgar, and rice. Add fruit juice or raisins to the pot while cooking. Good stuff!

*Can be purchased in frozen cartons in the freezer section. Veggies are in the egg mix.

3. Blend left-over fruit or ripe fruits with yogurt in the blender. Make gelatin using ½ of the water suggested. Fold in the fruit mixture when the gelatin is just beginning to set. Chill and serve.

Now try your own hand at mystery foods. When you serve them, you can play a game with your kids, trying to see if they can identify what you've mixed into the mysterious concoction.

■ *THE BETTER LIFE INSTITUTE FAMILY HEALTH PLAN*

Main Dishes

"What will I serve for lunch or dinner?" Here is an assortment of recipes that cut across a wide variety of Americans' favorite foods. I've tried to choose foods that always *sell well* at the Better Life Institute. I encourage you to learn how to adapt your own favorite recipes as shown on page 274. It will open the door to a wide variety of recipe ideas to help you satisfy your family. Good luck and happy cooking and eating.

Swedish Meatballs

Swedish meatballs are wonderful at parties and buffets, great for sandwiches, and make good "finger foods." And they are delicious when served with mashed potatoes. Good eating!

1 lb. ground turkey or very lean beef
1/4 cup onion, very finely chopped
1/4 cup parsley, very finely chopped
1 cup seasoned breadcrumbs
1/2 cup skim evaporated milk
Dash each nutmeg, ginger, and pepper

Use Modern Magic Meals™ Beef Flavored Spice Mix

Place breadcrumbs and skim evaporated milk in a bowl and mix well. Add the ground turkey (or beef) and mix well. Add the onion, parsley, and spices. Mix. Roll mixture into walnut sized balls and place on a vegetable food sprayed baking sheet. Bake in a 350° oven about 20 minutes or until done.

While meatballs are baking, make the sauce.

1 can chicken broth, de-fatted
1 cup water
1 tablespoon cornstarch

Mix ingredients in a small saucepan and heat until bubbly, stirring to dissolve cornstarch.

Place meatballs in a chafing dish or on a platter and pour sauce over the top. Serve very hot. Makes about 24 meatballs.

Meatballs in a Boat

French or Italian Roll
Cooked Meatballs
Meatball Sauce

Scoop out the center of a roll. Fill with meatballs and sauce. Heat.
Serve.

Enchiladas

For folks who love Mexican food, this is a staple. Anyone can
make enchiladas they're so easy to prepare. They can be made
the night before and kept covered in the refrigerator until ready to
cook. Try this recipe. You might surprise yourself!

1 lb. uncooked ground turkey, chicken, or very lean beef
1 16 oz. can Mexican beans in chili gravy
12 corn tortillas
2 pkgs. enchilada sauce spice mix
2 6 oz. cans tomato paste
2 cups water
12 slices skim milk cheese, cut in half

Sauté ground meat until no longer pink. Add the beans and mix
well. Remove from the heat. Spray a 9 x 13 baking pan with vegetable food spray. Spread the bean-meat mixture on the corn
tortillas. Add 2 half slices of cheese on each tortilla. Roll up each
tortilla and place side by side in the baking pan. In a pan mix
the enchilada sauce spice mix, the tomato paste, and the water.
Heat according to directions. Pour half of the sauce on the enchiladas and bake in a 350° oven about 25 minutes or until hot and
bubbly. Serve with extra sauce on the side. Very good!

I've found several different sauce mixes, both dry and prepared in a can. Some are
very spicy hot, some are not. I always choose the mildest I can find and then I offer
extra hot sauce for those who like their foods spicy.

  THE BETTER LIFE INSTITUTE FAMILY HEALTH PLAN

Let's Make a Taco

Tacos are fun fare. They taste good, are easy to make, and can be very healthy if prepared properly. And the kids love them. Here's how:

1 lb. uncooked ground turkey, chicken, or very lean beef
1 16 oz. can Mexican beans in chili gravy
12 corn tortillas
Mexican salsa
shredded lettuce
chopped tomatoes
chopped onions
Lite sour cream
Mexican spice mix, if desired

Sauté ground meat until no longer pink. Add the Mexican spices to taste. Mix. Add the canned beans and heat to a simmer. Spoon mixture into prepared taco shells. Add lettuce, tomatoes, onions, salsa to taste, and lite sour cream if desired.

Tortillas—Three Ideas

- For a "soft taco" heat tortillas in the microwave until soft and warm, about 10 seconds per tortilla. Fill and serve.
- For a "crisp taco," dry the tortillas in the oven by folding the tortilla in half (do not break) and placing in between the rungs of the oven rack. Toast in a 250° oven about 30 minutes or until crisp.
- The easy, quick way to do tacos is to purchase a package of dry taco shells already prepared. Fill, decorate, eat, enjoy!

Meatloaf

I've always loved meatloaf. Perhaps it is because Momma made it so well and in so many different ways. When I was raising a family, I soon found out that the kids could eat meatloaf without a lot of chewing (little ones have a difficult time chewing, so do kids with braces) and it was very inexpensive to make. I was always on a tight budget. So I served my Mystery Meatloaf once per week to my family, always coming up with variations. Now that my kids are all grown, they still love the stuff! Add baked potatoes, corn on the cob, and coleslaw, and you have a down-home meal!

Meatloaf—An Old-Time Favorite

2 lbs. uncooked ground turkey, chicken, or very lean beef
1 tablespoon minced dry onion
1 cup oat bran
4 egg whites
1/3 cup skim milk
1 tablespoon chicken or beef bouillon granules

Place the oat bran in a large mixing bowl. Add the egg whites, dry onion, and skim milk and mix well. Allow to "set" for 15 minutes. Add the granules and meat and mix well. Spray a 13 x 9 baking pan with vegetable food spray. Place the meatloaf mixture into the pan, pressing it firmly to make a loaf. Bake in a 350° oven about 45 minutes or until browned on top and cooked through. Serves 8. Great for left-overs and sandwiches.

Variations:
- Substitute spaghetti sauce for the milk and add 1 teaspoon mixed Italian spices.
- Substitute Bar-B-Que sauce for the milk.
- Substitute 1/2 cup applesauce for the milk. Add 1 tablespoon poultry seasoning. Different and good.
- Blend sautéed vegetables, i.e. red or green pepper, zucchini, etc., and add to the basic mix.
- Put the basic meatloaf mix onto a sheet of wax paper. Spread frozen mixed vegetables (defrost first) on the meatloaf mixture. Sprinkle with cheese flavored powder. Roll up

THE BETTER LIFE INSTITUTE FAMILY HEALTH PLAN

the meatloaf like a jelly roll and place in a baking pan. Bake in a 350° oven 1½ hours or until cooked through.
- Veggies and meat all rolled up together.

SOME GREAT CHICKEN RECIPES

Question: How can you take basic, good, healthy food items and make them different? Answer: With a little imagination and a spirit of adventure, you can do just about anything!

So here goes with the basics of a heart-healthy diet, chicken and fish.

Baking Fish or Chicken, a Basic Recipe

Clean, skin, and debone the chicken or fish of your choice. Spray a non-stick baking pan with vegetable food spray and sprinkle with spices of your choice. Squeeze the juice of a lemon over all. Bake in 350° oven until browned and cooked through.

SAFETY TIPS

1. Wash your hands in hot, soapy water before and after touching raw meat, blood, or juices from the poultry or meat.
2. Use a plastic cutting board to cut meat and poultry. Wash cutting board thoroughly before and after use. Wooden boards are porous and can harbor salmonella bacteria even after washing.
3. Do not use the cutting board for preparing foods without washing after preparing poultry or meat.
4. Thoroughly cook meat—red meat to 165° and poultry to 185°—to ensure any bacteria is killed.
5. Never eat raw eggs. Cook eggs until both white and yellow (if you still eat them) are firm, not runny.
6. Keep eggs refrigerated!
7. Use eggs within 5 weeks.
8. Wash hands before and after handling whole eggs.
9. Think twice before eating any foods with raw or partially cooked eggs, such as "health" drinks, hollandaise sauce, etc.

Marco Polo Chicken and Noodles

For a special occasion. This recipe takes a little more time and work, but it's worth it.

1 lb. chicken breast, skinned and boned
1 onion, sliced thin
1 red pepper, sliced thin
1 green pepper, sliced thin
1 clove garlic, minced
2 tablespoons peanut oil
1 tablespoon sesame oil
1 tablespoon fresh ginger, chopped

1/2 cup chicken stock, de-fatted
3 tablespoons rice vinegar
2 tablespoons low sodium soy sauce
1 pkg. EQUAL™ or sugar substitute
2 teaspoons cornstarch
hot red pepper sauce, if desired

Partially freeze the chicken breasts and cut cross-wise into thin strips. Put chicken in a large zip-lock bag. Mix the sesame oil, chicken broth, rice vinegar, soy sauce, sweetener, and cornstarch in a medium bowl. Pour over the chicken. Zip-lock and refrigerate 30 minutes. Heat a large wok and add peanut oil. Add the garlic, ginger, onion, and pepper and sauté until vegetables are softened a bit. Constantly stir to prevent browning and burning. Add the chicken and the marinade to the vegetables in the wok and continue to stir fry on high heat until chicken is cooked through, about 3–5 minutes. Add hot pepper, if desired and remove to a covered dish and keep warm.

Polo Noodles:

1/2 lb. thin spaghetti
2 tablespoons peanut oil
1 tablespoon low sodium soy sauce

While the chicken is being cooked, boil a large pot of water. Add the spaghetti and cook until tender but still firm (al dente). Drain pasta and toss with peanut oil and soy sauce. Heat the pasta in the wok over high heat until lightly browned. Form pasta into a ring on a large platter. Spoon the chicken mixture into the middle of the platter and serve to 4 people.

THE BETTER LIFE INSTITUTE FAMILY HEALTH PLAN

Chicken Dinner in Foil

This is a great recipe for everyone in the family to make. You might like to make the packs the night before and keep refrigerated until ready to cook. Fun fare!

Allow ½ chicken breast per person, approximately 5 ozs. uncooked. Brown chicken breasts in a sprayed non-stick pan. When browned, place each breast on a double-layered 12-inch square of foil.

On each chicken breast half, place:

½ cup frozen peas and carrots
1 slice onion
½ potato, cut into wedges
1 tablespoon white wine or broth
2 tablespoons meatless tomato sauce

Sprinkle over all:

garlic powder
onion powder
mixed Italian spices
lite salt and pepper to taste

Fold over the foil and seal tightly to keep juices in the package. Place packages on a baking sheet and bake in a 375° degree oven approximately 1 hour or until chicken and vegetables test done. Remove chicken from foil pack before serving. Also cooks great on the grill.

Curry Chicken

Lots of people like curry, so for those of you who do, here's a good one.

6 skinned and boned chicken breasts (approx. 5 oz. each)
1/2 cup each onion and green pepper, chopped
1 16 oz. can tomatoes, chopped
1/4 cup raisins

1/4 cup parsley, chopped
1 tablespoon mixed curry spices
1/2 teaspoon each nutmeg and pepper
1 tablespoon cornstarch
2 tablespoons water

Spray a non-stick skillet with vegetable food spray. Brown chicken. Add remaining ingredients except cornstarch and water. Bring mixture to a boil. Cover and reduce heat to a simmer. Cook 15 minutes or until chicken is tender. Uncover and cook an additional 5 minutes to reduce liquid. Mix cornstarch and water. Add to sauce to thicken. Serve chicken and sauce over rice. Serves 6.

Chicken in Wine Sauce

This recipe smells wonderful while cooking, and to boot it's great to eat!

4 chicken breasts, skinned, boned, and cut into large chunks
1 onion, chopped
1 clove garlic, minced
1/4 cup parsley, chopped
1 6 oz. can tomato paste

1/4 cup red wine
1/4 cup chicken stock
1/2 teaspoon mixed Italian spices
1/2 lb. mushrooms, sliced
2 tablespoons olive oil

Sauté chicken in olive oil in a non-stick Dutch oven type pot. When chicken is lightly browned, add the onion, garlic, and parsley. Continue to stir until onion is limp, but not browned. Add the tomato paste, wine, and chicken stock. Mix, cover, and simmer 45 minutes. Add the mixed Italian spices and sliced mushrooms. Cover and turn off the heat. Allow to "set" for 5 minutes, then serve. Wonderful with noodles or rice.

■ *THE BETTER LIFE INSTITUTE FAMILY HEALTH PLAN*

Bar-B-Que Chicken

Anyone can do this recipe. Anyone! I promise! And you can make a double batch to use in sandwiches the next day!

4 chicken breasts, skinned and boned, about 5 oz. each
1 cup prepared Bar-B-Que sauce (from your grocers)
¹/₄ cup water

Sauté the chicken breasts in a non-stick pan that has been sprayed with vegetable food spray. Brown chicken on both sides. Mix the Bar-B-Que sauce and water and pour over the chicken. Cover and simmer about 20 minutes or until chicken is cooked through. Serves 4.

Lemon Chicken

This lemon chicken recipe is very good served with rice and steamed carrots.

¹/₂ cup lemon juice
1 6 oz. can apple juice concentrate
1 tablespoon toasted sesame seeds
¹/₈ teaspoon cayenne pepper
4 chicken breasts, skinned and boned

Modern Magic Meals™ Oriental Spices give added zip to chicken recipes.

Mix apple and lemon juices, sesame seeds, and cayenne pepper. Marinate chicken breasts 2–3 hours in mixture, turning several times. Place chicken breasts on a sprayed, non-stick broiler pan. Broil until well browned on both sides, brushing on remaining marinade to keep from drying out. Serves 4.

Chicken Breasts with Orange Sauce

2 tablespoons grated orange peel
1/2 cup prepared orange juice
1 teaspoon lemon juice
1/4 cup low sugar orange marmalade
1/4 teaspoon dry mustard
1 1/2 teaspoons cornstarch
2 tablespoons water
4 chicken breasts, skinned and boned
lite salt and pepper to taste

Mix ingredients except chicken in a large zip-lock bag. Add chicken, shake gently to coat, and marinate 30 minutes. Broil chicken breasts on a sprayed non-stick pan until lightly browned on both sides. Baste breasts with the sauce while broiling until browned and well glazed. Serves 4.

Quick Dinner on Top of the Stove

When I say easy, I mean easy. This meal is a great after-the-holiday feast.

3 cups chicken stock
1 1/2 cups brown rice
1 4 oz. can sliced mushrooms, drained
1 2 oz. jar red pimento, diced
2 tablespoons minced dry onion
1 tablespoon dry parsley
1/2 teaspoon each onion and garlic powder
1 lb. cooked turkey or chicken, cut into cubes

Place all ingredients, except pimento, in a saucepan and bring to a boil. Cover and simmer until rice is cooked. Add pimento and toss lightly. Serve with a salad and bread sticks. Serves 4.

FISH DISHES AND A TIP

Often family members turn their noses up at delicious and nutritious fish dishes because they "smell like fish" and "taste fishy." Years ago my Momma Julia passed along to me the "secret" of what to do about fishy smells and tastes. She said, "Before you prepare or cook your seafood, rinse it in a cool water and pat it dry with paper towels. Then soak it in skim milk about 1 hour. Drain and cook. The milk will take away the 'fishiness,' so that you'll be able to enjoy this very healthy food. And don't forget to throw away the milk after soaking the fish, so it doesn't end up on your cereal in the morning!"

Stuffed Fish Fillets

Lots of cholesterol lowering qualities in this recipe!

6 fish fillets, sole, flounder, cod, etc. 5 ozs. per serving
1/2 cup mushrooms, sliced
1/2 cup green onions, chopped
1/2 cup onions, chopped
1 clove garlic, minced
1 cup oatmeal

2 egg whites, slightly beaten
1 tablespoon lemon juice
2 tablespoons olive oil or canola oil
1 small package chopped spinach, defrosted and well squeezed
1/2 teaspoon poultry seasoning

Sauté vegetables in oil in a non-stick skillet until lightly browned. Place oatmeal in a mixing bowl and add sautéed vegetables and remaining ingredients, except fish. Mix well. Place a spoonful of mix on each fillet and roll up. Fasten with a toothpick if desired. Place roll-ups on a non-stick baking pan that has been sprayed with vegetable food spray and spoon remaining stuffing around fillets. Sprinkle with paprika and bake in a 350° oven about 30 minutes or until fish tests tender and cooked. Serve with lemon slices and chopped parsley.

Baked Tuna Loaf

A variation on an old favorite. Notice we use oatmeal instead of seasoned cracker crumbs for those wanting to watch your cholesterol.

2 6½ oz. cans water packed tuna, drained and flaked
¾ cups each celery, onion, and green pepper, chopped
1 clove garlic, minced

1 tablespoon chopped red pimento
4 egg whites
½ cup skim evaporated milk
¾ cup oatmeal, uncooked
½ teaspoon lemon juice

Place oatmeal, skim evaporated milk, and egg whites in a mixing bowl. Mix well. Allow to "set" for 15 minutes. While oatmeal is setting, lightly sauté the celery, onion, green pepper, and garlic in a vegetable food sprayed non-stick pan. Add the vegetables, tuna, lemon juice, and pimento to the oatmeal mixture and mix well. Put the mixture into a vegetable food sprayed non-stick loaf pan. Bake in oven at 350° for approximately 45 minutes or until browned. Take out of oven and allow to stand for 5 minutes. Cut and serve.

Stir-Fry Vegetables and Scallops

For those who enjoy stir-fry, this recipe is a tummy-pleaser.

Oriental spices such as 5 spice powder are available in the Oriental section of your grocer's. Modern Magic Meals™ Oriental Spice is an excellent choice.

1 lb. bay scallops (or other firm fish)
1 each onion and green pepper, sliced thin
4 stalks celery, sliced diagonally
1 carrot, sliced diagonally
½ cup each bamboo shoots and water chestnuts, sliced

2 cloves garlic, minced
1 tablespoon cornstarch
2 tablespoons sodium reduced soy sauce
½ teaspoon dry mustard or Chinese mustard
1 tablespoon oyster sauce
1 cup chicken stock
Oriental spices to taste

Prepare a large skillet or wok with cooking spray. Heat for about 1 minute at highest setting. Add scallops and stir quickly until scallops are opaque. Remove with slotted spoon and set aside. Keep warm. Spray the pan again and add onion, green pepper, celery, carrot, and garlic. Stir to cook quickly and to avoid burning. When crisp tender, add the mixture of cornstarch, soy sauce, oyster sauce, chicken stock, dry mustard, and seasonings. Stir well. Add bamboo shoots, water chestnuts, and the scallops that were set aside. Toss lightly and serve over steamed rice.

Seafood Jambalaya

A wonderful meal in a pot. You control the "heat" by adjusting the spices.

1 onion, chopped
1 green pepper, chopped
1 stalk celery, chopped
1 clove garlic, minced
1 14¹/₂ oz. can Cajun-style
    stewed tomatoes
¹/₂ cup uncooked rice
¹/₂ cup chicken stock

1 teaspoon Cajun mixed
    spices
1 lb. shellfish, i.e., scallops,
    shrimp, lobster, or other
    firm seafood cut into
    chunks
Hot sauce to taste, if desired

Spray a non-stick Dutch oven with vegetable food spray and sauté the onions, green pepper, celery, and garlic until crisp-tender. Add the stock, tomatoes, rice, and spices and mix well. Bring to a boil. Cover and simmer about 20 minutes. Add the seafood and cook another 5 minutes or until seafood flakes. Serves 4.

Bouillabaisse

Pronounced BULL-YA-BAZE, it's a fancy name for fish stew. But it's not just ordinary stew. It is something very good to serve to and impress everyone! Enjoy!

3 bottles clam juice (from the grocery store)
2 cups chicken stock
1 cup white wine
1 16 oz. can chopped tomatoes
1 large onion, chopped
1 stalk celery, chopped
1 clove garlic, minced
½ teaspoon mixed Italian spices
¼ teaspoon fennel seeds
pinch of saffron threads
1 lb. firm fish cut into chunks, i.e., crab, shrimp, scallops, etc.
2 tablespoons olive oil

Heat olive oil in a non-stick Dutch oven and lightly sauté the onions, celery, and garlic. Add remaining ingredients, except fish, and bring to a boil. Cover and simmer 10 minutes. Add the seafood and cook another 5 minutes. Serve in soup bowls to 4 people with crusty French bread and a salad. Good eating!

PASTA AND SAUCES AND THE MANY VARIATIONS

It seems that everything I write has to have a section on pasta and sauce and other good Italian fare! Pasta, as we've come to know, is good food. It is high in carbos and relatively low in calories. Learn to enjoy all the different ways pasta can be used.

- Pastina, alphabets, ziti in chicken broth taste good!
- Wide noodles such as mostaciolli, rigatoni, shells of all sizes, spirals, tubes, dinosaur-shape pasta are all wonderful.
- The long skinny pastas, spaghettini, angel hair, linguini, fettucini, etc., can be eaten with sauce, in casseroles, in soups anytime!

I have some recipes you may enjoy trying. Use your own, if you have a special one, making it as healthy as possible.

Sauces

Good stuff bubbling on the stove that makes you feel wonderful when you walk into the kitchen and smell the good smells, that's what Italian sauces are. Here are some quick and easy recipes for you to experiment with.

The Easy Way Spaghetti Sauce

1 28 oz. can crushed tomatoes
1 48 oz. jar meatless spaghetti sauce
¼ cup white wine or chicken broth
1 tablespoon mixed Italian spices

Mix all ingredients in a pot and simmer 15 minutes. Serve over pasta of choice.

■ *Sauces made with Modern Magic Meals™ Spaghetti Sauce Mix and mixed Italian and Cajun spices are excellent.*

Quick and Easy Sicilian Pasta and Sauce

4 cups fresh tomatoes, chopped
3 tablespoons olive oil
4 tablespoons fresh basil,* chopped
2 cloves garlic, minced
1 lb. spaghetti

In a sauce pan, blend the tomatoes, olive oil, basil, and garlic. Heat until bubbly. Cook spaghetti as directed. Drain and pour sauce over the pasta. Toss to mix. Add salt and pepper to taste. Sprinkle with Parmesan cheese and serve to 4–6 people. Add a green salad with dressing, crusty Italian bread, and sorbet for dessert.

■ *Add sliced mushrooms to Italian sauce for extra taste and texture.*

Spanish Sauce

½ cup each sliced onion and green pepper
3 cloves garlic, minced
⅓ teaspoon Cajun spice seasoning
1 16 oz. can stewed tomatoes

Sauté onion, green pepper, and garlic in a sprayed non-stick pan until crisp tender. Add tomatoes and spice and simmer 10 minutes. Serve over omelettes, fish, chicken, etc. Store leftovers in the refrigerator.

*Please use *fresh basil* in this recipe. Most produce sections sell fresh herbs. It's worth it, believe me!

Quick Sauce

1 28 oz. can crushed tomatoes
1 tablespoon pesto (found in produce section of grocery store)
1/4 cup dry wine

Mix ingredients in a saucepan. Heat and simmer 5 minutes. Serve over pasta with a sprinkle of cheese.

Lasagna and Manicotti

Italian pasta dishes are quick and easy and very good to eat. When the children get involved, place newspapers or a sheet of plastic on the floor so that cleanup is easier. Children love to stuff manicotti shells. It makes them feel useful and helps to instill pride in a "job well done."

- Use the recipe for The Easy Way Spaghetti Sauce. Or use your own special sauce.
- For lasagna, purchase a 16 oz. package of lasagna noodles.
- For manicotti, purchase a package of 14 noodles.

Basic Cheese Filling Recipe

1 24 oz. container of 1% milkfat cottage cheese
1/2 cup grated Parmesan cheese
1 teaspoon mixed Italian spices

Mix all ingredients well. Cover and chill until ready to use in lasagna or manicotti.

Manicotti

Spread a small amount of sauce on the bottom of a large (9 x 13) baking pan. Stuff the *uncooked* manicotti noodles with the Basic Cheese Filling and layer in the baking pan. Spread any additional cheese filling on top of the uncooked noodles. Spoon 1/2 of The Easy Way Spaghetti Sauce on top of the manicotti. Place plastic wrap within the edges of the pan, and cover the pan with foil. Bake in a 350° oven about 1 hour or until fork tender. Serve with additional sauce and Parmesan cheese. Serves 6.

■ *THE BETTER LIFE INSTITUTE FAMILY HEALTH PLAN*

Lasagna

Spread a small amount of sauce on the bottom of a large (9 x 13) baking pan. Alternate layers of *uncooked* lasagna noodles, Basic Cheese Filling, and sauce, ending with sauce on top. Add enough liquid to cook the pasta. If you're using The Easy Way Sauce, use ¾ of the recipe in the layering and pass the other ¼ when you serve. Sprinkle the top with some additional Parmesan cheese. Within the edges of the pan, place plastic wrap, then cover the pan with foil. Bake in a 350° oven about 1½ hours or until noodles are fork tender. Serve with additional sauce and Parmesan cheese. Makes 6 generous servings. Freezes well.

Pizza Made at Home

No meat Spaghetti Sauce
Vegetables—onions; green or red peppers; mushrooms, sliced and lightly sautéed in vegetable food spray or a little olive oil
Parmesan cheese, grated
skim mozzarella cheese, shredded (optional)
turkey ham, bacon, or ground turkey, diced and cooked (optional)
prepared pizza crusts, purchased in the bread section of your grocers
OR
pita bread, English muffins, French rolls, etc.

Spread spaghetti sauce on choice of crust (bread or pizza crust, etc.). Layer vegetables, choice of meats (if desired), and cheeses on top of the pizza crust. Use the sauce and vegetables liberally and the meat and cheese sparingly. Place crusts on a baking sheet and bake in a 425° oven until browned on top. Quick and easy for anyone in the family to prepare.

Vegetables

Vegetables are the mainstay of any healthy eating program. The trick with vegetables is to season them to taste *without* butter, margarine, or any fat such as bacon grease. Use the new butter, cheese and sour cream, and onion powders to enhance flavor. Always remember that 1 tablespoon of butter or margarine has 100 calories.

THE WORD ON VEGETABLES:

- Serve boiled corn on the cob with butter powder, lite salt, and pepper.
- Cook green peas with cheese flavored and butter flavored powder.
- Carrots cooked and then seasoned with lite maple syrup and butter flavored powder make candied carrots!
- Children may not like cooked vegetables, but they'll eat raw carrot sticks, celery, cherry tomatoes, or mushroom caps when you serve them with Ranch Dip.
- Make candied sweet potatoes by adding lite maple syrup to cooked sweet potatoes. Sprinkle butter flavored powder on top and bake in a 350° oven until browned on top.
- Potatoes are good food. Serve with lite salt, pepper, and butter, cheese, and sour cream and onion flavored powders.

  Some tried and true, never-fail ideas:
- Scrub potatoes well and cut into wedges. Spray a baking sheet with vegetable food spray. Layer potatoes on the pan and season with lite salt and pepper. Spray potatoes with vegetable food spray. Bake in a 425° oven until potatoes are cooked and brown.
- Bake 4 potatoes. When touch-tender and mealy, cut in half and scoop out the insides. Mix with ½ teaspoon *each* butter, cheese, and onion flavored powders; 1 tablespoon Parmesan cheese; ½ cup cottage cheese; and lite salt and pepper to taste. Re-stuff the skins and place on a cookie sheet. Bake in a 350° oven 15 minutes. Delicious!

- Add vegetables, fresh or frozen, to soups and stews. Blend them when cooked and add to the broth or gravy. It's a good way to "hide" vegetables!
- Cooked cauliflower or broccoli tastes great with cheese flavored powders.

Desserts

Everybody loves "sweet stuff." Learning how to make it with less fat and sugar is a challenge, but we're up to it, aren't we? Here are some ideas and some recipes for you to try.

DESSERT TIPS AND IDEAS

1. Angel food cake with berries or with low calorie whipped topping and berries is always wonderful.
2. To make a "pie," sprinkle Grape Nuts™ in a pie tin. Prepare no sugar instant pudding according to directions. Pour pudding over Grape Nuts™ Sprinkle more Grape Nuts™ on top. Chill. Serve to 8 hungry people.
3. Marinate frozen peaches in brandy. Spoon into glass dishes. Place 1 teaspoon low sugar raspberry jam on the peaches. Top with low calorie whipped topping and serve well chilled.
4. Split an angel food cake into 3 layers. Spread low calorie whipped topping between layers. Wrap cake in plastic wrap and chill. Slice and serve with fresh fruit or chocolate pudding.
5. Wash, peel, and core baking apples, and place them in a baking pan. Drizzle lite maple syrup over the apples. Sprinkle with apple pie spice. Cover with foil and bake in a 350° oven about 35 minutes. Uncover and cool before serving.

Easy Cheesecake

1 cup Grape Nuts™
1 pint 1% milkfat cottage cheese
1 small can crushed pineapple in juice
1 large pkg. no sugar lemon gelatin
1 cup boiling water
¾ cup Grape Nuts™

Dissolve gelatin in boiling water. Mix well. Cool. Combine cottage cheese, pineapple, and gelatin mixture in the food processor and blend until very creamy.

Sprinkle ½ cup Grape Nuts™ in an oblong pan. Pour gelatin mixture over the Grape Nuts™ and spread to the corners of the pan evenly. Sprinkle remaining Grape Nuts™ on top. Chill 2–3 hours or until firmly set. Cut into pieces and serve with a dollop of calorie controlled whipped topping and a strawberry on top. Serves 6.

Yogurt Dessert

Low in calories. Easy to prepare. Good and healthy to eat.

1 small pkg. no sugar berry flavored gelatin
1/4 cup boiling water
1 20 oz. container nonfat yogurt, plain

Soften gelatin in boiling water. Cool. Place yogurt in a food processor or blender. Add gelatin mixture. Blend well. Pour into a glass bowl. Cover and chill. Serves 4 generously.

Twice Baked Cookies

2½ cups flour
1 cup sugar (or ⅔ cup fructose)
4 tablespoons canola oil
2 teaspoons baking powder
6 egg whites or equivalent
1 tablespoon anise seed, 1 teaspoon grated lemon peel, ½ tablespoon pumpkin pie spice, OR 1 teaspoon almond extract flavoring

Measure all dry ingredients into a large mixing bowl. Make a well in the center of the dry mix, and add liquid ingredients in the middle of the well. Mix with a wooden spoon until well blended. (Dough will be very stiff.) Divide dough in half. Wrap in plastic wrap and refrigerate for 1 hour. (Dough will become extra firm.) Preheat oven to 350°. Spray a large cookie sheet with food spray. Roll out ½ of the dough on a lightly floured board. Shape into a long loaf, about 10 x 2, and place on the cookie sheet. Repeat with other half. (Dough will not "spread" much on the pan.) Bake 20 minutes. Remove from oven and immediately slice each loaf, using a serrated knife, into ½-inch thick slices. Spray cookie sheet again and place cut slices on the sheet. Spray the top of the cookie slices and return the pans to the oven. Bake until lightly browned on both sides. Remove from oven and cool. Store in a zip-lock bag. This recipe makes about 2 dozen cookies.

Modern Magic Meals™ desserts are great. They're all calorie controlled (about 55 calories per serving) and made with Nutra-Sweet.™ They are desserts without guilt. Flavors include:

> *Cheesecake*
> *Chocolate Cheesecake*
> *Vanilla Pudding*
> *Chocolate Pudding*
> *Butterscotch Pudding*
> *Chocolate Mousse*
> *Lemon Mousse*
> *Whipped Topping*
> *Chocolate Cake*
> *Vanilla Cake*
> *Yogurt Desserts*
> *Fruit Whips*
> *Strawberry Mousse*

THE BETTER LIFE INSTITUTE FAMILY HEALTH PLAN

"Poke" Cake

1 baked no fat, no cholesterol cake, such as Entenmann's™
   Pound Cake or Angel Food Cake
1 cup boiling water
1 pkg. 4-serving-size no sugar gelatin, any color or flavor

Place cake on a serving plate. Dissolve gelatin in boiling water.
Cool. All over the top prick the cake with a very sharp 2-tined fork.
(Be careful not to break the cake.) Spoon cooled gelatin mixture
over the top of the cake. Chill at least 4 hours before serving with
a dollop of low calorie whipped topping. For a special occasion
garnish with fresh or frozen berries.

Brownies in 5 Easy Steps

1. Purchase a package of brownie mix that has 2 grams of fat.

2. Substitute low cal sour cream for the butter or margarine.

3. Substitute 2 egg whites for 1 whole egg.

4. Mix and bake as directed. Cut into 32 pieces.

5. Enjoy whenever the "urge" for chocolate calls!

Company Trifle

Purchase a no fat, no cholesterol prepared white loaf cake or
angel food cake (readily available at your grocer's). Break up the
cake and layer ½ of cake in a large glass bowl. Prepare 1 large
package no sugar vanilla instant pudding according to directions. Pour ½ of the pudding over the cake. Spread low sugar
raspberry jam over the pudding or layer fresh berries instead.
Continue to layer the dessert, cake, pudding, and jam or berries.
Cover and chill. Serve with a low calorie whipped topping. Wonderful!

Note: If you desire, sprinkle a little rum or brandy on the cake before you layer the pudding on top.

STEP INTO THE KITCHEN ■

Holidays and Snacks

Why is it that every time people get together, there's food around? People from every culture will entertain and offer their guests something to eat or drink. When it comes your turn, you may be in a dilemma. In this section of the book, we'll discuss foods for:

- Company Dinners—Entertaining with Style and Ease
- Cocktail Parties—How to Go to One and How to Give One
- Holiday Dinners for Family and Other VIPs
- Birthday Parties for Kids of All Ages

We encourage you to come up with your own ideas and have fun in doing so.

COMPANY DINNERS—ENTERTAINING WITH STYLE AND EASE

We do a lot of entertaining, and we keep it simple. Foods that can be prepared in advance and then quickly heated and served are ideal for the busy person. We always start with appetizers around the coffee table in the living room. It's a nice time to unwind and relax and get to know your guests. It also affords the hostess-cook time to slip in and out of the kitchen to "see how dinner is coming along." These sample menus are tried and true in our home. You'll want to use them too. You'll find the recipes in the recipe section. *Bon appetit!*

■

APPETIZERS
Turkey Ham Roll-Ups with Asparagus and Mustard Sauce
Pita Chips
Crudites (raw veggies) and Ranch Dip

■

MAIN COURSE
Chicken Broth with Green Peas and Green Onions
Marco Polo Chinese Chicken and Noodles
Pineapple Cheesecake
Coffee, Tea, Beverage of Choice

■

APPETIZERS
Swedish Meatballs
Bread Sticks
Crudites and Onion Dip

MAIN COURSE
Green Salad and Italian Dressing
Cioppino
French Bread
Berries and Cream
Coffee, Tea, Beverage of Choice

COCKTAIL PARTIES

How to Go to One

We all give parties, and we all like to go to them. Some of us just do it more than others do. Here are some tips for you if you're going to one and are apprehensive about it.

1. *Eat something before you go*—an apple, a salad, a fiber bar, etc. Don't go hungry!
2. Order a beverage when you get to the party and sip slowly. It will keep you busy.
3. Find the fruit, vegetable, or seafood tray and hang around. Don't hang around the chips and dips and peanuts. You'll find yourself munching away and not even be aware of it.
4. Compliment your hostess. Talk to those you know or like. Be nice to those you must be nice to and get away quickly. (Less stress!)
5. Have fun.

How to Give One

Cocktail parties can be fun to give, yet so many people shy away from having a party because they think that parties take too much time and effort. Here's a sample menu that is quick and easy. So if you're thinking about a party, try:

Asparagus-Ham Roll-ups with Cheese Curry Dip
Crab Canapés
Spicy Garlic Shrimp
Vegetable Antipasto
Turkey Meatballs in Bar-B-Que Sauce
Pesto Dip with Crackers
Salmon Spread with Crackers
Orange Wine from the Old Country
Non-Alcoholic Mango Punch
Strawberry Daiquiri Punch

And there's more.

STEP INTO THE KITCHEN

Lemon Punch

1 container lemon flavor Crystal Light™
3 cups water
1 bottle champagne or sparkling white wine, chilled
strawberries to garnish

Mix lemon flavor Crystal Light™ with water in a large punch bowl. Add ice and mix well. Just before serving, pour in the champagne or sparkling wine and serve with strawberry garnish. Serves 12.

Non-Alcoholic Mango Punch

2 ripe mangos, cut up
2 cups fresh orange juice
¼ cup fresh lemon juice
2 cups water
EQUAL™ to taste

Combine water, juices, and mango in a blender and blend well. Strain into a large punch bowl. Sweeten with EQUAL™ to taste. Add ice. Serves 8.

Strawberry Daiquiri Punch

4 cups strawberries
⅓ cup fresh lime juice
6 oz. light rum
EQUAL™ to taste
lime slices for garnish

Blend strawberries, lime juice, and rum in a blender until smooth. Sweeten to taste with EQUAL.™ Place a block of ice in a large punch bowl and pour berry mixture over the ice just before serving. Serve with lime slices. Serves 6.

Asparagus-Ham Roll-Ups

fresh asparagus spears
turkey ham, sliced thin

Wash asparagus and steam until crisp-tender. Cool. Roll up in turkey ham and arrange on platter. Chill well. Serve with Curry-Cheese Dip/Sauce.

Curry-Cheese Dip/Sauce

1 cup 1% milkfat cottage cheese
1 tablespoon cheese flavored powder
1 teaspoon curry powder

Blend cottage cheese and curry spice in a food processor or blender until very creamy. Add non-fat milk if mixture is too thick. Add spices to taste. Chill well before serving.

Crab Canapés

1 lb. fresh lump crabmeat, drained and flaked
1 cup celery, finely chopped
1/3 cup breadcrumbs
1/8 teaspoon dry mustard
1/2 cup lite mayonnaise
1 tablespoon pimento, chopped
1 teaspoon lemon juice
3/4 teaspoon Worcestershire sauce
1 loaf French bread, sliced, trimmed and cut into rounds or triangles.

Prepare French bread, cover, and set aside until ready to use. Combine remaining ingredients and mix well. Cover and chill 1 hour. Spoon crab mixture on bread pieces and arrange on a platter. Makes about 50 canapés.

Spicy Garlic Shrimp

2 lbs. large fresh shrimp
1/2 cup dry sherry
1/4 cup lemon juice
1 tablespoon olive oil

1 1/2 cloves garlic, minced
1 tablespoon Cajun seasoning
lemon wedges to garnish

Devein shrimp. Place in a shallow baking dish. Mix remaining ingredients and pour over the shrimp. Cover and refrigerate 8 hours or overnight. Broil shrimp 3–4 minutes in marinade. Serve on a platter with lemon wedges. Serves about 15.

Vegetable Antipasto

4 cups fresh vegetables, sliced (fresh mushrooms, cauliflower, pea pods, tomatoes, zucchini, carrots, etc.)
1/3 cup extra-virgin olive oil
3 tablespoons lemon juice
2 tablespoons Dijon mustard
1 1/2 lbs. turkey ham, thinly sliced

Place vegetables in a bowl with a lid. Combine oil, lemon juice, and mustard and pour over vegetables. Cover. Marinate in refrigerator 24 hours before serving, mixing occasionally. Drain vegetables and arrange on a platter with thinly sliced turkey ham. Serves 10.

Turkey Meatballs in Bar-B-Que Sauce

1 lb. lean ground turkey
1/4 cup oat bran
2 egg whites

1 tablespoon prepared barbecue sauce

Mix all ingredients well and shape into walnut-sized balls. Place on a baking sheet that has been sprayed with vegetable food spray. Bake in a 350° oven until browned. Serve with additional prepared barbecue sauce, such as Open Pit™ or Thick and Tangy.™

Pesto Dip/Spread

2 cups frozen spinach, defrosted and squeezed dry
1/2 cup Parmesan cheese
1/3 cup extra-virgin olive oil
3 cloves garlic, minced
2 cups fresh basil leaves
1/4 cup pine nuts

Blend all ingredients in a food processor until creamy. Chill well before serving. Serve with crackers.

Salmon Spread

1 15 1/2 oz. can red salmon
1/4 cup celery, finely chopped
1/4 cup onion, finely chopped
2 tablespoons lite mayonnaise
1 teaspoon lemon juice
1 teaspoon dill spice powder

Combine all ingredients in a food processor and process until smooth. Cover and chill several hours to "marry" flavors. Serve with rye or whole wheat crackers. This recipe yields about 2 cups of spread.

Orange Wine from the Old Country

2 lbs. oranges, peeled and cut into chunks (remove all the white membrane)
2 bottles dry white wine
1/4 cup cognac
sweetener of choice, to taste

Place wine and orange chunks in a jar. Cover and refrigerate 3 days. Strain and discard oranges. Add cognac and sweeten to taste. Chill well and serve with orange zest (skin strips). Delicious.

EXTRA TIPS AND IDEAS FOR A SPECIAL TOUCH

- Have a big bowl of luscious strawberries with a side of fruit yogurt on a table all by themselves. See how many people gather around the "berry table."
- Make bread sticks out of a refrigerator package product and place on your serving table by the dips and veggies. Everyone will think you've slaved away making them, but don't tell!

HOLIDAY DINNERS FOR FAMILY AND OTHER VIPS

Tips and Ideas
- Keep vegetable munchies around the kitchen for nibbling.
- Get the gang together and go for a walk before dinner. Walking helps you control your appetite! Honest!
- Eat a little bit of everything you like at dinner. You can always go back for seconds; however, when dinner is first served, your eyes can be bigger than your stomach!
- Take a walk after dinner and before dessert is served. Put space, time, and behavior between you and food!
- Share the leftovers with others. Give a care package to someone to take home.

■

SPECIAL OCCASION MENU
Turkey Ham Baked with Maple Syrup and Pineapple
Roast Turkey and Gravy
Mashed Potatoes
Candied Sweet Potatoes
Stuffing
Cranberry Relish
Green Peas and Onions
Corn
Rolls
Pumpkin Dessert Pie
Coffee, Tea, Beverage of Choice

Holidays and Party Extras
Holiday time can be healthy-fun time if you learn how to take the unhealthy out of a recipe whenever possible, and control your behavior when "what you see is what you'll wear" is on the table!

In our family we love holidays and look forward to family and friends coming together to share in the joy of life. Everyone gets in the kitchen to bake and taste good things, oatmeal raisin cookies, brownies, pound cakes. We make jams to give to our neighbors.

■ *THE BETTER LIFE INSTITUTE FAMILY HEALTH PLAN*

There's always noise and good smells and a house to clean up afterward. We wouldn't have it any other way.

Here's our basic holiday dinner that we've made for more people than we have grey hairs! (I guess that's more than ten or twenty or . . .) We hope you'll add your own twists and make a special meal for a special time for special people.

■

HOLIDAY DINNER
Turkey Ham with Maple Pineapple
Roast Turkey with Gravy
Stuffing
Mashed Potatoes
Candied Sweet Potatoes
Cranberry Relish
Pumpkin Dessert Pie

Turkey Ham with Maple Pineapple

Purchase a turkey ham at your grocer's. Decorate with canned pineapple slices and pour light maple syrup over the top of the ham. Stud with whole cloves, if desired. Bake in a 350° oven until browned on top. Cool 5 minutes before slicing.

Roast Turkey and Gravy

Purchase a turkey that *is not* fat injected or butter basted. Roast the turkey as directed on the package. Pour off all the juices in the roasting pan. De-fat the juices and make gravy using flour or cornstarch to thicken. Allow the turkey to stand for 10 minutes before slicing and serving.

Stuffing (or Dressing)

Prepare your favorite stuffing recipe as usual, only this time you're using a butter flavored food spray to sauté onions and celery. Also, moisten dressing with skim evaporated milk, skim milk, or chicken stock. Cook as usual.

Mashed Potatoes

Peel and boil potatoes until tender. Mash the potatoes using skim evaporated milk, butter flavored powder, and lite salt and pepper to taste.

Candied Sweet Potatoes

Boil peeled sweet potatoes or yams until tender. Drain and transfer to an oven-proof casserole. Cover with light maple syrup and sprinkle with butter flavored powder. Bake in a 350° oven until bubbly and browned on top.

Cranberry Relish

Prepare 1 pkg. (large size) raspberry gelatin according to directions. Mix in 1 16 oz. can cranberry sauce or relish. Mix well. Chill.

Pumpkin Dessert Pie

Prepare 1 package no sugar instant vanilla pudding mix using 1 cup skim milk and 1 cup mashed pumpkin. Add 1 teaspoon pumpkin pie spice. Mix well and pour into a prepared graham cracker crust. Chill well. Serve with a dollop of low calorie whipped topping.

BIRTHDAY PARTIES FOR KIDS OF ALL AGES

With as many children as we have, there have been a lot of parties around our homes. Parties for children are times of excitement, balloons, cake, kids, noise, and lots of cleanup afterwards! But we might add that it's all well worth it. Here are some party ideas from our home to yours. And kids of *all* ages enjoy a party!

■

MENU FOR A KID'S PARTY
Turkey Burgers* on Buns with Relishes
Chocolate Cake**
No Fat, No Cholesterol Ice Cream
Fruit Juice Punch

■

MENU FOR A BIG KID'S PARTY
Bar-B-Que Burgers or Sloppy "Tom's"*
Chips, i.e. Doritos Lights™
Brownies*
No Fat, No Cholesterol* Ice Cream
Iced Tea, Diet Sodas

■

NICE EXTRAS OR SUBSTITUTES
Bananas on a Stick*
Russian Tea*
Air-popped Popcorn—Sprayed and Spiced*

Party Extras

Here are 3 nice extras to make. The frozen bananas can be made ahead, frozen, and then stored in a zip-lock bag. When you get "a hankering" for a popsicle, just head for your freezer. A frozen banana has only about 130 calories and lots of vitamins, minerals, and other good things.

The recipe for Russian Tea is an adaptation from a long time ago. Make up this mixture and keep it in an air-tight container and use whenever you wish.

Keep popcorn around for snacking. This recipe is easy to "pop" and much less expensive than the microwave popcorn you buy all ready to go.

*See recipe section.
**Bake your favorite chocolate cake and ice it with lo-cal whipped topping. Sprinkle with colored sprinkles and add candles. Serve.

Bananas on a Stick

Peel a banana. Place a stick in the end carefully so as not to "break" the fruit. Dip banana in skim milk. Roll banana in a mixture of Grape Nuts,™ sweetener of choice, and cinnamon. Place on a cookie sheet and freeze. Eat and enjoy!

I've also rolled the banana in applesauce and then in Grape Nuts™ before freezing. Very good!

Russian Tea Mix

My children loved it when I'd make Russian Tea and cinnamon toast on Sunday evenings. Here is a modern version of that which I made the old-fashioned way many, many years ago!

1 "little tub" container of citrus blend Crystal Light™
1 "little tub" container of lemonade Crystal Light™
4 heaping tablespoons de-caffeinated instant tea
1 teaspoon pumpkin pie spice

Mix all dry ingredients in a covered glass or plastic container. Store until ready to use. This mix is enough to make 4 quarts of beverage!

To use: Boil water. Sprinkle (this mix is very potent, so a little goes a long way!) a bit of the Russian Tea Mix in a cup to taste and serve with an extra wedge of lemon or a cinnamon stick. Wonderful on a cold day!

This basic mix is also very good served over ice. Just sprinkle a bit of the dry mix (to taste) in a glass of water, mix, add ice, and enjoy.

Brands such as Kool-Aid,™ Summertime,™ or Active 8™ beverage crystals are great in Russian Tea mix.

Popcorn

Fun food. Good snack food if you choose the right kind. Some microwave popcorn is very high in added fat, so if you enjoy the convenience of a microwave product, choose the one with the least amount of fat. One cup of plain, air-popped popcorn has only 25 calories so use this figure as a guideline when purchasing a product. Or use this easy recipe.

1 paper lunch bag
¼ cup popping corn
Powdered seasoning

Modern Magic Meals™ Maple Syrup powder is great on popcorn!

Place popping corn in the lunch bag and fold over (leave lots of space for the finished product!) and seal with plastic tape. Microwave on high for 2½ minutes or until popping stops. Spray with butter flavored food spray and sprinkle with cheese, butter, or sour cream flavored powders. Or you might like to try Cajun or Mexican spices with cheese flavored powder!

Menu Ideas for the Single Non-Cooking Person

These suggestions are prepared with the minimum amount of work and stress for the non-cooking person. Cleanup is easy, also. Just make sure that you have all the necessary food items in the cupboard before you start cooking. Use biodegradable dishes and it's easier cleanup. And children will enjoy most everything on the menu idea list. We suggest that you review the menu and pick and choose the foods you and your guests (kids) will enjoy. Review the recipe (you'll find them in the recipe section), make a shopping list, and then cook! Have fun doing it.

■

MENU 1
Sloppy "Toms" on a Bun
Salad
Yogurt Dessert
Beverage

■

MENU 2
Pita Pizzas
Raw Veggies
Cookies
Beverage

■

MENU 3
Pasta and Sauce
Salad
Pudding
Beverage

■

MENU 4
Turkey Burgers
Relishes
Popsicles™
Beverage

■

MENU 5
Broiled Fish or Chicken
Baked Potato
Veggies
Berries and Cream

■

MENU 6
Dum-Dum Soup
Sandwich
Fresh Fruit
Cookies
Beverage

■

MENU 7
Quick Tacos or Tostadas
Fresh Fruit
Beverage

How to Adapt a Recipe

So many of you have great recipes from times past, recipes you and your family enjoyed. Now you're wondering how you're going to cook and please everyone (!?) on your new Better Life eating program! Do you have a problem? No way! Let me explain!

In life, to my way of thinking anyway, there are only situations and solutions! The solution to keeping meals and meal planning fun and enjoyable is to learn how to adapt old recipes to make them heart-healthy new recipes.

Difficult? you might say. Easy, I reply! You'll see in this next section four recipes I've taken from cookbooks of old, and the corrections I've made to make these recipes more heart-healthy and with less fat and calories. Try to adapt! Adjust your own favorite recipes at home and see what happens! Good luck and enjoy the challenge!

Quick Bistro Stew with Potato Crust

Original Recipe	Heart-Healthy Adaptation
4 medium Idaho potatoes, pared, cut into ⅛-inch slices	
¼ cup vegetable oil	vegetable food spray
1 pound sirloin steak, 1-inch cubes	very lean beef, chicken, or turkey
½ pound mushrooms, sliced	
1 medium onion, chopped	
1 clove garlic, minced	
1 cup beef bouillon	
1 tablespoon tomato paste	
½ teaspoon dried basil leaves	
½ teaspoon salt	Omit, not necessary
¼ teaspoon pepper	
¼ pound green beans, cut in half	
1 cup thinly sliced carrots	
2 tablespoons cornstarch	
¼ cup dry red wine	

In medium saucepan over high heat, bring potatoes and enough water to cover to a boil; cook 3 to 5 minutes or until crisp-tender. Drain; set aside. In large oven-proof skillet over medium-high heat, *heat 2 tablespoons oil.* (Omit oil and use vegetable food spray instead.) Add meat; cook 5 minutes or until browned, turning frequently. Add mushrooms, onion, and garlic; cook 5 minutes longer. Stir in bouillon, tomato paste, basil, *salt,* and pepper. (Omit salt.) Bring to a boil. Add green beans and carrots. Cover; cook 5 minutes. In a small bowl stir together cornstarch and wine until smooth; add to skillet. Stirring constantly, bring to a boil over medium heat and boil 1 minute. Remove from heat. Preheat oven to broil. Arrange potatoes over meat mixture to cover completely; *brush with remaining 2 tablespoons oil.* (Omit oil and use vegetable spray instead.) Broil 3 to 5 inches from source of heat 10 minutes or until potatoes are golden. Serves 4.

Apricot Pork Medallions

Original Recipe	Heart-Healthy Adaptation
1 pound pork tenderloin	**chicken or turkey breasts, thinly sliced, or very lean pork**
2 tablespoons butter, divided	**butter flavored vegetable food spray**
1/2 cup dried apricots, chopped	
2 green onions, sliced	
1/4 teaspoon dry ginger	
1 teaspoon wine vinegar	
2 teaspoons brown sugar	
dash hot pepper sauce	

Cut meat crosswise into 1-inch pieces. Flatten each piece slightly with heel of hand. Heat *1 tablespoon butter* (use butter flavored food spray) in large skillet over medium-high heat. Brown medallions, about 2 minutes on each side. Add remaining ingredients to skillet with remaining *tablespoon of butter.* (Omit butter and spray contents of skillet with butter flavored vegetable food spray.) Cover and simmer 3–4 minutes. Remove medallions to serving platter, spoon sauce over. Serves 4.

Warm Cabbage Slaw

This is just as good cooked on the stove in a tightly covered skillet.

Original Recipe	Heart-healthy Adaptation
5 cups shredded or coarsely chopped green cabbage (1/2 of a 2 lb. cabbage)	
1/2 teaspoon salt	salt substitute
1/4 teaspoon freshly ground pepper	
1/2 tablespoon rice wine vinegar	
2 tablespoons unsalted butter, cut into bits	butter flavored spray

In medium glass bowl toss the cabbage with the *salt* (salt substitute), pepper, and vinegar. *Spray with the butter spray* and cover tightly with microwave plastic wrap. Cook on high power until heated through but still crunchy, about 7 minutes. Remove from the microwave and let stand for 2 minutes. Uncover, toss, and serve hot. OR, in a large non-reactive saucepan, melt the butter over moderately high heat. Add the cabbage, *salt* (salt substitute), and pepper; toss to coat and cook for 5 minutes. Add vinegar and cook until the cabbage is wilted but still crunchy, about 3 minutes more. Serves 4.

Granola Muffins

Original Recipe	Heart-Healthy Adaptation
1 cup flour	
1 teaspoon soda	
1 teaspoon salt	
1 cup bran	
1 cup granola	
½ cup milk	**½ cup skim milk**
½ cup molasses	
1 egg	**2 large egg whites**
¼ cup raisins	
¼ cup chopped nuts	**Omit (very high in fat and calories)**
¼ cup apricot jam or orange marmalade	**low sugar jam spread**
Cinnamon and sugar	

Mix flour, soda, and salt together. Add bran, granola, molasses, milk, and *egg* (egg whites). Stir until just mixed. Do not beat or over-stir. Add raisins. Fill custard cups only ½ full and make a dent in each one. Fill indentation with 1 tablespoon *apricot jam or orange marmalade* (low sugar apricot or orange spread). Shake cinnamon and sugar over top, if desired. Let stand 10–15 minutes. Place in microwave oven and heat 4–6 minutes, or bake in conventional oven for 30–40 minutes at 375°. Yield 12 muffins.

See . . . I told you it isn't difficult!

Quick Calorie-Counting Guide

For those of you who are not familiar with calories, and few people are, we're including a basic calorie count for healthy foods. There are excellent calorie-food books available at the library or in the local bookstore. We suggest you check them out if calorie counting is important to you. The U.S.D.A. "Handbook No. 8" is the best reference, and probably the most difficult for the non-professional to understand. *Food Values* by Jean Pennington is current and easy to read and understand.

This information is based on data in U.S.D.A. "Handbook No. 8" and product information available.

ANIMAL PROTEIN
Chicken, Beef, Turkey, Seafood, Game, Etc., Cooked

	SERVING SIZE	CALORIE VALUE
Chicken Breast (no skin)	3½ oz.	175
Turkey Breast (no skin)	3½ oz.	175
Lean Ground Turkey	3½ oz.	175
Flank Steak	3½ oz.	250
Venison	3½ oz.	200
Swordfish	3½ oz.	150
Filet of Sole	3½ oz.	150
Filet of Cod	3½ oz.	150
Trout	3½ oz.	150
Shrimp	3½ oz.	100
Lobster	3½ oz.	100
Crab	3½ oz.	100
Clams	3½ oz.	140

BEANS AND PEAS

	SERVING SIZE	CALORIE VALUE
Garbanzo Beans	½ cup cooked	110*
Split Peas	½ cup cooked	110*
Lentil Beans	½ cup cooked	110*
Black Beans	½ cup cooked	110*
Kidney Beans	½ cup cooked	110*
Pinto Beans	½ cup cooked	110*

*Approximate value.

DAIRY

	SERVING SIZE	CALORIE VALUE
Skim (1% fat or less) Milk	8 oz.	90
Low Fat (2% fat) Milk	8 oz.	145
Nonfat Yogurt, plain	4 oz.	60
1% Fat Cottage Cheese	4 oz.	70
2% Fat Cottage Cheese	4 oz.	110
Buttermilk	8 oz.	90

FRUITS

	SERVING SIZE	CALORIE VALUE
Apple	medium	70
Orange	medium	70
Banana	medium	100
Pear	medium	70
Grapes	½ cup	50
Strawberries	½ cup	35
Cantaloupe	¼ melon	40
Grapefruit	½ fruit	40
Applesauce	½ cup	55

GRAINS

	SERVING SIZE	CALORIE VALUE
Rice	½ cup	110*
Noodles (pasta)	½ cup	110*
Barley	½ cup	110*
Corn Meal (Grits)	½ cup	110*
Hot Cereals (oatmeal, etc.)	½ cup	110*
Cold Cereals	½ cup	110*
Bagel	1 each	180
Whole Wheat Bread	1 slice	75
Lite Bread	1 slice	40
Sourdough or Italian Bread	1 slice	75
Pita Bread	½ pocket	70
French Roll	1 small	75

*Approximate value.

VEGETABLES

	SERVING SIZE	CALORIE VALUE
Lettuce	unlimited amount	FREE
Tomatoes	medium	25
Onions	½ cup	25
Green Peppers	½ cup	15
Celery	½ cup	10
Cauliflower	½ cup	15
Broccoli	½ cup	25
Zucchini	½ cup	15
Carrots	½ cup	15
Green Peas	½ cup	50
Beets	½ cup	25
Potatoes	medium	100
Sweet Potatoes	medium	150

Family Circle Suggestions

FUN LEARNING AT FAMILY CIRCLE

Before you go to the store, you *must* learn how to read a label. And label reading is fun when everyone gets involved. This is what we suggest.

1. Everyone old enough should have a pad and pencil and be ready to do some math. Little ones should have buddies who read.
2. Each person should get a packaged product out of the cupboard to practice with—a product with the nutritional analysis printed on it.
3. Someone must be in charge and that person should go over all the material related to reading and analyzing labels prior to Family Circle so that he or she can teach each family member and be able to talk about what they're going to do.

Here are some other Family Circle activities that focus on the family's food:

1. Check out the foods-recipe section and ask everyone what meals/dishes they'd like to try.
2. Plan brown bag lunches and snacks to have around the house.
3. Make a grocery shopping list.
4. Choose the "shopping team."
5. Ask for a volunteer who will become familiar with the label reading section and teach all other family members. This is a *BIG* one!
6. Make a responsibility list:
   Who shops.
   Who helps put away groceries.
   Who prepares meals.
   Who makes lunches.
   Who is on the cleanup committee.
7. Plan a time to debrief, to make changes, to incorporate suggestions, etc.
8. Ask for volunteers who will collect restaurant menus to take home and review and discuss. Many restaurants have throw-away menus you can take out. Choose menus from fast food emporiums, Chinese, Mexican, and Italian restaurants, and coffee shops.
9. Get together to plan special dinners, parties, and holidays and make a responsibility list.
10. Have fun! Remember our friend Lulu? She always says, "If it's not fun, it ain't worth doing."

FAMILY CIRCLE HOLIDAY AIDS

1. Always eat breakfast on the day of the big feast.
2. Snack on fruit during the day.
3. Eat a smaller portion of everything at "the feast" and go back for seconds if you're still hungry.
4. While helping in the kitchen avoid nibbling the goodies. Chew on carrot sticks and drink diet beverages or iced tea.
5. Plan a family walk before *and* after your meal. The *before walk* will help you in controlling your appetite and the *after walk* will help you burn off some of what you've eaten.
6. Have dessert a couple of hours after dinner. S-T-R-E-T-C-H those calories.
7. Always enjoy yourself.

■ *THE BETTER LIFE INSTITUTE FAMILY HEALTH PLAN*

Healthfully Ever After: How to Maintain Your Family Health Program

■ ■

Welcome to Fantasyland

The Universal Studios Tour hosts tens of thousands of visitors in Hollywood and Florida every year. A video tape welcomes visitors to "a world where things that seem what they are . . . aren't." For a few blissful hours adults and children let their fantasies wander and dream of knights and dragons, swashbuckling swordsmen and distressed damsels, Rambos and killer sharks. And at Disneyland, at both the Anaheim and Orlando versions, wide-eyed visitors are treated to the wonders of Mickey, Donald, and Goofy, the awesome world of Captain Hook and his pirates, and the fantastic meanderings of Tinker Bell. These escapes from reality into a world of make believe don't happen just at places like movie studios and theme parks. We seem to balance a good amount of time and energy spent on the nitty-gritties of life with leisure-time activities meant to rejuvenate both our spirits and our bodies. While we focus attention on diet, exercise, and lifestyle, we also put in a good bit of couch-potato time, our eyes glued to the tube.

It's no surprise to us then, when perfectly mature men and women, experienced in the ways of life, express surprise and disappointment over their eating and exercise habits. Why does all the enthusiasm for a healthier lifestyle that roared into their lives when they read about the need to improve, talked about change, and decided to make drastic changes fade away to a wimper in the months that follow? Perhaps it's because we live in a world that believes in "magic," "the Force," heroes, heroines, and *miraculous change*. It stands to reason that sometimes we want to believe the Force will make us want to eat turkey and broccoli and get us out of bed early to exercise.

The people who expect a change in eating and exercise habits to simply happen to them are the very same men and women who believe their success in business and family life is not due to magic or the Force, but to hard work, persistence, flexibility, and patience. People are complex, and while they use logic and common sense to guide them in certain aspects of their lives, they sometimes rely on magic and the Force in other areas. The business executive or auto mechanic who uses precise, logical procedures to solve problems at work, will arrive home and immediately place his health in jeopardy by eating food that will have the worst possible effect on his body and making excuses to avoid exercise. The trick is for him to transfer the logic and common sense he uses when operating his office computer or repairing an engine to his family health program. Sounds impossible? Of course it isn't. We're here to show you it is indeed very possible. Just step into our office, please!

THE VIEW FROM BEHIND OUR DESK

For an example, let's take a sober and calculating look at the work world and family lives of two men, a business executive and an auto mechanic. Each has been at his job for many years. Each has learned his skills on the job through continual practice day after day. It took more than a few weeks to build the skills, experience, and successful know-how that their customers want. They have practiced for years. Every minute, every hour, every day has presented new challenges. Slowly and steadily, they perfected their skills. At first they made many mistakes. But they learned from their experiences and improved, ready for the next time. Essentially they built a new set of work and business habits that were different and improved.

Actually it's not unusual that these two men, whose business successes are the result of years of hard work, are surprised that they cannot maintain proper eating and exercise habits at home and with their families. We all have a little bit of "the Force" feeling in us. On one hand, we believe that hard work and persistence are essential for business success and building a good family life. But, on the other hand, we also believe that some kind of "magic dust" will be sprinkled on our health habits to keep us motivated to pedal away on our exercise bikes and eating turkey and broccoli with enthusiasm. Just as the business executive and auto mechanic practiced

284   ■ *THE BETTER LIFE INSTITUTE FAMILY HEALTH PLAN*

their business skills and need to apply the same consistent practice to their family health habits, we all need to practice the changes we want to make to our lifestyles.

Practice Makes Perfect

Our lives are filled with examples of accepting the value of hard work, trial and error, and continual practice as a basis for success. Try hitting a golf ball straight and true after not playing for three years. Or how about skiing down a Gold Double-Diamond trail on your first day on the slopes after a ten-year layoff? If you haven't touched your computer for a few years, could you expect to remember the basic command keys? What about that language you learned last year? Did it mostly disappear from your mind when the class was finished? How much of your high school algebra is still with you? Who remembers which years Louis XIV ruled (now be honest), or when the planet Pluto was discovered? Are you thinking, "Of course I don't remember all those things. I learned them and then never used them again. If I were a golf instructor, I'd be good at golf. If I were a math or history teacher, I would still be good at math or history because I would use the information every day." That's exactly the point. The more you use a skill or a habit, the more you practice, the more you profit from your mistakes, the better and stronger that skill or habit becomes. After a few years it is simply a way of life. You use it naturally without "batting an eyelash."

The exact same conditions apply to your family's new eating and exercise habits. The fact that you know they are good for you and you *ought* to do them won't guarantee you will. Learning algebra, history, or the fundamentals of golf, was good for you, but learning once didn't make you retain what you learned when you stopped using it. Why then should "ought to" work for eating and exercise? Practice is the secret.

Some people think eating vegetables and taking a daily aerobic walk are easy because they look easy. After all you don't really have to learn any new skills. You already know how to eat and how to walk. You don't need a degree from Harvard to know how to put vegetables on your fork or to place one foot in front of the other. What we all forget is that new health habits are really *new*. You already have a set of *old* health habits. You may not see them as health habits per se, but they were the eating and exercise habits you practiced and lived with every day. Think of all the meals, holidays, restaurants, and vacations you and the family have enjoyed. And what about all those years when your heart was young and your body was tireless (before you were married)? Think of all the mornings, evenings, and weekends when you have practiced diligently being a couch potato instead of exercising regularly. The couch-potato "moves" are automatic now and familiar. They even give you pleasure. It will take much, much more than good intentions and a few chapters in a book to change decades of living habits. *Old habits die hard.*

REPLACING THE OLD WITH THE NEW

There's both good news and bad news in the fact that old habits die hard. The bad news is that changing them requires hard work and persistence. The good news is that the longer you work at building your *new* eating and exercise habits—with hard work and persistence—the more likely they will replace your *old* eating and exercise habits. In other words, after a few months you will have a new set of automatic, familiar, and pleasurable "moves." It should be obvious that you already have the skills to integrate these "moves": hard work, persistence, patience, and the ability to profit from your mistakes. Now you just need to roll up your sleeves and apply your working skills to healthy eating and exercising, to lifelong family health!

HEALTH HABITS NEED CULTIVATION

If you accept a new lifestyle as a *challenge,* rather than a problem, there will be changes in your family's lifestyle and overall health. The challenge translates into changes in the life of each family member at home, at work, at school, and at play. An important aspect of the challenge is to cultivate, and nourish the changes. If you just throw grass seed on a dry lawn, you don't really expect much new grass to grow. You may get a few green sprouts, but if you don't continually cultivate, water, and nourish, the sprouts that do appear will wither and die.

Making changes in your family's eating and exercise habits is, in a way, no different from taking proper care of your lawn. New health routines also require continual nourishment and cultivation if they are to become lifelong habits. The best dietary and exercise recommendations, heart-healthy recipes, and advice about equipment and Family Circle will not grow and thrive unless you continually feed, nourish, and support them. They have to be practiced and continually adjusted as need dictates. They have to be used every single day. They have to be *lived* on the weekends, during holidays, and at school. They should be anticipated and enjoyed as a natural and desirable part of family life. Even such basic household routines as cooking, grocery shopping, and housekeeping must utilize your new eating and exercise habits. What the family eats at school, at work, when traveling, or in restaurants must support your commitment to health.

WE'RE IN THIS FOR LIFE

Your new habits should become as natural as brushing your teeth or taking a shower. Family health must become a routine part of family life. When this is accomplished, and it will take a little time, the family will truly have a new permanent lifestyle—a healthy lifestyle. It will never again be something *special*. It will be *routine* and as easy to live with and enjoy as any thing you've been doing for years. Thus, your goals are not to just memorize new eating and exercise habits. Your goal is to practice, practice, practice, creating a new family lifestyle that will support, cultivate, and nourish a new way of lifelong living for the family. You must believe *we're in this for life*.

A Lifestyle for a Lifetime

THE BASICS

Accentuate the Positive

It's one thing to have a worthy health goal for your family. It's another thing to achieve the goal and make it a part of the rest of your lives. As you've probably guessed by now, there is no single, permanent, "etched in stone" diet, exercise, or living pattern. A healthy lifestyle for a lifetime is a continually changing process, rather than a specific pattern you acquire by reading a book. The first basic of this evolutionary process for healthier family living is a very obvious one that is necessary for all aspects of our lives: a positive "can do" attitude.

No Problems

How many times have we heard ourselves or members of our families say, "I have a problem"? The word *problem* places a negative value on the situation. There is also a sense of passivity and hopelessness about a problem. It means, "This bad thing has happened to me," and often it's something you can't do much about it. And if you could, it would take an enormous amount of effort to "dig yourself out of this hole."

Just Situations and Solutions

By exchanging the word *problem,* for the word *situation* you immediately feel different. A *situation* is not necessarily bad. There is no negative value attached to *situation*. It is merely a given set of circumstances that is neither good nor bad. Now something that was bad has become neutral. What is even better is that for every *situa-*

My boys often used the word con-version when they talked about cars. Fast cars, old cars, racers, were con-verted and became something different. When it came time for me to change my lifestyle I began to use the word conver-sion, which means to turn around, to change one's mind, to change the way something works. My boys understood when I said, "I con-verted this recipe from an old one grandma gave me," or "I'm thinking of converting the base-ment into a room for exercise, television, and family fun." Somehow change was threatening, but conversion wasn't!"

Mother of nine

tion you face, there is a *solution*. Problems just sit there and continue to be problems. Situations get solved.

Think Positive

We suggest you begin to see the family health challenges facing you and your family as a series of *situations with solutions* never *problems*. A situation with a solution embodies a *can do* attitude. Instantly you have a positive mindset. Whatever has happened is no longer hopeless or insoluble. Similarly, your youngster's reluctance to exercise is not a problem, but a temporary situation with a solution. This is a wonderful attitude to instill in your family. It causes less stress, evokes less anger and frustration, and sets a positive "can do" approach for all of your lives. A "situations with solutions" approach has long-term staying power, and that's what is needed for family health. *Think positive!*

IF IT AIN'T LIVABLE, IT AIN'T A LIFESTYLE

At the Better Life Institute we are emphatic about the absolute importance of selecting livable and enjoyable eating and exercise habits. In their efforts to improve health most people attempt to adopt overly restrictive, unappetizing diets and overly aggressive exercise programs. They want a fast and dramatic change that will "knock the socks off" their friends, relatives, and associates. Others attempt to prepare food requiring much chopping, steaming, and time. These kinds of efforts are probably doomed from the beginning.

Initial change is easy during the excitement period when something is new and different. There usually is a "honeymoon" of about two weeks when whatever you do will work just from the momentum of having initiated something new. This will carry you along for a few weeks. And then the best of intentions runs out of steam and your program starts to fall by the wayside. The reality of having to live with what you are eating and how you are exercising sets in. That's when the going gets tough, and suddenly, you can't keep going.

A "lifestyle of family health" means practicing healthful living all day and every day. The food that is cooked at home must be very tasty and prepared easily and quickly. If it's not, if preparing healthy food for the family just requires too much work or will power to continue, you're likely to use the first excuse to stop doing it. Also, an exercise program that is very difficult because of the effort and time it requires or the inconvenience it causes will also be abandoned very quickly. Exercise must be fun and convenient if it is to become a permanent part of your family's lifestyle. It must become a regular part of everyday life just as your new eating habits must be.

The exact same conditions apply to Family Circle. If it is too long, too argumentative, or uninteresting, the family will start to make excuses and find reasons not to attend.

Behavior Is Not by the Numbers

Most people have an idea of how long it will take to lose a certain amount of weight, jog a mile, or get the family going steadily on a health program. We aren't sure where these notions come from. There certainly are no numerical formulas or tables that predict how speedily these kinds of changes will take place. Thinking you can lose ten pounds in three months seems realistic, but bodies do not respond to changes in diet in the same way. Just as one person can build up the stamina and muscle strength to jog a ten-minute mile five times a week within a relatively short period of time, others will require longer to reach that goal.

Our experience is that most people tend to expect too much too soon. They want and expect more from their new habits than they can possibly get in a short amount of time. When they don't get the results they expected, they are discouraged and have difficulty continuing their programs. However, this situation can easily be avoided!

The investment you and the family make in health should be evaluated in terms of new habits and not the number of pounds lost or miles walked. There is a logical relationship between the work you do to improve your health and the visible results, of course, but the results may not show as quickly for you as you would like. There are good scientific reasons why you can't predict the rate and extent of physiological change in your body or in anyone else's.

The Relationship Between "Dose" and "Response"

Each person has an individual sensitivity to a given diet or exercise program. It's called a *dose-response* relationship. For example, if you give a grain of aspirin to twelve people with the exact same headache and wait twenty minutes to see if the headache is gone, you will have a wide variety of reaction. Two people will still have the headache with no change whatsoever. Eight people will have experienced differing amounts of relief, but more or less they will still have the headache. The remaining two people will be headache free.

This is true for diet and exercise changes as well. Each body has its individual rate of response and progress and timetable for change. That's why the family should focus on behavior or habits instead of numbers. If the habit has existed a long time, the effect of changes could be dramatic. But, always there will be differences in response. For some a great change will occur, for others only a moderate difference. But as time passes, everyone catches up and experiences significant change.

You should explain this in a simple way at Family Circle. Use the "different strokes for different folks" concept. It's important to support efforts to change rather than talk about statistics. At the Better Life Institute, we never congratulate people on the weight they have lost or on the number of points their blood cholesterol level has gone down. We always ask how they are doing on the program. We congratulate and support them for their habits and not for the manner in which their bodies respond to their habits. They have no control over the psysiological response of their bodies, just as you and your family cannot control the ways your bodies will respond to your new behavior.

NOTHING SUCCEEDS LIKE SUCCESS OR FAILS LIKE FAILURE

We think of changing family health habits as a positive and joyful experience, not one to be regarded as "medicine." Heroic acts of will power, sacrifice, and deprivation make wonderful subjects for movies and books, but they don't work well in real life—unless there is a life-or-death situation. In the case of family health particularly, will power, sacrifice, and deprivation neither work nor are they necessary. Your program is doomed if you attempt to change eating and exercise habits melodramatically.

The challenge is to design a program that allows each person to work toward behavioral and health goals slowly. With slow and steady progress, each family member is more likely to find the program easy to do and enjoyable. Each one will feel successful and success is a remarkable thing. It tends to breed a positive attitude and that leads to further success. With that in mind, if you doubt you or the others can live comfortably with a certain eating or exercise change, you should suggest an easier program and gradually build to something more aggressive. This way the family will have positive and encouraging experiences to report at Family Circle. Never express disappointment with the rate of progress of any of the others and don't allow anyone else to say anything about a family member that isn't positive and supportive. A "can do," "we have confidence in you" attitude is absolutely essential for everyone.

You don't throw an old habit out the window. You have to gently coax it down the stairs and out the door.

Mark Twain

A Straw Bends in the Wind, But Does Not Break

We usually remember the happy, past experiences of our lives in terms of absolutes: "I graduated from college, it was a snap." "I loved having my baby." "Last summer was a blast." But if we could go back to the time of each of these experiences, we might find some "raggedy edges" or setbacks we don't remember now. It's human na-

■ *THE BETTER LIFE INSTITUTE FAMILY HEALTH PLAN*

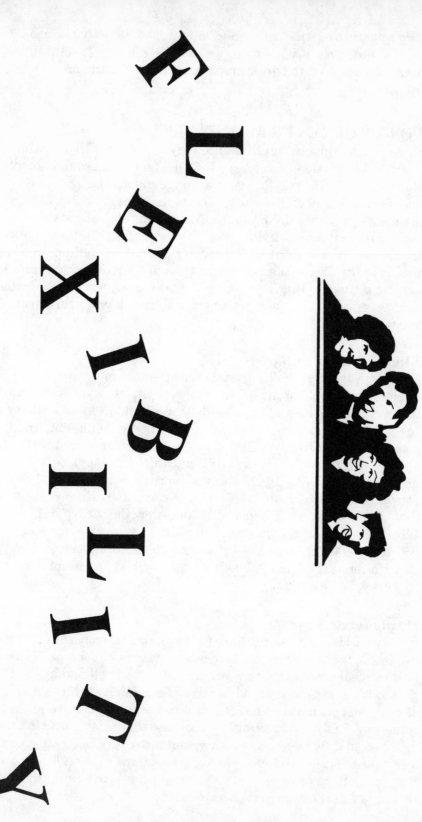

FLEXIBILITY

ture to gloss over the "split ends" and remember only the good things. But, even if it's sometimes painful, it's very helpful to look back into our past to better prepare ourselves for the present and future.

DON'T WORRY, IT'S ADJUSTABLE

Some people naively feel that once they've changed their eating or exercise habits, they won't have to make any further adjustments. But that is not the way it works. Change means there will be ups and downs. You need to be prepared to make modifications and adjustments in the family program. As your family enters a new way of individual and family living, you will encounter situations, not problems, disasters, or signs that you can't "cut it"—situations with solutions. Family Circle is an excellent time to "inoculate" the family against setbacks. Talking about and making adjustments, because of your experience, is a very healthy way to create new solutions to unforeseen situations.

I Wanna Get Off da Bus!

Even with the best of circumstances, we sometimes want to quit. It's impossible to understand all the reasons why we want to "throw in the towel," but now and then we do. You shouldn't forge a lifestyle of "getting off the bus" because quitting can become a habit, and it is not a good habit to have. But, if it does happen once in a while, relax and go with it for the *shortest time possible!* Just don't beat yourself up about it, or try to psychoanalyze yourself. When you feel this way your attitude is too negative for you to come up with any answers at that time to the "what happened?" question. Just leave it alone. When you "get off the bus," just chalk it up to experience and tell yourself you'll take a peek at it when you're feeling better. Then get on with the rest of your life as soon as possible. We promise you'll "get back on" eventually.

Family Circle Support

Family Circle is an opportunity to normalize the concept of "throwing in the towel." A simple, supportive statement such as "I know how you feel since I feel that way sometimes" is all it takes to tell a person it's okay and you and the rest of the family are there to help and support each other. You can also ask others if they've felt the same way. But it's important to recognize that this feeling is perfectly normal for everyone—both young and old. When you take the sting out of such a common emotion, you allow that person to concentrate on getting back on track. And don't try to minimize the situation or laugh it off, or permit anyone else to do so. Ask if there's

THE BETTER LIFE INSTITUTE FAMILY HEALTH PLAN

SET
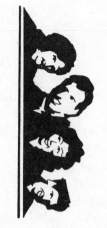
BACKS

anything the family can do and check back during the rest of the week to see how the person is feeling.

The Pause That Refreshes

A lifestyle for family health means the family members plan their lives in ways that support their eating and exercise habits. Weekends and vacations are wonderful times to combine fun and relaxation with healthy living. There are many delightful family outings your family can plan right in your community which contribute to healthy living: picnics, walks in the park, boating, biking, watching sporting events, dinner in a restaurant. We all need a break from our daily routines. We may enjoy what we do every day, but the repetitious aspects of so much of our lives produces a sense of tedium. We all need to take a "pause that refreshes."

There are great ways to combine a family vacation with healthy living. Camping or outdoor vacations are excellent examples of activities that strengthen family ties and have exercise and a bit of physical work associated with the fun. Many resorts provide an assortment of family activities as well as activities just for children. And the good news is that at most resorts today there is ample opportunity to plan for healthy eating. You just have to know how to do it. Don't forget about the many spas or health and fitness resorts throughout the country. Many also provide programs for children. Fond memories can be built around healthy family vacations. Start those memories now with an outing next weekend.

THE PERMANENCE OF CHANGE

Everything that is worth doing for a long time will at times have to be adjusted. Everyone's needs and priorities change. Your children are living in intense, turbulent years of development. Each school year does indeed present situations and solutions. As they grow, there are developmental and maturational situations and solutions. Your family health program *must* have a "thermostat" to continually adjust daily actions to new realities. Life offers an inexhaustible supply of "situations and solutions," and it can happen any hour of every day.

At the Better Life Institute, we teach people to change their health habits by isolating a specific situation and "drawing a line around it" so it can be managed and solved. For purposes of change we help them to see their lives as a sequence of situations and solutions. We don't mean to imply that family life or life itself is that simplistic. This method is just a practical way to start to solve something. We do this in business all the time. A businessman solves a poor sales situation by identifying the specific situation and the solution. Is the situation defined as a poor product? Is it the price of the product or the advertising? So what is the solution?

We don't mean to tell you what your situations and solutions should be, but we'd like to provide some examples of those we feel are very common. We offer no pat solutions or formulas in the following situations, but merely an idea of how to approach certain common situations and solutions for family health. The key points to remember are:

1. Keep a positive attitude all the time.
2. Always try to see the situation from the other person's point of view.
3. Ask everyone in the family who is capable of offering advice to participate.
4. Don't forget that little minds grow into big minds. Get everyone possible in the act.
5. Always phrase comments or suggestions in a supportive manner.
6. Everyone should feel accepted and important.

Family Circle should always have a "situations and solutions" time.

"SURVIVAL OF THE FITTEST" PARTY-GOER

Many families who come to the Better Life Institute have the feeling that good health habits mean avoiding all festive occasions. They believe they can't attend a party where the food and drink runs counter to their new eating habits. Nothing could be further from the truth. This is a situation with a solution. You can "survive and thrive" at any party if you're prepared in advance.

Family Circle is an excellent place to solicit constructive suggestions about eating at parties. A discussion of what parties and celebrations are coming up in the following week should be routine. Make sure you mention the meetings and events that are part of your work schedule. They can be excellent examples for the rest of the family. Undoubtedly, as the family discusses situations and solutions that concern you, you will learn some new tips from the most unlikely source!

The worst enemy of health habit change is the unexpected. The more a person can anticipate situations, the easier and less stressful are the solutions. Discuss what the party will be like and what general types of food and drink will be available. Everyone will have some solutions when the situation is described properly. The trick is to take a positive stance and discuss what can be done—never what can't be done. And for health's sake, don't go to a party when you're famished; it just gives you an excuse to eat everything in sight. One solution is to eat something before you go.

Practice Makes Perfect

Plan some parties together and give the entire family the opportunity to discuss what the foods should be. The recipe section of this book re-invents the term *junk food* in a way that allows you to eat fun food that won't hurt you. You might call it *good junk*. There are other recipe books that describe ways to prepare good-tasting, festive party dishes you can serve with pride and without guilt.

Trips to the movies or family picnics and outings are other excellent opportunities to learn by doing. On a long car trip you should provide proper snacks, whether you take them along or come to a consensus in quick-stop stores. And Family Circle "situations and solutions" is a great time to discuss "television food"—what do you eat while watching the "tube"?

When you or your children entertain at home, try not to impose your new eating habits on others. It is perfectly fine to provide many different foods for everyone to enjoy. Try to remember that the family's eating habits are the family's, not the guests'. You want to avoid any possibility of making your guests uncomfortable about food. Discuss with the family what you should provide when entertaining your friends. It's a good way to include everyone in family decision-making and learning about food.

There may be certain situations, such as a kid's birthday party, where there appears to be no solution. Everything served is loaded with fat and sugar: birthday cake, soda pop, hot dogs, potato chips, cole slaw, and ice cream. There *always* is a solution. We offer some in another part of the book. In some situations, where no acceptable alternatives are available, the solution may be to "punt." It's just one party. Nothing disastrous will happen if your child eats what the other kids eat. This would usually be wiser than requiring your child to eat different from the other children at parties. Causing your child to stand out could create some social difficulties. The family should recognize and accept that there may be certain situations when they should just "go with the flow." This, in itself, is a good lesson in living. Teach everyone that flexibility is a wonderful approach to many situations. You must also emphasize the importance of getting back on track afterward. (Remember the teenager described in the "Let's Grow Healthy Kids" chapter and how he did it.)

Teenagers face a tremendous amount of peer pressure to drink and use drugs at parties. Family Circle is an opportunity to show them that they can talk about the pressures they face without threat of criticism. They'll learn by the way everyday subjects are discussed at Family Circle that the very troubling subjects will be discussed in

■ *What food has more nutrition and fiber in it, ounce for ounce, than any other plant food?*

■ *It contains almost twice the USRDA for Vitamin C.*

■ *It contains half the USRDA for Vitamin A.*

■ *It contains over 20% of the USRDA for calcium.*

■ *It contains 10% of the USRDA for iron.*

■ *It contains many other vitamins and minerals.*

■ *And it has only 45 calories in a half cup.*

■ *It's . . . Broccoli!*

■ *THE BETTER LIFE INSTITUTE FAMILY HEALTH PLAN*

the same way. The family's support and understanding will encourage them to share their concerns with you. They'll remember this when they have something personally important to discuss. It's very important to them and to you that lines of communication always remain open and that you use the opportunity to explore when it's all right to "go with the flow," when it isn't all right, and how to handle those not-all-right times. One of the most important things you can do for your teenagers is help them practice handling the tough times before they happen.

A GUIDING LIGHT

"As the twig is bent, so grows the tree" goes the saying. We agree with this approach. We believe that as the young child is nurtured, so grows the adolescent, the teenager, and ultimately, the young adult. Life should be fun, but one doesn't have to abandon the principles of good health to have fun. Since there are only "situations and solutions" in life, every person should recognize the exception and then get back on track at the earliest possible moment. We love our children, just as you love yours. We love them so much we are willing to take a stand on experiences that we think are essential for health, growth, and a long life.

Making Your Weekends "Wild"

Use Family Circle to plan an occasional family "wild weekend." Plan a "mystery weekend" and surprise the family with an outing in a nearby city. Try associating it with exercise or an activity that is physically oriented. And plan to include the grandparents as well. Most hotels have an exercise room and a swimming pool. Take some snacks along with you. And keep a bowl of fruit in the room. Of course, hiking and camping are very good family activities and can bring out the best in people.

There's lots of family things to do: ride horseback, teach mom how to play miniature golf, or go to a square dance, a rodeo, or the circus. There's so much out there to do. Just stop and think about it.

Vacations that provide family time are preferred. Try to avoid those situations where everybody splits up and goes their separate ways. Plan to have some special private time with each child instead of spending all your time with the entire family. And don't forget about time alone with your spouse! If necessary, get a babysitter. Engage in activities that refresh, rather than exhaust you. Reading, walking, listening to music, knitting, golfing, and dancing are examples of refreshing activities. Come home refreshed instead of coming home needing a vacation from your vacation.

It's prudent to check out the contents of your water supply, since you and your family cook with it and drink it. Water utilities test water at its source, not from your pipes. Contact a local lab to analyze your water. You can call the EPA Water Hotline (1-800/426-4791) for help in understanding your report. You may want to consider some sort of filtration system. Buy a unit that has been certified by the National Sanitation Foundation (NSF).

We hardly consider a family evening at home with some enjoyable video movies a "wild weekend," but it's a wonderful way to spend time together. There are many family movies available. Select two or three movies and have a movie marathon on the weekend. Many family movies present some interesting ideas for discussion at Family Circle.

KEEPING THE "BLEACHER BUMS" AT BAY

We suggest a very simple rule of thumb for all situations relating to potential conflict with friends about health habits: There is no need to pit one way of life against another. Friendship is far more valuable than the differences that may exist between friends concerning how they live their personal lives. Friends are very important and health is important. Two lifestyles can live side by side without one sacrificing the other. This is another situation with a solution and you just have to develop strategies to make it work. Inevitably you or your family will encounter friends with different points of view about health, ranging from total ignorance or rejection of a particular issue to strong alternative points of view. If you have an open mind and are able to see the opposing view, everyone can live happily in spite of the differences.

Remember, it takes two people to succeed with a wisecrack about your health habits—the person making the wisecrack and the person receiving it. Don't bite at the hook. Let it go right past you. Give the person a smile and say something like "different strokes for different folks" or "that's why Baskin-Robbins has 31 flavors." Tell your friends that they have their personal style of living and you have yours. And why shouldn't everyone live as they wish? There's no reason why you can't be friends with everyone. Their eating and exercise habits are not the basis of your friendship. Avoid debating with others over the merits of your lifestyle. And don't become "holier than thou" just because you've "seen the light" for better health. Know deep down that you and your family are on the correct path without having to convert anyone. Your friends may emulate you when they see how much better you look and how much more energy you have.

Make sure you bring this type of situation up for discussion at Family Circle. Your children will appreciate help in learning how to handle other kids who might poke fun at them.

GUESS WHO'S COMING TO DINNER?

When you're on your own turf, you can call the shots. But, when you're a guest at someone else's home, it's their call. Most people evaluate the success of their entertaining by the food they serve to their guests. The next thing they focus on is how much their guests

"Jack Spratt could eat no fat, his wife could eat no lean. But betwixt them both, you see, they licked the platter clean."

Think about that . . .

■ *THE BETTER LIFE INSTITUTE FAMILY HEALTH PLAN*

eat. Both these factors can place you in potentially difficult situations. How do you cross these potential mine fields?

You can take the initiative and compliment your host and hostess on the wonderful food they are serving. Try a few bites in a very public manner and eat a little bit of everything. Usually there are many choices available at a party or dinner. Do the best you can and pick foods that are as supportive as possible to your new eating habits. Avoid making statements that the hostess may perceive as challenges to her hospitality. As a guest in someone else's house, you shouldn't debate "good food" versus "bad food." It's too threatening to the host and hostess. If there are questions about why you have changed your eating habits, answer them in private and be sure that what you say is not critical of your hosts' hospitality.

Buffets are very simple to manage. You can eat what you wish quietly without talking about the choices of food. And remember, the purpose of parties and dinners is to have fun and relax. As we mentioned in a previous section regarding children's birthday parties, there may be times when you just have to eat what is served. Although it may not be as palatable now, the food will not harm you. Just get right back on the program at the very next opportunity.

The exact same principles hold true when you eat with friends in a restaurant. Just relax and order the food you wish without making comments about the food selections that your friends make. And please shrug off with a smile any comments they might make about your choices. It takes two to make an argument.

Don't think all learning comes through traditional homework. Let your children help you make a meal, for instance. They'll learn a lot about measuring and fractions.

Walk Softly and Carry a Big Stick
We remember when our children asked what they should tell their friends who had "bad" eating habits. We went through an elaborate explanation, describing the merits of teaching by example rather than by lecturing and criticizing. One of them interrupted and said, "You mean keep your mouth shut and just do it?"

That's exactly what we mean. People pay more attention to your actions than your words. They will watch you very carefully and learn more than you realize without anything ever being said.

I Still Don't Like String Beans
Parents can turn grey worrying that their little child will not like the healthier food choices that the family is trying to adopt. In fact, this phobia holds true for any family member. "I don't like it!" is indeed a powerful statement. It has an aura of finality and emotion that says, "I don't want to negotiate!" The child that says, "I don't like my lunches; everybody has stuff they like, why can't I?" indeed has a situation. But, there is always a solution.

An opportunity exists here to teach children and adults to think positively instead of resorting to an automatic "I can't" or "I don't want to." Give the family a chance to suggest "can do" solutions. Instead of bologna, perhaps turkey bologna will be just as tasty. Tuna salad with light mayonnaise may be just as good using full-fat mayo. There are many whole grain breads available that are more tasty than white bread. Suggest that the family pick out a few at the supermarket and try them. Ask the family if they have any suggestions on more healthy lunchbox snacks. Sometimes an opinion from an older child will be more influential with your younger child than your opinion. It's important to get the whole family to think as a team for one family member.

A Supermarket Safari

"Situations and solutions" provides an excellent opportunity for the family to take a trip to the supermarket. Everybody can walk around together and pick out lunch foods and snacks that they think will "fill the bill." A walk through the supermarket will open everyone's eyes to new foods and ideas for meals and snacks. It's a good idea to plan such a trip before starting your new family eating program. You might add to this adventure a trip to the local health food store.

Exercise: A Tie That Binds

There are certain activities that provide far more benefits than the activity itself. Exercise is essential for health, but it also is a wonderful basis for fun and relaxation. It's impossible to consider changing eating habits without planning an exercise program that includes family activities and individual exercise. Exercise provides immediate benefits to each person and helps maintain the new healthy lifestyle. The sense of vigor, relaxation, and self-esteem that results from aerobic exercise provides a firm foundation for new eating and exercise habits and gives individual family members pride in their accomplishments and a real desire to continue. Every family member should have an enjoyable and livable exercise program. There should be no exceptions made for little children, grandparents, or even the dog.

LET'S BE BUDDIES

A number of Better Life families use a buddy system. Family members pair up and agree to help and encourage each other. If you consider this approach, we suggest you pair a child and a parent whenever possible. The buddy system can strengthen relationships because two family members are working together toward a common

Exercise Safety Tips

■ **Dress to be seen** *if you exercise outdoors in the early morning or evening. Use reflective tape on clothes and shoes.*

■ **Never exercise outdoors alone** *in the dark. Always bring a friend.*

■ **Stay away from dimly-lit isolated areas.**

■ **Carry a quarter** *in your shoe so you can make an emergency phone call if necessary.*

■ **Always carry ID** *when you exercise away from home.*

■ *THE BETTER LIFE INSTITUTE FAMILY HEALTH PLAN*

goal. There is the sense of being partners and equals, which goes a long way toward building parent-child relationships that last for a lifetime. Think of the enjoyment your younger child especially will have in being your "exercise buddy," and what both of you will learn when you work together. This kind of support system may not be comfortable for some families, and it is not essential to a family health program. You must use your own judgment in deciding whether to use it.

It is impossible to avoid feelings of competition, jealousy, or envy in any family. Changes in eating and exercise habits may be difficult for some and easy for others. There may be differences in rates of progress that can cause emotional reactions. Close emotional and blood relationships are very complex. We really can't figure them out and don't expect that you can either. But there are ways to deal with such situations in order to find very positive solutions.

MORALE BOOSTING

Sometimes family members feel envy, jealousy, or competition among themselves. These feelings are natural and stem from the human need to compare. Even when there is love, caring, and a close relationship among people, the desire to compete is destructive. You can use Family Circle to tell the family about the naturalness of these feelings. You will not be encouraging the feelings, but trying to avoid some of the self-destructive fallout that occurs when a family member has such feelings and keeps them inside.

A smile doesn't cost you a penny and it goes a long way. When things are unpleasant and tense, a smile, no matter how difficult the effort, can soothe the waters.

One of the best ways to "normalize" everyone's internal feelings is to set an example. Discuss a past situation when you were jealous of someone in the family or of a friend and ask the others to describe similar situations. A simple, honest, supportive discussion can defuse potentially harmful situations that could jeopardize your health program. More importantly, the discussions will help the family understand it's okay to have these feelings. Family Circle will also provide each person with opportunities to consider solutions to their situations. Jealousy over someone else's weight loss or successful exercise program can be converted into a constructive discussion about exactly what is causing the jealousy, how the person can change the situation, and how the family can help.

Do to Others As . . .

Emphasize that no person in the family is in competition with anyone else. As we mentioned earlier, it's the *effort* that should be applauded, not the results. Praise and recognize commitment, honesty, coping with difficulties, positive attitude, and family support. These are personal qualities that every family member, regardless of age, can acquire.

The goal of Family Circle is not concerned with statistics. The overriding consideration is *family unity*. Start to look at this experience with eyes that recognize and praise the personal qualities you value in yourself and your children. That is the true purpose of Family Circle. Never let a family member toot his own horn and never support such behavior. Ask the person how he would feel if someone else were bragging about their success. It always brings people back to earth when you ask them how they would feel in the other person's shoes. "Do unto others as you would have them do unto you" is still the *golden rule*.

KEEPING THE BALL ROLLING

When you think of family lifestyle instead of merely diet and exercise, you will have a very different way of approaching your family health program. Whether you realize it or not, you already have a lot of experience in thinking this way. For example, the way you approach your marriage relationship is more "lifestyle" than reacting to one isolated event. Every time you discuss where you want to vacation, the type of restaurant where you'll eat, where you want to live, the decor of your house, you are not making isolated decisions. You and your spouse approach what seems to be simple, everyday, sometimes inconsequential decisions from a long-term relationship point of view which generally asks, "how are we going to live together with this?" This is family-lifestyle thinking. It is a view toward long-term enjoyment, livability, and an enduring relationship.

Think the same way about family health. Think of family health as your opportunity to reinforce all the family values you and your spouse cherish: love, respect, health, security, spirituality, joy, . . . *healthfully everafter*.

YES, I CAN!

- I can find a new interest or hobby that I can work on together with my child.
- I can put aside five minutes each day to talk privately and quietly with every other person in the family about "just things" without any lecture.
- I can say every day to each individual member of the family, *"I love you!"*

FAMILY CIRCLE HINTS

Set a strong example for your children when they are doing their homework. Ask them how you can support them. We have some suggestions:

a. Children are very impressionable and will appreciate your support if you stay near them while they do their homework. Ask them if they want to do their homework in an area where you are sitting.

b. Rather than watch television while they are doing homework, read a book, or do some office work near them. It's a great time to do budgets, pay bills, read the newspaper, and write letters. It shows them you are actually there with them and not just occupying the same room.

c. Sit next to your children and express an interest in their homework. Avoid giving them criticism unless they ask for it. Children always feel wonderful when their parents express surprise at the "difficulty" their kids can master with their homework. "I didn't know you could do that already!" makes them feel good.

Spirituality and the Power of Family

■ ■ ■ ■ ■ ■ ■ ■ ■ ■ ■ ■ ■ ■ ■ ■ ■ ■

The Family and Survival

THE BEGINNINGS OF "FAMILY"

Historically and anthropologically the family is the center of human life. Thousands of years ago the huddle of people called *family* was what today we call the "extended family." It was multi-generational and held together by economic necessity rather than biological kinship. The perpetual struggle for food and shelter made collective effort necessary. Each individual, as well as each nuclear family unit, could survive as a part of a large, cohesive group which provided safety, security, food, and shelter for all its members. The nuclear family—a father and a mother and their children—could not survive on its own.

SURVIVAL OF THE FITTEST

With each advance in science and technology, the family's ability to survive improved. Consequently, over the span of years the shape of the family slowly changed. Each advance meant that the number of people who had to huddle in order to survive could be smaller. Slowly, steadily, as man's technological abilities improved, the basic biological unit consisting of parents and their immediate children evolved. The forerunner of today's nuclear family, this family unit included others who were biologically related and for one reason or another did not have separate families of their own. Still, the object was survival.

SURVIVAL GETS EASIER

During Feudal times the family required the support and protection of small collectives called *Manors*. The families of the Manor earned their support by working the land that belonged to a feudal lord who in turn allowed them to live on his land and join together to help each other and protect themselves.

As technology gradually progressed, man was freed from surviving solely on the land. With the establishment of towns and commerce, small cottage industries and newly developed machinery created a lifestyle that allowed the family to survive by its own labor.

FOR SOME, SURVIVAL IS STILL TOUGH
Historically the capacity to survive has played a dominant role in the evolution of the family. As our scientific and technological capacity to meet life's needs has increased, the size of the family has decreased. However, there are many different forms of family in the world still today. In the Third World, for example, family structure is often dictated by economic necessity. In those poorer nations, extended families with more children and kin still "huddle" in order to meet life's basic needs.

HEY BEAV, WALLY, JUNE, AND WARD
In our country from the middle of the Eighteenth Century forward, the basic biological family not only survived, but thrived. It gradually decreased in size as its members' ability to survive without the help of other "kin" increased, until by the middle of the Twentieth Century the nuclear family had become the norm. The 4.3-member-family consisting of working father, stay-at-home mother, and 2.3 children had come of age. We can describe this kind of family structure as the "Leave It to Beaver" family or the "Ozzie and Harriet" family of television sit-com fame.

Traditional couples with young children comprised 27 percent of all households in 1990, down from 32 percent in 1980.

THE NON-TRADITIONAL FAMILY APPEARS
Since the 1950s the structure of the American family has changed again. Modern technology and social welfare seem to have reduced the need for a mother, father, and children to live together beyond the biological act of creation, for the physical survival of individuals is no longer dependent upon the survival of the biological family. The Leave-It-to-Beaver, Ozzie-and-Harriet type family has become the exception. Young adults still marry, establish homes together, and have children, but often these families break apart after a few years and re-structure in less traditional ways. Today more than one in three children lives in a single-parent family. Most dramatic of all, however, is that about 70 percent of families in America are not the traditional family with two biological parents.

THE BETTER LIFE INSTITUTE FAMILY HEALTH PLAN

Beyond Physical Survival

The story of the family is much more than the story of man's age-old struggle to survive physically. While economic necessity shaped the size and form of the family as a unit, it did not totally insure its survival and had little effect on the happiness of its members. Since the dawn of history the group that huddled around the warmth of a fire did not have only economic needs. Each member had the need for emotional support and companionship as well. They had feelings for each other. They "belonged" to each other, cared for each other, and supported each other.

The family provided purpose and meaning to life. There was a special sense of comfort and security within the family that did not exist between unrelated individuals. As centuries passed and the economic importance of family size diminished, love, caring, support, comfort, psychic security, and purpose were the glue that kept the family together.

It is fair to say that both economic need and affluence have shaped the contemporary American family into a group that is far different from anything it has ever been before. But always there has been that same glue, the "tie that binds." This too has made a difference. It has not only contributed to physical survival, it has helped to make life happy and has given it meaning.

Throughout history the power of economic necessity has ebbed and flowed, and undoubtedly will continue to fluctuate. Still regardless of nomadic, feudal, cottage, factory, or corporate conditions, there has always been caring, love, support, comfort, respect, and companionship in a family. These values transcend the shifts and changes of time and fortune. Simply stated, they *are* family. Without them the family unit withers. When this happens there is an erosion of love, caring, purpose, hope of life itself.

OUR NEW VALUES

Materialism, productivity, and profit have led to magnificent technological advancement and consequently vast improvement in our way of life. We agree that these modern changes have been very important and have made our daily lives easier. However they seem to have become the dominant forces in our lives. In fact the changes have begun to overshadow and to undermine many of the values that families have always thrived upon. Love, caring, support, morality, companionship, psychic security, and trust are not a part of "high tech." Instead the language of the modern technological world revolves around profit, productivity, speed, convenience, credit, expedi-

■ *Single mothers were the heads of 8 percent of all households in 1990, up from 7.5 percent in 1980.*

■ *Up from 1 percent in 1980, single-father households made up 1.5 percent of all households in 1990.*

■ *A new Census Bureau report states the number of single-father households has grown 82 percent since 1980, faster than any other type of household.*

ency, and immediacy. One unfortunate consequence of modern times is that in the minds of many, traditional *morality*, what has been defined as "right" as opposed to what is "wrong," has been replaced by legality, convenience, and the everybody-is-doing-it mindset.

Throughout history what was considered our second language, the language of economics, for many is now the primary language. Over time, the means of survival has slowly become the purpose of survival. The impact of the modern age on the human values that are the glue of family life has presented the American family with an unprecedented challenge.

"These are the times that try men's souls," those immortal words of Thomas Paine, have been applied to many situations since he first used them to describe our country's struggle for independence. Never before, however, have they so aptly described the situation facing the American family. We can paraphrase Paine's words to make them even more revealing: *These are the times that try families' souls.* We must each reach deep into every available resource if we are to meet this challenge.

SPIRITUALITY AND FAMILY VALUES

Throughout history a sense of spirituality has been the rallying point for family values. Every major religion in the world, whether Christianity, Judaism, Islam, Hinduism or Buddhism, places the value and unity of the family at the core of its beliefs. These religions all emphasize family values as the basic building blocks of personal and community life. Through the family, religion has attempted to provide to individuals moral guidance, psychological support, and a purpose for living.

In January 1988 *Better Homes and Gardens* magazine published a special report entitled "Are American Families Finding New Strength In Spirituality?" The purpose of the study was to assess whether spirituality and religion are important and relevant to families. After giving a questionnaire to a cross section of American families, the magazine discovered that religion and spirituality were indeed alive and well in American families. The major reasons the participating families gave for their desire for spirituality can be divided into four general categories:

1. A religious or spiritual life emphasizes the importance of the family and strengthens family bonds.
2. A religious or spiritual life provides guidance to all family members on right and wrong and how they should live and conduct themselves at home and away from home.
3. A religious or spiritual life gives the family members personal values that improve their character and personality.

4. A religious or spiritual life provides psychological security and a purpose in life.

Our Wellspring of Life

The spiritual person of modern times sees the family as the wellspring of life, the same perception of family as the nomad, feudal serf, tradesman, and factory worker of the past. For the spiritual person, the value of *family* is non-negotiable. It is the origin of feelings, experience, cooperation, honesty, a sense of value—all that is important in shaping the lives of the children. The family teaches faith, trust, compassion, self-respect, courage, forgiveness, gratitude, reverence, humility, purpose, brotherhood, and morality.

It is the basis for building every important personal quality for all members of the family. It is the basis for parents and children to learn how to live in this world. Everything that is truly important in life is learned in the family.

Everything that is truly important in life is learned in the family.

A Language of Spirituality

The challenge facing the American family today is to once again emphasize and live by the *first language* of life, the language of individual, family, and societal values. As the *Better Homes and Gardens* survey indicates, many families find religion and spirituality desirable guides for living in the modern world. For these families and countless others in America and the rest of the world, nothing new has to be created. We just have to start speaking and living a language of spirituality.

We can affirm the importance of family through our renewed commitment to a religious and spiritual way of life. Obviously there are other alternatives and we are not implying that one must, of necessity, be religious or spiritual in order to have a strong family life. But we think it ain't a bad idea! After all, it's been right in front of our noses for thousands of years.

Spirituality and Health

A BROAD SWEEP OF THE BRUSH

Several years ago we visited the Sistine Chapel at the Vatican in Rome, to see Michelangelo's fresco, "The Creation of Man." This brightly refurbished, centuries-old painting has inspired the spiritual imagination of millions, whether Christian, Jew, Muslim, or Buddhist. One cannot look at this scene on the chapel ceiling and not be struck by its overwhelming power. As we looked at it and tried to imagine the mind and the skill of the man who painted it, we became convinced this was one of the most inspired of all the world's art treasures.

The Hand of the Master

Michelangelo portrays the moment of creation when God reaches out and with a touch of His finger gives the spark of life to Adam. The expression in Adam's eyes is kindly and thankful and expectant of guidance. God's eyes are loving, firm, and purposeful. If you stand back and carefully study the eye contact between these two giant figures, you begin to understand that the mind of God is revealed along with his intent for Man. God is communicating his expectations to Adam about how Man should live and conduct himself on Earth. God seems to be saying, "I created you, but there's much more that I expect of you." The expression in Adam's eyes seems to be one of agreement, "I know, I'm thankful, I will try." There is no scene on earth that says so much about how Man should live than the one Michelangelo painted on the ceiling of that chapel in Rome over five hundred years ago.

I Expect Much More

Let's explore some of the expectations that God might have had of Man. We all agree that He was very specific about our personal relationships with Him. It would seem logical and consistent with God's intentions for Man to expect He had some thoughts about how Adam should take care of the physical body that God gave Adam in which to spend his earthly life. We can assume it was never discussed because it was so obvious. Who would think Man would not take care of the bodies God provided! It seems impossible to consider yourself a spiritual person unless you care for and cherish the body God gave you.

MAN'S WILL

If you look carefully at Adam's physique, you will see he is lean and well muscled. He does not have a pot belly or a double chin. And Eve, whose creation is depicted in another part of the fresco, does not have cellulite. God did not tell Adam and Eve or us to devour a 2,000 calorie brunch after going to church or synagogue. He did not intend for us to huff and puff after climbing two flights of stairs. It is not part of God's plan for us to die twenty years before our full natural, biological, God-given lifespan. In our opinion, it is not *God's will* that you smoke, have high blood pressure and too much cholesterol, be twenty pounds overweight, and die prematurely of a degenerative disease. All of that is your lifestyle—not His will! We are not saying that you have purposely decided that you will be unhealthy and sick, but that you have not decided you will be healthy! There's a *big* difference. We have not carried out the promise that shines in Adam's eyes on the Sistine Chapel ceiling: "I know, I'm thankful, I'll try."

Perhaps this interpretation of "The Creation of Man" associates your spirituality with your own and your family's health in a new way. A family life consistent with spiritual values is a challenge today in more ways than you might think. Practicing good health habits is more than a personal and family responsibility. It is a spiritual responsibility. We will take license and say that the family that eats and exercises together also, in a sense, is a family that prays together.

At the moments of our own creation, each of us has essentially looked into the mind and eyes of God. And, as He did with Adam, God has looked back at us and said, "I created you, but there's much more that I expect of you." So don't forget the health portion of your spiritual life. The gift of Creation has some moral and physical strings attached! You were given a strong, lean, and healthy body in top-notch working order. It is your spiritual responsibility to keep it that way—*healthfully ever after*.

> ■ *The family that eats and exercises together is, in a sense, a family that prays together.*

BODY, MIND, AND SOUL

Fifteen years ago any scientist discussing mind-body relationships was considered someone who was "out on the fringe." More than that he had to be very careful about what he said or he would be dismissed as a kook. But Psychosomatic Medicine with an emphasis on the relationship between mind and body had been an accepted field of medical practice for quite a few years. This branch of medicine treated asthma, headaches, and back pain. Studies had documented that these ailments improve with stress management treatment. There were also some reports that suggested the remarkable impact of Eastern Oriental meditation techniques on blood pressure and pain reduction and tolerance, but these methods were too unorthodox to be accepted by mainstream medicine. The field of Holistic Medicine was still considered "fringe" medicine.

The Mind-Body Connection

Ten years ago the late Norman Cousins, former editor of *The Saturday Review,* wrote the book *Anatomy of An Illness*. Mr. Cousins described how he used laughter to cure himself of a deadly form of inflammatory disease. At about the same time Dr. Kenneth Pelletier wrote *Mind as Healer, Mind as Slayer,* a remarkable book describing the power of one's mental state to cause, magnify, and cure illness. Since the early eighties the notion that our thinking affects our health has been well accepted. Today the science of Neuroendocrinology studies the fascinating chemical and hormonal changes that occur in the body as the result of emotions. Most scientists and physicians now accept the idea that our state of mind is directly related to our physiological status, our health.

The Healer and Killer Within

Exactly what does this mean to us in our everyday lives and how are mind-body relationships related to spirituality? It is quite simple. The moment we experience anger, stress, despair, or frustration, a complex cascade of chemical and hormonal changes race through our bodies. The adverse impact on our hearts, livers, brains, muscles, and other tissues causes them to tighten, spasm, constrict, elevate, and become inflamed. Conversely, when we experience joy, rapture, laughter, inner peace, and calmness, our bodies relax, feel soothed, reduced, and loosened. The mind can indeed, in the words of Dr. Pelletier, both "heal and slay."

The Internal Doctor

Mary Baker Eddy founded the Christian Science Church over one hundred years ago on a very simple belief: A deep faith and complete trust in God and a life lived in accordance with this faith, is enough to prevent or treat disease and to promote health. She had discovered the power of spirituality and faith as they relate to healing and promoting health. We might argue with Mary Baker Eddy about the extent to which she applied her beliefs, but we certainly do not find fault with her overall philosophy. Dr. Albert Schweitzer, Nobel Laureate and devout Christian, apparently would agree. Over fifty years ago, he noted that many people in his Lambarene, Gabon, missionary hospital got well without any known medical explanation. He said, "We must allow the doctor inside of them to help them get well."

We have already discussed the significant impact that leading a spiritual life can have on your family. Love, caring, support, hope, joy, comfort, and belonging are among the many emotions that are part of the everyday spiritual experience. These are very positive experiences that are relaxing, soothing, reducing, and loosening. It is hard to perceive how a sense of inner peace, rapture, purpose in life, security, and nurturance can be anything other than positive.

Today no one argues about the importance to family health of proper eating and exercise. The potential contribution that leading a spiritual life can make to health is equally significant. And let's not forget the double dividend you and the family receive—spirituality strengthens family ties. Living more spiritually does not require lots of fancy equipment, blinking screens, shiny stethoscopes, and modern medicines. Spirituality means a commitment to time-honored basics: in lifestyle, in relationships, in human conduct, and in how we live with each other. It's real, but it's just not "flashy"!

■ *THE BETTER LIFE INSTITUTE FAMILY HEALTH PLAN*

Health and "The Good Life"

MORAL LAW

C. S. Lewis, Oxford University Don and Cambridge University Professor of Medieval and Renaissance Literature, states that we all believe in some standard of behavior that stands above routine convention and is universal. In his book *Mere Christianity*, Lewis says that all people, regardless of race, culture, or ethnic origin, have subtle differences in their moralities, but the similarities far outweigh the differences. Lewis intended *Mere Christianity* to be an explanation of the basic concepts of Christianity. However, he also made a solid case that in the minds of all people there is "some kind of Law or Rule of fair play or decent behavior or morality or whatever you like to call it" about which we all really agree and by which we all try to live. This moral standard, what we could call a "higher law," is an integral part of the great religions of the world. Each is guided by a code of conduct found in their "written word," and, as Lewis points out, the higher laws of each religion are quite similar to those of all the others.

Everyday we hear ourselves or someone else say, "It's not fair," "That's wrong!" "I don't like what he is doing to that customer!" We often make these statements in connection with what we perceive to be inappropriate behavior, for there are many rights and wrongs in life. Some, however, are merely social convention. We have rules for the way we dress, our manners, how our children should behave, and other arbitrary rules for daily living. But all cultures agree there are some "rights and wrongs" that are not merely for convention but are actually necessary for people to live in safety and security. They are usually fundamental parts of spiritual and religious moral law.

Laws of Human Nature

These moral laws are what Professor Lewis calls *Laws of Human Nature*. People should not steal, should not lie, and should be fair. It is important to have courage, self-discipline, and will power. Honesty is right and cheating others is wrong. It is good to love, honor, and cherish, to have gratitude and reverence, and to be humble. We teach our children to be kind, considerate, and caring, and to respect their elders. The subtle differences in the ways different cultures apply these laws of human nature do not diminish their universality. We all know there is a Law that holds above and beyond all the little circumstances of our lives. It is there. We know it is there. And we try to obey it. We teach the law to our children and we expect others to live by it too. There are behavioral and social consequences when we do and when we don't. There are also physiological and health consequences.

HEALTH: IN THOUGHT AND DEED

Endocrine specialists have studied the physiological and health consequences our thoughts and actions have on our bodies. This fascinating area of scientific study has revealed that each time we do or truly intend to do something that we know is "good," wonderful responses happen inside our bodies. When we obey the Laws of Human Nature, our greater sense of right and wrong, we trigger a cascade of healthful chemical and hormonal reactions in our bodies which soothe, calm, relax, and "open" us. Each time we do or truly intend to do something that we know is "bad," the action or thought causes anxiety and stress. The consequent cascade of chemicals and hormones inflame, constrict, tighten, and "elevate." Since a strong, living sense of spirituality or religion encourages us to strive to live by our "rights" and avoid our "wrongs," we have continuous opportunities to improve our health or threaten it.

By affirming moral law in our daily decisions, we affirm the responses our bodies make that favor good health—a triple dividend of mind, body, and soul.

Spirituality places standards and judgments on how we live our lives every day. Regardless of our religion or spiritual calling, we have opportunities every day to live according to our basic moral beliefs. The wonderful thing about these opportunities is that they are present in all life situations. Every moment of our lives, we and every member of our families are faced with challenges and decisions relating to "right" and "wrong." Each thought we have and action we decide to take provides us a new opportunity to decide in favor of "right" or moral law. By affirming moral law in our daily decisions, we affirm the response our bodies make that favor good health.

The "Natural Juices" That Can Save Lives

Spirituality teaches us there are consequences to all our actions. We just have never thought the consequences reach everything we experience! But they do. Soon the science of Endocrinology will be able to detect these subtle positive and negative changes and the ways in which they affect our health. (Certainly God has always been an Endocrinologist—we're the ones who are just beginning to catch on!) The bottom line is that we just can't escape or hide from the emotional responses of our bodies. Our sense of spirituality and the sense of each family member is always with us controlling our "juices." Get those "juices" going in the right direction, toward improved health. It could save your life and give you a wonderful day at the same time!

You can't go wrong by affirming your own and your family's spiritual life—at home, work, school, and play. The basic principles and teachings strengthen and enrich family life. In fact they are the very foundation of family life, and the extra bonuses are more than just bonuses. They are "lifegiving"! Spirituality and the experience of living closely to moral truth leads to more healthful physiological

314

conditions. Did you ever buy a share of stock and find out the next day it tripled in value? Well, that's just what will happen to you. Besides being spiritually rich, you will also be healthfully rich!

SPIRITUALITY: FIRST THOUGHT, THEN DEED

The good news about leading a spiritual life is that it provides us endless opportunities for happiness. All we have to do is strive to live by our most treasured personal values. We don't wear, buy, or negotiate spirituality, we live it. It is inside of us all the time. It is a way of seeing, feeling, and acting. Every living moment is an opportunity for you to live or deny your spirituality.

The bad news is that there's nowhere to hide from spirituality because it focuses first on your thoughts and motivations and *then* on your deeds. Every action, every thought, every moment of your life is a reflection of your "being." Others may never know, but you cannot escape your own innermost judgments of how every thought and action of your life affirms or denies Moral Law. What a wonderful opportunity! What a wonderful gift!

We mentioned earlier the mythical *Star Wars* version of "The Force," a state of mind and being within Luke and Obi Wan Kenobi. To use "The Force," they had to allow themselves to "feel it." You should consider your sense of spirituality a living megaversion of "The Force," your "Spiritual Force." It is there inside of you wherever you go, whatever you do. Every moment of your life presents you a new opportunity to use it. It is in you always.

As an example, suppose you gave twenty dollars to a community charity. On the surface this seems to be a spiritual act, but it may not be "spiritual." A spiritual act depends first on motive and then on behavior. The spirituality of your donation depends on a number of factors:

- Whether twenty dollars is a little or a lot of money to you.
- Whether you gave it with love or gave it grudgingly because you "had to."
- Whether the motive was that you cared or that you wanted a tax deduction.
- Whether the charity was important to you and you felt part of its "community."

Living a spiritual life never lets you "off the hook." Since spirituality teaches that thought is primary and deed is secondary, there is forgiveness if the deed goes astray. It's your motivation and your intent to live by your higher law that counts. Others may not know, but

Few children grow up remembering the house was always spotless, but they do remember the good times and the bad times. They remember the holidays and vacations and special times when the family laughed, danced, and enjoyed one another. Build a positive legacy for your children and begin today.

you always know what motivates you. Because the thought-deed quotient always applies, you must constantly face and correct the inconsistencies between your values and your actions, and you'll likely do better because of it. Spirituality provides a fail-safe system for peace of mind and self-respect—it's a true source of happiness.

Live and Teach Your Family: Do the Right Thing

Make sure you discuss the thought-deed aspect of spirituality with your children. Since it may be a difficult concept for little children, we ask that you discuss it many times. Always ask young children, "What did you *really* think when you did it?" Help them explore their motivations and intents in a supportive manner. Make sure you do not leave them with the impression that their thoughts are "bad," but that they need to improve a little at times just as you do. It's really quite wonderful when spirituality becomes your lifestyle. And like everything that's good in your life, you will need to give it all of your support. Just like your new eating and exercise habits, your new spirituality needs continuous discussion and nurturing.

The "Ten Suggestions"

We have several practical suggestions for daily living that we provide the Better Life Institute families. We call them "The Ten Suggestions." We know there could be many more depending on your personal views and faith, but from our years of experience, these ten seem to "hit the nail on the head" for both parent and child. We cannot overemphasize the value of discussing these ten points with your family. They contain some immensely important general principles. They will bring on lively discussions if presented during Family Circle. The best part about these suggestions is that they require you to practice actions you already have used many times in your lives. You and your family will not have to read any books or learn anything new or complicated.

I

FORGIVE YOURSELF AND OTHERS.

Most people don't let go of their mistakes and regrets very easily. We have spent many hours with people who have not forgiven themselves for a significant mistake. They can't stop punishing themselves for something that happened in the past. The psychological motivation for holding on is less important than the spiritual rationale for letting go. Spirituality teaches us to analyze less and be more forgiving and accepting of our own imperfect natures. Forgiving yourself may not come easily at first. Practice it. You'll like the results. You'll be liberated to move on with the rest of your life. Once you've learned to forgive yourself, you'll need to learn to forgive others for the mistakes they have made. It is equally as important.

Our past work at Hospice has given us the opportunity to help terminally ill people prepare for what lies beyond the illness. During these very precious last moments of life, differences, feuds, and deep hurts involving loved ones are forgiven. We fully understand why this happens at that time, but it strikes us that if one is willing to forgive and forget during the last moments of life, how about doing it a few hours before that? or a few weeks? or a few years? or right now? Our spirituality teaches us that family, relationships, understanding, and compassion are far more important than the reasons for a disagreement or a feud. Spirituality helps us to see the truth and meaning of our lives.

The next time you have the opportunity to forgive and forget a past mistake you have made or when you believe someone has wronged you, put this suggestion to practice. Ask at Family Circle if there is anyone who has forgiven something or some one this past week or if anyone would like to be forgiven. Remind everyone that "He who is without sin [imperfection] should cast the first stone." You won't be chucking them at others and you can bet you won't get hit by any other person's stones. The quality of forgiveness does not come overnight. It will take a while so you might as well start today. You might be surprised at the results!

II

HAVE REVERENCE FOR LIFE AND NATURE—USE YOUR SPIRITUAL EYES.

What do you *see* when you sit down to dinner with your family? You see the roast chicken, of course, and the salad and mashed potatoes. You see the kids with food on their faces. You see your spouse across the table talking to you. While we all can see with our eyes, spirituality teaches to see with our hearts.

At the dinner table your spiritual eyes *see* a precious moment: the mind, body, and soul of your family sitting down together to break bread. Spiritual eyes help us *see* the immeasurable value of what is simple and readily available in our lives. Even an argument between two loved ones is seen differently through spiritual eyes as a natural expression of "I care." Your spiritual *touch, smell, taste,* and *hearing* can bring vastly different and exciting experiences to family life. Think of how the air would taste and smell, the birds would sound, and the touch of your child's hand would feel at the moment you awaken after life-saving critical surgery when you are grateful that these sensations are still yours to have. There are some marvelous things—even miracles—in our lives right now every day. You just need to see them.

Tonight at your family dinner, take a few moments and practice this new way of seeing. Look carefully at everyone in your family and ask yourself, *What does this evening meal really mean to me and everyone in the family?* Ask each member of the family what they truly see. And why not use all of your senses? Start to practice this kind of super-aerobic seeing, smelling, touching, tasting, and hearing and you will begin to notice all the incredible sensations life offers. It could do more for your health than exercise.

III

VALUE INNER GROWTH.

Far too often people equate personal growth with the size of a bank account, the mastery of a foreign language, or a valuable job skill. We agree that these aspects of life are important, but there are many aspects of personal growth that are often overlooked when winning the "rat race" gets out of perspective.

Spiritual values emphasize the need for inner growth. All the values we have discussed in this section are part of your spiritual growth. And, as with your bank account, golf swing, or sewing skill, inner growth requires time, attention, and practice. Think of your commitment to inner growth as taking on another hobby, but instead of looking down at a golf ball or a sewing needle, you're looking inside yourself. You've no idea what pleasant surprises you may find!

Take a pencil and pad and jot down one inner-growth quality you'd like to practice for the next week. Opportunities for practice will present themselves at every moment of the day, you just have to see them. This is a wonderful activity for Family Circle as well.

IV

LIGHTEN UP—PEOPLE ARE FUNNY.

In his book *Anatomy of an Illness*, Norman Cousins called laughter "internal jogging." Humor, smiles, and laughter release many chemicals and hormones that relax your body. We know how wonderfully relaxed we feel after laughing at a good joke or watching a funny film, but sometimes people think that laughter or a giggle is childish behavior and not appropriate for adults. Most of us place a high value on trying to be a serious person, but there is nothing inconsistent with adulthood or a serious approach to life and including a lot of laughter every day. Let that little kid hidden in you come out once in a while. The little kid in you might enjoy cavorting with your own children. Let loose, play a little, and get your hands deep in the sandbox of life.

The place to begin to see some humor in life is with yourself. Perhaps you are lucky enough to have a spouse or kids who see the humor in things you do everyday that don't seem funny to you. Stand back and take a look at what they see in you that they think is funny. Remember, instead of laughing *at you,* they are laughing *with you* if you will allow yourself to laugh. Many of our personality quirks are very humorous. You just need to allow yourself to see them. When you let your family see that you have a sense of humor about yourself, they will begin to see themselves in the same way. Some of the most wonderful and memorable experiences we can have are to learn laughter and good-natured humor from our children.

Teach your children to enjoy the lighter side of life. Practice with them. Make a point to "lighten up" the atmosphere when Family Circle gets a little "heavy." Everyone will learn from the experience. We also suggest you rent funny video tapes for family evenings at home.

V

BE IN THE PRESENT—DON'T LIVE YOUR LIFE ON HOLD.

Our society is very future oriented. Most of us are so busy planning for the future that we forget about where we are right now. We ignore or don't notice the wonderful experiences we have everyday because we're thinking about what we'll do when we retire, or how we'll spend our next vacation, or how wonderful it will be to have grandchildren, or how we're going to get a promotion. Living only for the future instead of being in the immediate present is an easy habit to fall into, especially when we see our everyday lives as routine. If we take for granted what we have now and habitually dream of what is coming down the pike, we miss the joys and satisfactions of being alive, and we miss the opportunities we have today that we may not have in the future. A spiritual life places value on planning for the future, of course, but it places a greater value on living to the fullest in the present.

We once knew a wonderfully talented woman who kept putting off the things she could do for herself and for her community and friends until there was a better time. She thought the better time for her would be when her children were in college. She had so much to give to so many worthwhile projects, but she said all of that would occur in just a few more years. She was waiting, always waiting. She was living her life on hold. Tragically she died young of a brain tumor. Not only was she never able to fulfill her destiny, she was never able to begin to try. By living her life on hold, she cheated herself, her family, and the surrounding world of her gifts as a human being. Unfortunately many people live their lives on hold, waiting for this situation to be finished, that goal to be reached, some circumstance to change.

Do you share the habit of listening to your children or your spouse with only one ear while you think about a few other things? Does the phrase "You're not listening to me" sound familiar? Practice listening to your family, regardless of whether you already know what they'll be saying. Listening to people you care about conveys an important message to them. It says, "I value you as a person enough to listen and pay attention to you." It also teaches them to approach others in their lives in the same manner.

Settle down, perk up your ears and mind, and just tell yourself at Family Circle, "I'm going to listen to my family members despite the fact that I've heard it all before." You may hear familiar words, but we guarantee the experience will be very different for all of you. And talk to your family about planning for the future while living in the present.

VI

ALLOW YOURSELF TO TRUST.

One of the unfortunate facts of life is that people sometimes hurt our feelings, violate a personal confidence, or do things to us that they know are not in our best interests. Let's step past the psychological reasons for why we feel hurt or why someone hurts us because spiritually we must consider our options based upon these experiences.

We can either never trust any part of ourselves to another, or we can place such a high value on trust that it doesn't matter if that trust is violated. Never trusting leads to a negative and hostile view of life. The second choice, which is based firmly upon spiritual teaching, leads to a positive view of life and of people. Trust is an absolutely essential ingredient in the experience of a sincere relationship. Without trust, a personal relationship becomes impersonal.

When you trust you expose yourself to the risk of having your

THE BETTER LIFE INSTITUTE FAMILY HEALTH PLAN

trust violated, for if there were no risk, the term *trust* would have no meaning. The basis of spirituality is to live in a spiritual state of mind about yourself and about others, and it is practiced in spite of whether it's deserved or earned by others. Trust is accepting and valuing people as they are, not as you would like them to be. It is a quality we are born with that we begin to use at the moment of birth. Sadly along the way some of us lose it.

Unqualified trust in others is probably the most difficult personal quality to acquire. Trust requires "a leap of faith." It is basic to a spiritual way of life!

VII

PRACTICE SELF-DISCIPLINE AND EARN SELF-RESPECT.

Living a spiritual life requires living with values and actions that may not be the easiest, most convenient to practice. The real challenge, however, is that self-discipline includes both mind and deed. Every day throughout our lives we are faced with countless opportunities to practice self-discipline at home, work, school, and play. The opportunities for practice exist whether you are facing a just-baked chocolate chip cookie or a cold, dark morning for exercise. Remember the old saying, "He who conquers himself is worth more to God than he who conquers a city"? The speaker was referring to the difficult practice of self-discipline, and he was right. A self-disciplined person is a spiritual person and a tribute to God.

The practice of self-discipline leads to two very important personal experiences: self-respect and personal freedom. The act of making your actions consistent with your personal values is the only way you can acquire self-respect. And only through self-discipline are you able to do what you feel is important to you. These acts of self-discipline lead to your personal freedom. No one can give to you or take from you your self-respect or your personal freedom. You're the only person who can earn them and you're the only one who can lose them. Because self-respect and personal freedom are so vital it is particularly important that we teach self-discipline to our children. They need inner guidance for the how, when, and why to say "No" to potentially dangerous or unhealthy situations.

Improving eating and exercise habits are wonderful opportunities for you and your family to acquire self-respect and freedom through self-discipline. At Family Circle you can ask each member of your family if they can recall a moment during the past week when they had to use some self-discipline. It's a precious gift that goes a long, long way in life.

VIII

CALM YOURSELF—DON'T DO, JUST BE.

We often ask the question, "What is the most important consequence of living a spiritual life?" The most common reply is "inner
peace." In their spirituality, many people find a sense of security,
being taken care of, restfulness, and ultimately peace. It is a settling,
calming, and wonderfully revitalizing feeling to experience. Usually,
however, we don't experience these feelings while driving in traffic or
shopping in the supermarket. We have to deliberately take time
away from our harried days and revitalize ourselves with our own
sense of spirituality.

Americans place great value on doing, achieving, and striving.
While these traits are important, there are other less aggressive
traits that should hold an equally important value for us. Someone
once mentioned to us that the way to comprehend the concept of
calming is to understand the difference between "Don't just stand
there—do something!" and "Don't do something—just stand there."
Begin Family Circle by asking everyone to imagine for a few minutes
a quite relaxing scene. It is when we calm ourselves that we get a
spiritual refueling. For some, calming is prayer. For others, it is lying
in bed before the alarm clock goes off, a walk in the park, a favorite
tune on the radio, or a quiet moment with your eyes closed. The nice
part about spirituality is that you don't really have to learn it or buy
it. Your spirituality is always there. You just have to "see" it and
allow it to fill you up!

IX

BE GRATEFUL AND PRACTICE HUMILITY.

Did you ever think that maybe, just maybe, you are a guest who
only participates here on earth? Could you ever conceive of the notion
that you aren't the epicenter of the universe and of life in general?
It's a worthwhile attitude to consider. One of the easiest ways to give
this some serious thought is to walk outside on a night when the sky
is filled with stars and just gaze at them for a while. It sort of puts
everything into perspective, the kind of perspective Steven Hawkings
has about himself. A noted astrophysicist and discoverer of black
holes, when asked about his uniqueness Hawkings remarked casu-
ally, "The earth is a small planet in the solar system of a minor universe in a small corner of a galaxy in a million million galaxies."

Sometimes, we're so busy with ourselves, other people, and other
things that we loose our perspective. We don't stop and take time to

THE BETTER LIFE INSTITUTE FAMILY HEALTH PLAN

smell the roses as the saying goes. Stand back for a few moments and be an observer. You could be looking at a butterfly, or the rain, or a newborn baby, or maybe even the Space Shuttle. When you let yourself really "see," you begin to contemplate the wonder of all things and of all people, and your sense of spirituality deepens. A sense of spirituality provides you and your family with additional perspective on what our place is in the scheme of things. This perspective builds humility in human beings.

Family Circle can focus everyone on gratitude. Ask a simple question to each member of the family: "What are you thankful for this week?" We all have something to appreciate every day of our lives, but most of us have to practice noticing these things. Parents, teach your children by example. Be thankful for life, for love, for family, for friends, for the beauties of nature. Appreciate it all because we don't have it forever. And, give thanks.

Spirituality implies that there is "something" higher and greater than all of us. It implies more meaning to the wonder in our lives. All of this tends to dwarf the day-to-day experiences that seem so important at the time they happen. Because of this wonder, we cannot help but feel gratitude and humility for being allowed to be here for a while to see and participate. Gratitude gives you some perspective on the importance of a football game, a new car, or the lawn your son didn't mow in relation to the brief moment in time that we visit this spot "in a million million galaxies."

X

DO AS YOU WOULD BE DONE TO.

We do not live by ourselves. We live in our parent's families. We live in our own families. We live in our community and work families. We live in America. We live in the Family of Man. Our sense of spirituality tells us we live in relationship to all others and all things. We have obligations and responsibilities since we're "all in the same boat," and others have the same obligations and responsibilities to us. Hundreds of years ago Sir Isaac Newton said, "Every action has an equal and opposite reaction." He was not the first to observe that every action has some kind of result, he was just the first scientist to discover the "opposite reaction" part.

With no exceptions, our sense of spirituality should provide each of us with very specific guidelines for how we should live in all of our families. One of our basic non-negotiable rules of conduct is what we have known all our lives as the "Golden Rule": "Do unto others as you would have them do unto you." In this simple statement lies the meaning of the worth of the individual and of all things. If we value the idea of loving, honoring, and supporting ourselves, we must also value the concept of loving, honoring, and supporting others. Sometimes the other person's reaction is not the one we expected. However, it's your reaction that is your spiritual objective. In the final analysis all people and things depend upon each other for existence. When we break the "Golden Rule," we risk our personal existence and the existence of everyone and everything else.

Perhaps this sounds a bit melodramatic to you, but we don't think it is. Consider the importance of the "Golden Rule" to you and to your family. "For every action, there is an equal and opposite reaction" applies to your family, community, and country—to the world. Whatever you give, whether it's from mind or deed may take a little longer to get back, but what goes around indeed does come around. When you talk to your child, spouse, parents, friends, business colleagues, or even your pet rock, you should take care to do as you would be done to.

There are two simple questions that everyone in the family should learn to ask: "How does the other guy feel?" and "Would I like the same thing done to me?" Remember, we're all in the same family!

AMEN

If there is any common thread woven among the "Ten Suggestions," it is to *see, touch, taste, smell* and *hear life* with highly attuned senses. A strong sense of spirituality is the special ingredient that magnifies your senses. As you sense life more deeply, everything in your life seems to change for the better.

It has not been our intent to convert you to any specific religious or spiritual calling. However, we do not wish to hide our personal and strong commitment to a spiritual way of life. We feel that if you haven't thought about it already, such a potentially significant experience in family life merits another "peek." A young mother who was a respondent in the *Better Homes and Gardens* survey, echoed our sentiments precisely when she said, "I was content to explore my own spiritual and religious needs and beliefs at a relaxed pace until I took on the job of modeling life for two little people."

We have deliberately avoided any theological discussion and have concentrated on generic spiritual concepts that strengthen the family unit. That was not because of our lack of commitment to a belief in God or religion but because we want to respect the individual religious differences of our readers. We have observed, however, that just as the belief in God creates a sense of inner peace for the individual, it also provides the same experience for the family. And, regardless of your diet and exercise habits, adherence to the values of your religion can also bring to you a special sense of self-esteem and respect. Remember those soothing, relaxing, and reducing effects of the endocrine system!

We think spirituality can be a significant, enriching, enlightening force in your lives. We are convinced that very few people are totally lacking in a sense of spirituality. We know it evokes a great deal of emotion in people, both positive or negative. We also believe a sense of spirituality can contribute a great deal to your family's future. It would be nice to provide your loved ones with a legacy of values to anchor them in this stormy sea of life. A spiritual and religious life is one way to accomplish that.

YES, I CAN!

- I can help our children develop new interests and skills by encouraging them to try a new activity, book, food, or audio tape each week.
- I can try to make our home a happy home by doing some simple things each week. I can remember to smile at my children at every possible opportunity regardless of whether there is a reason.
- I can ask everyone in the family "How did your day go?" every day.

FAMILY CIRCLE SUGGESTIONS

Ask each member of the family to tell the rest of the family how he or she did over the past week keeping personal promises.

One of the sayings in a Chinese fortune cookie says, "Get your mind set and aware. . . . Your actions will follow." Ask the family what this means?

Ask if there is anyone in the family who would like to tell the rest of the family about a moment in the past week when he or she really trusted someone.

Family Health: 2000 A.D. and Beyond

■ ■

Several years ago the Senate Select Committee on Aging and the House of Representatives Special Committee on Aging impaneled a commission and instructed its members to try to predict our scientific and medical capability over the next thirty years to increase health and length of life. About twenty eminent scientists were named to the commission. Each of them represented one of the nation's most distinguished medical institutions and had been involved in research on health and longevity for at least the previous fifteen years.

This was the first time in history the United States government had commissioned a study of this kind. These medical scientists were asked specifically to predict future health challenges in America as well as to define our ability to effectively treat the challenges of the degenerative diseases we now face. These diseases significantly effect the health of American families and we know the effects will continue. Today's parents face degenerative diseases in the immediate future, and the current generation of children will have to deal with these diseases in twenty, thirty, or forty years.

What can the American family expect of science and medicine in the year 2000? What will be our capability to improve health and extend life in twenty years, or in thirty years? Will our children suffer from these diseases as much during their adult lives as adults do now?

The commission's report states that our ability to improve the quality and length of life through science and technology is rapidly increasing every year. According to the commission, we will be able to conquer degenerative disease in the next twenty years. When we enter the second decade of the twenty-first century, Americans can look forward to living up to and beyond one hundred years of age. But these achievements will require a radical departure from current medical practice. Why will the "new" science and the treatment of traditional degenerative diseases so radically depart from current medical practices? A part of the answer is found in the history of the development of knowledge of all kinds.

Science Then and Now

Humans began to use a written language about 3500 B.C. when the Sumerians and the people of the Indus Valley City States first wrote on tablets. The term *etched in stone* truly describes the writings of these ancient civilizations. For the first time man had the ability to record thoughts, daily activities, ideas, and feelings.

Just think how different life was before there was a written language. All knowledge had to be trusted to memory. Only with spoken word could people exchange ideas and fact. This indeed placed severe limits on repeating what was done or learned during a day or the week before. It was difficult to improve upon what was thought about the day before or to share those thoughts with others either for enjoyment or for information. Before written language the only way to preserve ideas, the development of skills, or the knowledge of tradition was to personally relate them to others from memory or carry them into the future in the form of pictures, songs, or stories.

HEY, TELL ME THE NEWS

We are so accustomed to our written language that we take a great deal for granted when we read the newspaper, the Bible, or a book such as this one, or write a letter to a friend. Remember that the bicycle you bought for your child last Christmas had a picture and the phrase "easy to assemble" on the label? Would you like to try to assemble it without the instruction booklet? And without a written recipe, how would you prepare that wonderful recipe from Italy for "Chicken alla Pappagallopecorinofortissimo" or something else truly delectable?

A record of what others have learned helps us when we want to do the same thing or have a need to know the same kind of information. Otherwise when we want to assemble bicycles or prepare dishes that are new to us, we would each have to "re-invent the wheel" so to speak by starting at the very beginning and learning all over again by trial-and-error what someone else has already learned.

While putting together bicycles and cooking Italian chicken dishes does not seem so important in the overall scheme of things, the same kind of accumulation of knowledge is of enormous value to the areas of investigation that can affect health, longevity, and qual-

■ *THE BETTER LIFE INSTITUTE FAMILY HEALTH PLAN*

ity of life. The accumulation of knowledge is what allows scientists and specialists to take the next steps toward unraveling the mysteries of physical health.

THE MARCH OF SCIENCE: A ROLLING SNOWBALL

After the development of written language, life was altered forever. Societies could retain, transmit, and improve knowledge in every area of life. Historians estimate that just before we developed the written word, it took about ten thousand years for the accumulation of human knowledge and skill to double. With the development of written language, the amount of time needed to double scientific and technical know-how was reduced to one thousand years. With each succeeding century both the accumulation of knowledge and its rate of growth has increased. By the time the printing press was developed in the fifteenth century, it took about one hundred fifty years for the accumulation to double. Today with computers and almost instantaneous communication with anywhere in the world, the fund of scientific and technical knowledge doubles every two-and-one-half years!

We don't rely only on pen and paper or simple machines anymore to communicate. We use computers and electronic devices and in a few years communication will be almost entirely through fiber optics and laser beams. And the speed of communication is directly related to the accumulation of knowledge and consequently, the amount and rate of increase continually snowball. It is estimated that by the year 2000 scientific knowledge will double in only two years. This staggering amount of information will need to be handled carefully for already scientists have difficulty keeping up with the wealth of new knowledge available. We have to spend hours each week reading abstracts and reviews of articles and reports. Most of us subscribe to computer search systems to help us obtain the information we need. Truly the world is in the midst of a mega-information explosion.

A Nation of Older People

In what way is this science and technology explosion important to you and your family? It directly affects the quality of your life in the future. In 1980 about 30,000 people lived to be one hundred years old. Today there about 50,000 centenarians. By the year 2000 we will have about 100,000, and we estimate that in the year 2050 there will be over one million people who are 100 or older. There is, however, a problem with these estimates. They were made in 1990 with 1990's scientific and medical knowledge. As the speed at which we accumulate and develop new knowledge continues to increase, what will be our estimates of the expected number of centenarians with 2000 science and medicine, or with 2010 or 2025 science and medicine? Keeping up is like trying to catch a shooting star.

THE "GRAYING" OF AMERICA
Percent Change of Total Population from 1980

AGE	IN THE YEAR 2000	IN THE YEAR 2020
20–39	−1%	−10%
40–64	+44%	+70%
65+	+25%	+52%

Number of 100 Year Olds

1980	1990	2000	2050
30,000	50,000	100,000	1,000,000

United States Public Health Service, 1990

A Bigger Snowball
Do you remember your high school science and biology courses? When we were in high school we were amazed at the fantastic world we saw under those simple microscopes. We studied the cell walls of onions and memorized the periodic table of chemical elements, but today's high school students have a different science curriculum. They discuss RNA and DNA, genetics, and the molecular structure of living cells. Our science fiction was Captain Video, Rocket Man, and men from Mars. Theirs is *Star Wars,* quark and neutrino particles, outer galaxy probes, and Black Holes. It took thousands and thousands of years to accumulate the knowledge we have at this moment in science and medicine, but it will take only about two years to double that knowledge!

THE TIMES THEY ARE A CHANGIN'
The families of the past faced different health challenges from the ones we face today. And healthwise our children's families will live in a far different world. But one thing's for sure: There are going to be many more one hundred-year-old grandmas and grandpas around when your grandchildren are growing up! The degenerative diseases that we face today will be treated more effectively and cured more frequently. We won't be able to totally prevent degenerative disease because we won't be able to prevent old age. But it's likely we will delay the onset of old age until we are well into our eighties.

■ *THE BETTER LIFE INSTITUTE FAMILY HEALTH PLAN*

The Scientific and Medical Triumphs
of the Past

In the year 25 A.D. Seneca, who was Emperor Nero's tutor, said, "Man does not die; he kills himself." What this famous Roman philosopher meant was that at that time, 25 A.D., we killed ourselves by virtue of the manner in which we lived. The basic challenges to health of food, shelter, exhaustion from hard work, or infectious disease did us in before we could get to be old. By 1940 science and medicine in the Western World had all but eliminated the traditional killers of adults and children. The threats of cholera, typhoid fever, the poxes and plagues, intestinal diseases, infections, infested water, and lack of food had been conquered. Our scientists and physicians had used the accumulation of knowledge of drugs and surgical procedures to virtually wipe out these killers. Public Health officials had vastly improved our sanitation facilities. Our babies were given inoculations and vaccinations against diseases that had routinely killed thousands of children only a few decades earlier and our farmers provided us with ample food for our tables. We survive and live longer now because we do not die from those factors that have killed people prematurely since the beginning of time.

Degenerative Disease and the Realities
of the Present

As people began to live longer, our bodies began to age and to acquire the illnesses of aging that we call degenerative disease. In what seems to be a peculiar turn of events, we are privileged to be the first generation in history to die routinely of something other than trauma or infectious disease. But our drugs, surgical techniques, and other high tech procedures, no matter how complex or electronically dazzling, are not curative. They cannot do to degenerative disease what we were able to do to infectious disease. Seneca is still right. We don't die; we kill ourselves. We just kill ourselves in different ways.

Science and medicine are moving at blinding speed into a future when these diseases of premature aging will be better treated and ultimately their onset can be delayed. They will not be cured, but they will be significantly postponed. It's difficult, perhaps impossible, to cure a person of old age. Since we can be certain that people will continue to live longer lives, we want to focus on the quality of life we will have during those years. Quality of life—in a nutshell that's what this book is about.

The Future: Truly, a World of Wonders

Already we have the glimmerings of our medical future. Several years ago there was a popular television show, "The Six Million Dollar Man." The hero was a pilot who was so severely injured experimental medical procedures were used as a last recourse to save his life. He was equipped with bionic parts that replaced his arms, legs, eyes, and even parts of his brain. In the fine tradition of Superman, the bionic man could truly run fast, see through metal, and "leap tall buildings in a single bound!"

Even though the six million dollar man was a made-up story, it was not entirely foolish. Today biomedical engineering has made the replacement of certain organs and functions a reality. New materials replace damaged artery walls, heart valves, and worn out hips and elbows. Special alloy screws, plates, and wires are commonplace in severe trauma surgical procedures. Corneal implants, cardiac pacers, and insulin pumps are synthetic systems that are routinely placed in our bodies. Our children are part of an emerging age where actual organs can be transplanted. Now that heart and kidney transplants have become routine, we are replacing livers and lungs and may soon be able to do even more. We can honestly say the prose has been written, but the real poetry and music have yet to be sung.

THE CUTTING EDGE OF SCIENCE
In the late 1950's two scientists, James Watson and Francis Crick, raced to discover the genetic secret of human life. In their book *The Double Helix*, they describe the blow-by-blow scientific adventure that changed the course of our biological world. They had discovered the structure of RNA and DNA which is the basic "stuff" that carries the genetic code—all the information that every living cell needs to maintain and reproduce itself. From that moment our understanding of life processes was fundamentally changed. Subsequent decades of basic scientific research have brought us to the cutting edge of the useful application of our knowledge of RNA and DNA to human health and disease treatment.

At this very moment, medical researchers are attempting to treat children with severe genetic-based disease by inserting corrected genes into their blood cells. The implications for this type of approach to the treatment and prevention of disease is profound. The results will change the course of medical treatment forever.

A BRIDGE BY ANY OTHER NAME

What does this mean in terms we can all understand? In prehistoric times if a tribal chief came to a large river, he and his followers would have to find a narrow place where they could wade or swim across. In 3500 B.C. if an Etruscan or Sumerian king came to the same river, he could cross the river by building a bridge with a log that reached from bank to bank. If the river was too wide for one log, they could put support posts in the river bed to extend the bridge. Many centuries later if a Roman emperor came to the same river, he could instruct his workers to build a stone bridge with an arch. King Richard and Napoleon could use the same techniques. However, if the river was too wide for one arch, they would have their workers build several arches supported by stone pillars.

If Teddy Roosevelt came to the same river, he could have his engineers span it with metal girders and pillars made of concrete. Franklin Roosevelt, John F. Kennedy, and George Bush could span it with metal and cables suspended from either side. This high-tech bridge would use lighter and stronger alloys than the materials used to build earlier bridges. We may want to call the new, improved bridge by some modern name, but it's still a bridge. It would be recognized by the tribal chieftain, Etruscan, Roman emperor and everyone else as a bridge. The only difference is that it is a better bridge.

The same is not true of our future medicine. No one from any former era would recognize the medicine and treatments we are on the verge of using. We are at the dawning of a new age which will encompass a completely different approach from any ever applied before to disease treatment and health. Future medicine will not use new drugs and better materials, stick artificial things into our bodies, or transplant parts from one person to another. Those improvements are the same as building a better bridge, for no matter how modern or sleek, a bridge is still a bridge. But the new Golden Age of Medicine is just around the corner. And the bridge it will build will be a very different kind—in fact, it won't be a bridge.

The Golden Age of Medicine

In the new era just ahead scientists will be able to influence basic life processes by changing the actual behavior of cells and genes. The medicine of the future will not blast, cut, burn, patch, replace or "nuke." It will harness the very powerful processes of biological life itself to improve health and cure disease. Medical scientists will be able to instruct our natural disease-fighting systems to destroy or cure a budding or existing disease process. New drugs will mimic our immune systems or replace parts of them. Hormones exactly like those in our bodies will be substituted for older, tired ones. Genes that are defective or destined to cause certain diseases will be detected at birth, snipped out, and replaced with healthy ones. Many diseases that have eluded treatment are about to topple with these new approaches. Imminent breakthroughs for cystic fibrosis, Tay-Sachs disease, and certain inherited blood diseases are the first candidates to herald in this Golden Age of Medicine.

We will be able to harness and program the very processes of life itself to give life, improve life, and extend life. If we compare this magnificent advance to our analogy of a bridge, and the ways in which people of various times would build one, the medical advances possible in the golden age will be like standing on the banks of the river and causing the earth and stones on each side to grow up and span and "birth" a natural bridge. Parents who could not otherwise conceive will be able to have children. Infants who would normally enter life with severe defects will have these defects corrected before birth and have healthy long lives. Adults with diseases that usually have been terminal in nature will be cured and able to play with their grandchildren once again.

LIVING TO THE RIPE AGE OF 100

The precious gift we call *health* will be with us for a far longer time. We will not only live longer, but we will live those additional years with more youth and vigor. Besides having more hundred-year-olds, we will have people who live ten to twenty years beyond one hundred. Right now, the length of our lives is determined more by the degenerative diseases that kill us prematurely than by our biological potential for life. Rarely has anyone reached his or her biological potential, but new medical advances will close the gap. Those of us who are alive and, better still, those of us who are "well" will be able to take advantage of these new wonders.

Beyond the horizon even more dramatic advances loom. We will be able to identify the genes that determine the rate at which we age. The potential to influence our biological clocks exist in theory today; very soon it will be fact. The natural lifespan of a human cell and thus a human being will be altered, and Seneca's statement, "Man does not die, he kills himself," will take on a dramatically different meaning. In 2010 many of us will truly be able to reach our biological potential. And our children? God only knows!

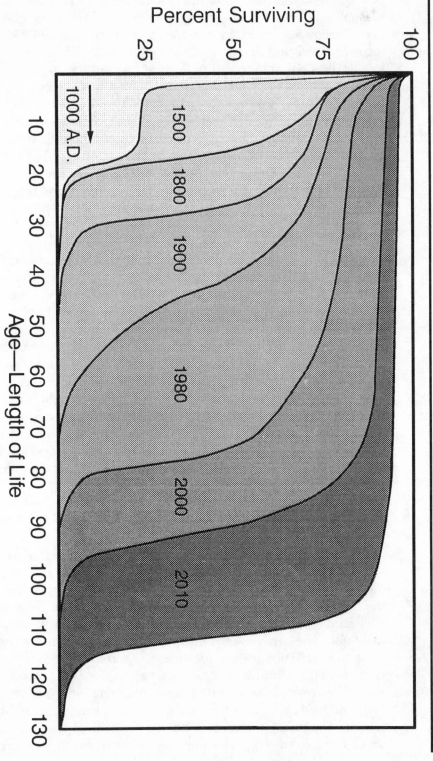

The Increasing Survival Curve

The Increasing Survival Curve figure illustrates two important points. First, the "length of life" value demonstrates how long the lifespan has been for most of the population during the historical periods shown. Second, by combining the percentage of people living (percent surviving) in the vertical values with the horizontal lifespan values, it is possible to estimate what percentage of the people were alive at any given age. Notice how lifespan has increased over the centuries. But more important to us today, notice how in each succeeding period a greater percentage of the people were alive for longer lifespans. As the curve becomes rectangular, it indicates a greater percentage of people alive at the extreme end of the lifespan. By interpolating the survival curve, we can expect a greater percentage of people to have an increased lifespan and a greater percentage to be alive at the upper end of the lifespan.

A NEW LEASE ON LIFE

In a previous chapter we mentioned that your notion of how long you probably will live is guided by two factors: your genetic history and your lifestyle. We hope you are convinced now that you have greater genetic potential than you thought and that you will want to take steps to reach your potential. Your parents, grandparents, and earlier ancestors, whether they "lived long" or "died early," probably never came close to their full life potential, but you are a member of the first generation to have a chance to achieve biological potential. Our discussion of proper eating and exercise habits should have whetted your appetite for a better daily menu of eating and exercise because a longer and healthier life is out there waiting for you and your children. However, we're just on the fringes of new discoveries. Medical science hasn't yet reached its potential either. What does this mean for today's families? We must all strive for health.

Health is a state of complete physical, mental, and social well-being and not merely the absence of disease or illness.

World Health Organization

How, Then, Should Our Family Live?

You can now appreciate the fact that we live in a unique moment in the history of medical science. But with all of our medical advances, we still die prematurely. We don't get from life what we are biologically due. The array of current medical treatments is not yet sufficient to effectively prevent all diseases or treat and cure them. Genetic and molecular medicine as a specialty is a decade or more away. We are still faced with considerable challenges if we are to live long and well. We are in the midst of a long journey fraught with treacherous turns in the road, but we are still on the road. Now we've come to the edge of a dark forest. We can see light on the other side, but we still have to find our way through the woods in order to get to the other side. It would be delightful if we could just be whisked to the other side. Unfortunately we must walk slowly and carefully to get there.

LIFE DOESN'T COME WITH A WARRANTY

There are no guarantees in life. We cannot know about in advance or influence everything that will effect us. Daily cause and effect is not entirely in our hands. It is not definite that when you start out for work you will get there. It is not definite that your hard work will pay off, and you'll get that long-awaited promotion. It is not definite that a strong family life will lead to strong, secure, healthy children. It is probable, however, that good will come to us and our families if we work at it. Living in today's world is infinitely complex. There will always be factors beyond our ability to control because we do not know the absolute secrets for a long and healthy life. But we do have some valuable tools we can use to help ourselves.

■ *The best esti-mates are that the medical system (doctors, drugs, and hospitals) influences about 10 percent of the factors affecting our health.*

Aaron Wildavsky, M.D.,
University of California
School of Public Health

ACCENTUATE PREVENTION AND MINIMIZE RISK

Unfortunately there are some people whose attitude toward their health is summed up by: You can get hit by a bus anytime so why should I worry about change? These unenlightened souls don't real-ize that the know-how is out there right now to lengthen their fam-ily's lifespan. It just is not available in the form of a magic blue pill. Since the know-how is available, it is everyone's responsibility to be-come aware of what is considered high risk and what is an effective course of prevention. High on the prevention list are nutrition and exercise. Smoking is a very powerful risk factor. So are stress and excess alcohol intake. And, from our chapter on spirituality, you now understand the relationship of your state of mind to your biochemical and hormonal systems.

Aging is inevitable. But today the rate at which the family ages is definitely negotiable. The thesis of this book is to present methods to slow down the aging process as much as possible and give you the ability to negotiate. When you and the members of your family enter the twenty-first century, medical science will have far greater capa-bilities to influence your health and life span, and it goes without saying that it will be better for you to be there, rather than not be there, when all these wonderful things happen. But it also stands to reason that the healthier you are, the more Golden Age Medicine can do to treat, cure, and ultimately prevent disease for you and your children.

Finally, and probably more importantly, you have the opportu-nity to build a healthier, happier family—one with heart-healthy eating and exercise habits. Lifestyle improvements will lead to immediate and especially to long term health benefits, and you'll get the bonus of behavior benefits as well. It's like putting money aside for your children's future education and buying life and health insurance for those future potentially rainy days. Think of the Better Life Institute Family Health Program as both health insurance for and the building of health and behavioral equity in the family's future.

Family, the Most Important Risk Factor

Scientists are the first to admit that as a method of inquiry and understanding science has its limitations. Science can only examine what can be studied by scientific methods. In our discussion on the importance of spirituality in our lives we have tried to make the point that there are other quite powerful ways of knowing. Scientific investigation is not the only way to understand life. As the foundation of our discussion of the power of spirituality we have used considerable effort and time in emphasizing the importance of family to health and happiness. Family is the source of life experience for you and your children. All that is "seen" during childhood and after (and, perhaps, in the hereafter) is "seen" through the eyes of the family experience. It's impact on eating and exercise should by now be evident. We have also suggested that through living a spiritual life, the family can acquire a state of mind that affects health.

Whether or not it is a part of scientific discourse, *Family* is also a risk factor for health and happiness. When the family is strong, its members have a lower risk of premature health problems and a higher chance of happiness and long life. If a family has weak ties, there is usually an increased risk of degenerative disease and less happiness, fulfillment, sense of purpose, and peace of mind. This observation may not hold when subjected to the rigors of scientific analysis, but it certainly holds when held under the light of our life experiences and common sense. In the final analysis family may make a more significant contribution to health than blood pressure, cholesterol, exercise, or smoking.

A NEW FAMILY FOR A NEW WORLD

There will be many unknowns out there in the years ahead. The integrity and existence of the family itself will be challenged. Already parents and children face unique forms of stress as they try to adjust to an increasingly fast-paced lifestyle. These forces, along with economic factors that foster more independence for adults, will continue to change family relationships, the need for the institution of marriage, parenting techniques, and traditional roles for men and

■ *THE BETTER LIFE INSTITUTE FAMILY HEALTH PLAN*

women. A new world awaits us, offering new challenges for adults and children—for families. Whether it will be a better world is up to each of us and to the traditions and experiences we provide for our families.

HEALTHFULLY EVER AFTER

You and your family are standing at a crossroads in life. It is impossible not to make a decision about family health and happiness because every moment in life either contributes to or diminishes the factors related to health and happiness. Life in America can be either increasingly hazardous or increasingly beneficial to the health and strength of your family.

We have tried to show you that the tools to improve family health and family strength are one and the same and you have them right now. The experience of using these tools is livable and even enjoyable. But, as with everything that's worthwhile in life, success requires some work. It's up to you now. It will always be up to you *healthfully ever after!*

Where to Go for More Information

■ ■ ■ ■ ■ ■ ■ ■ ■ ■ ■ ■ ■ ■ ■ ■ ■ ■ ■ ■

There's no lack of readily available, easy-to-read information on eating and exercise. Every newspaper and magazine has useful tips. The trick is to use the information in your total Better Life Institute Family Program.

When you read about an interesting family activity or recipe, you can think about the big family picture. The family should have a plan by now. It should not be a hodge-podge of hit-and-miss activities depending upon what does or does not catch your eye that day.

Since there are so many sources of information, you should try to be selective in your reading. We suggest your local newspaper as a starter. Sometimes you can pick up tips on television and radio programs. Remember the suggestions you listen to should come from a person with some experience and credibility in the nutrition and exercise area. Try to avoid sensationalist types as sources for information. Stay with the pros. It's your health and that of your family at stake, and you want responsible, tried-and-true suggestions.

We have reviewed several popular sources of information that are available for you and your family.

National Associations

National and governmental associations are organizations that often are governed by consensus, which requires compromise with all the varied interests involved in decision-making. Usually these organizations involve a blend of conservative and liberal elements, young and old, business and science, pro-government and anti-government, big-interest and little-interest groups, scientists and practitioners, urban and rural, and so forth. Government organizations are also vulnerable to powerful special interest lobbies and political interests.

The net result of this interplay is a moderate, safe stance. It is not overly aggressive, yet it contains nothing that is not safe and well accepted. This is, generally, a practical and appropriate strategy for you to follow. Look for and seek guidance from these organizations. You can't go wrong. Other local public organizations that have safe-sounding names or appear to be objective can be more advocacy- or special-interest oriented. You may learn valuable information from them too. But, you still must use your common sense when making the final decision.

SUGGESTED NATIONAL HEALTH INFORMATION SOURCES

The Center for Science in the Public Interest
The Center for Consumer Medical Education
American Heart Association
American Diabetes Association
Juvenile Diabetes Association
American Cancer Society
American Institute for Cancer Research
National Cancer Institute
National Heart, Lung, and Blood Institute
National Institute of Children's Health and Development
The Childrens Better Health Institute
The President's Council on Physical Fitness
Public Citizen Health Research Group
American Health Foundation
National Institutes of Health (NIH)
Food and Drug Administration (FDA)
Department of Health and Human Services
Center for Disease Control (CDC)
American Association for Retired People (AARP)
Your family physician
All the national medical specialty associations: Pediatrics, Family Medicine, Obstetrics and Gynecology, Sports Medicine, Preventive Medicine, Gerontology, Cardiology, etc.

Avoid national or community associations that are funded by corporate interests. The "payload" on their recommendations usually is positioned so that it does not "disinvite" people to use certain products. If you call an organization for advice, ask what their funding sources are.

NATIONAL HEALTH NEWSLETTERS
There are several national monthly health newsletters that can also provide guidance. These newsletters are usually sponsored by major

universities or health institutions. As with any periodical, they are not totally objective because they select editors and reviewers with a particular point of view. But as with our national consumer organizations, their recommendations are moderate and safe. Examples of such newsletters are:

Harvard Medical School Newsletter
Tufts Nutrition Newsletter
Berkley Wellness Newsletter
Mayo Clinic Newsletter
Better Life Institute Longevity Digest

Health Magazines

Health magazines are funded by advertisers and usually have a point of view that is supportive of these advertisements or the editor's sense of consumer interest. One would like to think these magazines are guided by a philosophy based upon impartiality and that they select advertisers who support this approach, but that is not what usually occurs. Many of the articles are timely, interesting, and practical; however, they may be more advocacy than unbiased science. There is a place for these magazines in your strategy to get current information. Just be aware that the articles are screened for audience suitability, practicality, and interest level (regardless of their objective factual base) and advertiser support.

We suggest you read bodybuilding magazines with discretion. Bodybuilding is not a desirable activity for children or for most adults. These magazines often suggest foods and exercise activities that are not designed for health and fitness but for building muscles. All such magazines are sponsored or published by companies that produce bodybuilding products.

There are several children's health magazines that can be very helpful to you and also motivating to your children. They translate the topic of health into content that is enjoyable and practical for children. The Children's Better Health Institute, a subsidiary of the *Saturday Evening Post,* located in Indianapolis, Indiana, publishes a series of magazines for children geared to specific age levels. They are:

Humpty Dumpty
Jack 'n Jill
Turtle
Child Life
Children's Digest
Children's Playmate

Examples of adult magazines are:

Heart Healthy Living—a new magazine for family health
Prevention Magazine—general health information
American Health—general
Runner's World—oriented toward fitness buffs
Longevity Magazine—oriented toward ways to increase longevity
Women's Health—general
Reader's Digest—general
Saturday Evening Post—general
and many, many others geared to specific people, or health topics.

General Reference Books

The Better Life Institute suggests you purchase several general reference books that offer general home/family health guidance. You can't go wrong with books published by major American associations or universities. They are good foundations for your family health programs. Don't forget to purchase a home medical and safety book. It can save a life in an emergency. Every general bookstore has these books, and they are too numerous and similar to recommend one over the others. Get one that suits your budget, eye, and format. The general areas to cover are: home safety, accidents, poisoning, CPR (cardiopulmonary resuscitation), and nutrition. Children's health reference books are also important to have available.

SPECIFIC REFERENCE TOPICS

It's a good idea to purchase several nutritional reference books and cookbooks. All nutritional reference books provide you with accurate nutritional data. They all use the USDA Handbook #8 as their "bible." They merely adapt this basic reference information to more practical interests such as brand names, portion servings, or specific nutrient analysis (protein, carbohydrate, fat, cholesterol, and vitamin and mineral "counters"). Select recipe books that provide you with low fat, low cholesterol, and low sugar recipes or teach you to adapt your own recipes to new, more health-oriented concerns.

In summary, we suggest your family health library contain the following:

A monthly newsletter
General health reference books on:
- home safety
- accidents, poisoning, CPR
- general nutrition and exercise guidance
- children's health care

- several nutrition analyses books
- several recipe books
- one adult health-oriented magazine
- one child health magazine

Other Sources of Health Information

HEALTH FOOD STORES

A health food store is in the business of selling you *health foods,* or more appropriately *special consumer interest* foods. Quite often the foods sold have no added advantage for health purposes but appeal to a special segment of people. You can usually find similar foods at your supermarket at cheaper prices. The information disseminated at the health food store is based on sales promotion, even though it appears objective. BLI suggests that you not rely on this information to guide your decisions. The owner of the health food store is exactly that, the owner of a business. Owners usually are not professional experts, nor do they have the license or perspective to guide you in your decisions about food purchases. Always read the labels on everything you buy. Never assume that a product is "healthy" just because you bought it at a health food store.

FOOD LABEL AND PACKAGE INFORMATION

The label on a food package contains three elements:

- specific ingredients in descending order of weight
- specific nutritional content by serving size (optional)
- graphics and advertising claims

You have to be very careful of the claims that food companies make for their products. They are in the business of selling you their products, and nothing more. Quite often their statements in advertisements or on the package may be legal but misleading. You must learn to read the ingredient and nutritional content portion of the label and interpret the information yourself. Advertising claims often lack credibility. Ask an independent source if you are in doubt.

Most American homes have a dictionary, a first aid book, cookbooks, perhaps a set of encyclopedia, and various magazines. Enlarge your library to include several health reference materials such as a children's health magazine, a similar publication for yourself, and a general health reference book or newsletter. There's no lack of printed material. Just be selective and use publications from well-established organizations.

Words You
Should Know

■ ■ ■ ■ ■ ■ ■ ■ ■ ■ ■ ■ ■ ■ ■ ■ ■ ■ ■

Many of the health terms you and your family will come across in this book already are familiar to you. There will be other less familiar words and terms that we think are important enough for you to understand more fully. Health requires action, and action requires knowledge. We have prepared a short list of words that we think are important for you to understand.

There's a difference between recognizing a familiar word and truly understanding what that word means. The terms we have selected are important enough for you to understand rather than just be familiar with them.

We have grouped these words under general subjects that should be of interest to you, but there may be terms that we have overlooked. Every bookstore has a simple consumer medical dictionary. You might consider adding one to your library.

Exercise

Aerobic Dance: This form of exercise is a wonderful way to have fun and exercise at the same time. It is usually done to music and you get to move every muscle in your body, even some you didn't know you had! Low impact aerobic dance is preferable to high impact aerobic dance because there's less hard pounding on your hips, knees, and ankles.

Aerobic Exercise: Aerobic exercise is simply exercise that provides a lot of blood and oxygen to your cells, organs, and tissues. Aerobic exercise results in increased blood circulation and involves most of the larger muscles in your arms and legs. This type of exercise involves repetitive activity such as biking, stair-climbing, walking, jogging, swimming, aerobic dance, and cross-country skiing. Activities such as racquetball, tennis, golf, and shopping are not aerobic because there's a great deal of "down" time, unless you're of Olympic caliber and a "shopper" like the co-author of this book!

Basal Metabolism: We hear this term a great deal because it's associated with weight control. Your basal metabolism is the energy or calorie intake required by your body to meet its basic maintenance needs. Aerobic exercise tends to increase your basal metabolism and caloric needs. The more body fat you have the lower your basal metabolism.

Conditioning Activities: These are activities that force the muscles involved into using large amounts of oxygen because they are working very hard. As you gradually improve your exercise ability, your muscles learn to gulp more oxygen and use it better. The result is less muscle fatigue. You also get the same amount of work from your muscles with a little less oxygen. That's why athletes can run very hard for a long time. They're "in shape," or in condition. Their muscles gulp more oxygen and give them more work for the same amount of oxygen. Otherwise their heart rates would be dangerously high. Don't confuse "iron pumping" with being in condition. Some bodybuilders believe in conditioning from an oxygen uptake point of view along with their weight-lifting regime. Others do not.

Exercise Electrocardiogram (EKG):   Sometimes it is called an "exercise stress test." This test evaluates the performance of your heart and your pulse rate and blood pressure while you exercise. We recommend this test before any adult over thirty-five starts a regular aerobic exercise program.

Target or Training Heart Rate (THR):   Your THR is a number that represents the number of heart beats that is safe for you, yet vigorous enough for aerobic exercise. The THR is never one number. It is a zone, or a range, such as 125–135 beats per minute. You should take several minutes to reach your THR. Once in your zone, check it every ten minutes or so. If you are experiencing any difficulty, use your physical comfort level *not* the THR to guide your exercise program. If you are out of condition, it might take several months to be comfortable at your THR.

Always check with your physician before you start any aerobic exercise program and please re-read the chapters on exercise for additional information.

The Fat Family

There are dozens of fats used in foods and food processing. We will highlight the fats that are commonly used in your foods or related to your health. Every year we learn more about fats and become more concerned about them. The national dietary recommendations suggest you restrict your intake of dietary fat to less than 30 percent of your daily calories. Your daily caloric intake of mono-unsaturated, polyunsaturated, and saturated fats should be about equally divided, or about 10 percent each or less.

Cholesterol: The most famous of the fat family, your level of blood cholesterol is related to the risk of blood vessel or heart disease. Cholesterol is a waxy, fatty substance produced by your liver. Of course you can increase your blood cholesterol by eating foods high in cholesterol such as animal foods, dairy foods, and saturated fats. Your blood cholesterol level should be below 190 mg/dl.—the lower the better.

High Density Lipoprotein (HDL): This is the member of the fat family that removes cholesterol from tissue. It is a cleanser or scavenger. The higher your level of HDL, the lower your risk of heart disease. Ideally, your HDL level should be above 60 mg/dl.

Low Density Lipoprotein (LDL): Cholesterol is carried through the bloodstream on another substance called LDL. Thus LDL is a risk factor for blood vessel disease. In fact, it is more predictive of the risk of heart disease than cholesterol. Your LDL level ideally should be below 125 mg/dl.

Mono-unsaturated Fats: These fats are present in vegetables, especially olives, peanuts, general mixed vegetable oils, and canola oil. They tend to slightly lower cholesterol and LDL. But they are still fat and should be used carefully. Of all the types of cooking oils and fats, these are the safest.

Mono- and Diglycerides: Technically these are fats, but they don't have the adverse health effects of fats. They are now being used in "fat free" foods to give you the feel of fat, but without the calories or adverse health effects.

Polyunsaturated Fats: Formerly called the "good" fats, these oils have since lost some of their luster. They were considered desirable because they tend to lower cholesterol. But now their safety is in question and food companies are switching to mono-unsaturated fats. Corn, safflower, sunflower, cottonseed, and soy oils are high in polyunsaturated fats. Use them sparingly.

Fish Oil (EPA/DPA): This type of polyunsaturated fat in small amounts tends to improve circulation and reduce both cholesterol, triglycerides, and LDL. It has an anti-inflammatory effect in the bloodstream and prevents blood clotting. It's also called "Omega 3" fatty acid. Eat fish as your main entrée whenever you consider animal food.

Saturated Fats: Everyone agrees that these fats are generally not healthy. They tend to elevate your blood cholesterol more so than eating foods high in dietary cholesterol. They also elevate your LDL, the "bad" cholesterol. Meat and dairy products can contain high amounts of saturated fats. Coconut, palm, and palm kernel oils, called Tropical Oils, are very high in saturated fats and are usually present in sauces and baked goods.

Triglycerides: If someone pinched your fat, they would be pinching your triglycerides, your common fatty tissue or oil. The white fat on meat is very obviously triglycerides. The fat, or oil, in your blood is called blood triglycerides, a risk factor for heart disease and diabetes. Your blood triglycerides should be below 125 mg/dl. Blood triglycerides affect the sugar level, viscosity, and sludginess of blood, and thus circulation.

General Health Terms

Arteriosclerosis: This term is used to refer to hardening or calcification of the artery. The artery tends to crack and scar when it hardens, which causes blockage in the blood vessel. Sometimes this condition is called "aging of the artery."

Artery: A large blood vessel that carries blood with oxygen to all your cells is the artery. A small artery is called an arteriole. An artery has four layers of live tissue: the endothelium (inner layer of cells through which blood flows), intima, media, and adventitia. Your arteries are not made of naugahyde, so take care of them!

Atherosclerosis: The clogging of arteries with fatty deposits, cholesterol and blood clots is referred to as atherosclerosis. The subtleties between atherosclerosis and arteriosclerosis are not important. Try to avoid both for as long as possible.

Blood Pressure: The fluid pressure your blood exerts on the sides of blood vessel walls as it is pumped through your body is your blood pressure. It is measured by a pressure meter placed on your arm that senses maximum and minimum pressure in the vessels. *Systolic blood pressure* refers to the maximum pressure from blood flow. *Diastolic blood pressure* refers to minimum pressure during blood flow. In general, the lower both numbers are the less wear and tear on your blood vessel walls and consequently the healthier they are. A healthy blood pressure ranges from 65mm to 85mm diastolic and 100mm to 125mm systolic.

Cancer: This is a term that describes the presence of rapidly growing cells that destroy tissues and organ function. These cells, for some reason, have leaped beyond their normal growth constraints. They wander through the body and if they stop and congregate in a certain area, there's trouble. Certain substances called carcinogens are associated with the development of cancerous cells.

Cardiovascular Disease: *Cardio* refers to heart and *vascular* refers to blood vessel; thus the term *cardiovascular* simply means blood vessels related to the heart. The heart is a muscle. Heart disease is usually blood vessel or cardiovascular disease because these blood vessels clog and choke off food and oxygen from the heart muscle.

Claudication: When blood vessels in the legs start to fill up with deposits, it is often called claudication. Irregular blood flow is called intermittent claudication.

Diabetes: Some people cannot properly metabolize sugar (simple carbohydrates). This causes metabolic problems and also injury to large and small blood vessels. There are two general types of diabetes:

Type I, or juvenile onset diabetes, is caused by a genetic defect or an injured or diseased pancreas. The pancreas is responsible for producing insulin, a hormone necessary for metabolizing sugar in the bloodstream. Type I diabetics require insulin injections. Quite often, but not always, this disease strikes when young. That's why it is called juvenile.

Type II, or adult onset diabetes, is not associated with a diseased pancreas. The person has enough insulin, but it is not being used properly. The disease is often associated with people who are over forty years of age and are overweight, but not necessarily so. The Type II diabetic may or may not need insulin to control blood sugar. Sometimes the Type II diabetic uses drugs that improve use of sugar in the bloodstream. Most of these diabetics can control their disease simply by improving their eating and exercise habits and stopping smoking and drinking.

Glucose: Your level of blood glucose, or blood sugar, is an indicator of your risk of diabetes. The higher the glucose level above 125 mg/dl, the greater your risk of blood vessel disease. A high glucose level is evidence that your body cannot properly metabolize glucose and thus it accumulates in the bloodstream. Blood glucose levels are affected by genetic capability, sugars, fat, and alcohol intake and aerobic exercise. Your glucose level should be between 75 and 125 mg/dl.

Both Types I & II diabetes result in heart disease and small blood vessel disease. Small blood vessel disease is associated with poor blood flow leading to gangrene and eye, kidney, or leg circulation problems.

Myocardial Infarction: This is another name for a heart attack. *Myo* means muscle, *cardio* means heart, and *infarct* means muscle damage or no function.

Stroke: When blood vessels to the brain get clogged, cracked, or hardened, the effect on the brain is the same as on the heart. Its food and oxygen supply gets choked and brain cells die or malfunction. Sometimes it's associated with cerebrovascular disease or a transient ischemic attack (TIA).

Vein: These blood vessels carry blood away from cells and dump waste products. Their structure is different from an artery, and they are not as affected by fats and cholesterol as arteries. There's also less turbulence and blood pressure in a vein. It's a "return" vessel.

Label Terms

Note: The Food and Drug Administration is currently working on new food label laws. However, until these new laws are enacted, the following definitions are accurate.

Lean: No more than 10 percent fat *by weight,* not by percentage of calories.

Extra Lean: No more than 5 percent fat by weight, not by percentage of calories.

Leaner: At least 25 percent less fat by weight than the original product.

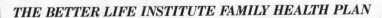

Dietetic: One or more ingredients has been changed, substituted, or restricted, usually salt or sugar.

Sugar-free/Sugarless: Contains no sucrose (table sugar). The product may contain other sugars such as fructose, corn syrup, honey, or sorbitol. These terms do not mean "low in calories."

Very Low Sodium: No more than 35 mg of sodium per serving.

Low Sodium: No more than 140 mg sodium per serving.

Reduced Sodium: At least 255 mg less sodium than the original product.

No Salt Added/Salt-Free: No salt is added in the food processing, but the food may be high in natural sodium or sodium from other sources such as soy sauce, MSG, or hydrolyzed vegetable protein.

Hydrolyzed Vegetable Protein: A flavor enhancer containing sodium, sometimes used in place of MSG.

Enriched: A process of replacing nutrients lost in the manufacturing process. It does not mean nutrition value added to the food over and above its natural content.

Fortified: The addition of nutrients to foods that did not originally contain them. Milk is often fortified; so are cereals and salt.

Hydrogenated: Refers to a special process vegetable oils are subjected to that makes them thick and solid at room temperature. Corn oil that is liquid in a bottle is hydrogenated to change it to margarine, which is solid at room temperature. Creamy peanut butter has hydrogenated oil in it. Natural peanut butter doesn't. That's why the oil rises to the top at room temperature. The process of hydrogenating oil is currently under investigation. The "changed" oil may have some properties that make it a health risk when used to excess. We suggest you avoid the controversy, and stop smearing fat on your bread!

Nutrition Terms

Artificial Sweetener: This is a term used for sweeteners that are manufactured and don't have a plant food base. Because they are artificial they must be labeled as such. If there is any known health hazard associated with them, it is necessary by law to disclose it. Technically they are used only for special dietary or health needs, but their use has extended to the general population. They contain no calories or an insignificant amount. Please check with your doctor if you have any questions about artificial sweeteners. There are a number of them:

> *Saccharin:* a common sweetener found in a variety of foods that we consume daily. It is the only artificial sweetener that can be heated.

> *Aspartame:* the most common artificial sweetener available today. Despite skepticism by certain healthy-food advocates, aspartame has no known health hazards except for those associated with a very rare disease called Phenylketonuria. It has been approved for use with pregnant and lactating women, infants, diabetics, and for weight control. It's called Nutrasweet™ in liquid form and Equal™ in crystal form. Aspartame has amino acids that are commonly found in many foods.

Calorie: To most it means *danger,* but it truly is just a measure of the energy value of a particular food. Calories come in the form of the four nutrients. Protein has 4 cal/gm., carbohydrate has 4 cal/gm., fat has 9 cal/gm., and alcohol has 6 cal/gm.

Carbohydrate: This is the basic nutrient of foods. It is the nutrient that should comprise most of your calorie intake. Plants are very high in carbohydrate.

Simple Carbohydrate: The sweeter the plant food, the more simple the carbohydrate. Fruit is a simple carbohydrate, as is honey and all sugars. The simple carbohydrate is usually accepted as a primary source of immediate energy. For some people too much simple carbohydrate at one feeding could lead to "sugar blues"—giant mood swings.

Complex Carbohydrate: These are found in plants that have complex sugars. They are not sweet, but your body can break them down and get the sugar from them in a very safe, moderate manner. Beans, peas, lentils, brown rice, most vegetables that aren't sweet, potatoes, and whole grains are excellent sources of complex carbohydrate.

Crude Fiber: This is another term for the cellulose and bran present in all plant food. It adds bulk without calories and is excellent for weight control and preventing constipation. Fiber is only present in plants. It is not in animals.

Fat: A nutrient found naturally in all foods, fat helps metabolism, synthesis of hormones, and growth and is a secondary source of energy. There is increasing evidence that all excess fat intake regardless of its type is a risk factor for all degenerative diseases. High fat intake also increases the risk of obesity for obvious reasons.

Protein: A nutrient that provides the amino acids required to sustain muscle, bone, and organ cells, meat, chicken, fish, beans, and peas are high in protein. Too much protein is not good for your health.

Vitamins and Minerals: Technically not nutrients, vitamins and minerals are necessary for all essential life processes to take place—growth, metabolism, reproduction, etc. Sometimes they are called "micro nutrients" or "catalysts." Recent research suggests increased intake of certain vitamins and minerals may promote health and prevent certain diseases.

Water Soluble Fiber: These gooey, gummy fibers are technically called gums, mucilages, and pectins. They add bulk to food without calories and aid in preventing constipation. Some scientists think water soluble fiber tends to lower cholesterol. Beans, peas, lentils, rice and oat brans, and some fruits have high levels of water soluble fiber.

Whole Grain: If it doesn't have the term *whole* in front of it, you're not getting the whole grain. Whole grains are the largest source of dietary crude fiber available. A diet high in crude fiber is considered a healthier diet.

Weight

Weight loss and weight gain are basically controlled by calorie intake. If you eat more calories than you expend, you will gain weight. If you expend more calories than you eat, you will lose weight.

Body Composition: Probably the most accurate assessment of your weight status, body composition consists of both your lean body mass and your fat body mass. In general, the best weight control strategy is to reduce fat body mass and increase lean body mass.

Fat Body Mass: The total weight of fat on your body, the fat body mass is sometimes expressed as *percent of body fat*.

WORDS YOU SHOULD KNOW ■

Ideal Body Weight: A standard weight formulated by health insurance companies to assess your lowest health risk, it's often used by physicians as a benchmark as well. The calculation takes into account your sex, height, weight, and body frame.

Lean Body Mass: The total weight of your body, minus the fat weight is the lean body mass. The greater your percentage of lean body mass, the easier it is to control weight and the lower your overall health risk.

Obesity: This term is defined as having a total weight of 15 percent above ideal body weight, or a body fat that exceeds the ideal by 20 percent for men and 30 percent for women.

Overweight: You are overweight if you exceed your ideal body weight by 10 percent.

"Guardian Angel" Letters

■ ■ ■ ■ ■ ■ ■ ■ ■ ■ ■ ■ ■ ■ ■ ■ ■

Everyone needs a buddy, a support person, or a Guardian Angel. An "angel" can help you through difficult times or provide you with a gentle reminder of what you had promised yourself you would do.

At the Better Life Institute we ask our graduates to write themselves a "what will I be like and where will I be in a few months?" letter. We call them Guardian Angel letters. It's helpful to set a few practical and attainable goals for your immediate future. It's also helpful to read your own letter describing your goals a few months later. Measuring your performance against your own stated ambitions is a great motivator. You can't blame anyone else if you haven't reached your goals. You set your own goals, and it's written in your own hand to you—and to no one else! A "Guardian Angel" letter can continue to motivate you and the family in the programs to improve family health.

We suggest you and each family member write a "Guardian Angel" letter. Send it to the Better Life Institute in a self-addressed, *stamped* envelope. We will mail it back to you in a few months at an unexpected time. It can help each person continue efforts to improve their health.

Our address is:

The Better Life Institute Guardian Angel Program
220 Lyon, Suite 100
Grand Rapids, MI 49503

The letter should be personal and informal. We suggest you write it in confidence, but you will have to help children who can't write on their own. Encourage everyone to write a "Guardian Angel" letter and put each letter in a separate stamped envelope that is addressed to the writer. Put them all in one large envelope and mail it to us. We'll take care of the rest. We'll even send you a little surprise to help each of you continue on your Better Life Institute program. If your child can write at any level, help him write his letter to us. We have some sample "Guardian Angel" letters to help you and your family get started on your own letters.

Tommy is eight years old:

Dear Tommy,
This is stupid but,
1. *I promise to eat my broccoli—but not too much.*
2. *I'll help mom set and clean up the table.*
3. *I'll throw away the garbage and won't drop it all over the floor unless Chad starts to tease me. Then I might drop it so Dad makes Chad pick it up! Ha! Ha!*
4. *I will brush my teeth everyday when I remember.*
5. *I will say my prayers and go to church with Grandma and Grandpa.*
6. *I will feed Skippy and clean up his mess.*
7. *I won't slug Jimmy, unless he takes my mitt like he did today and I had to bleed his nose.*
8. *This is stupid, but everyone is doing a letter and I had to.*
You're the greatest!

Love me,
Tommy

Chad is sixteen and he is Tommy's big brother:

Dear Awesome Chad,
  By the time this letter arrives, I will be running in the School 10K!!! If I can get Dad to go with me, it will be good for both of us. We'll be a team and do it together.
  I will make enough money mowing lawns to buy a weight set so my muscles will be rad and impress you know who.
  I'll offer to carry out the garbage for Tommy so I won't have to clean up after him. I hate the kitchen stuff, but I'll take charge on pizza, burgers, and spaghetti. I'll sweet talk Mom! I'll try to do better in Algebra and get a tutor earlier this year, if I need one!
  I'll spend more time with Gramps and Grams because they're old and they love me and I love them. I'll try to be nice to Leslie, even though she's a pain and I can't stand her.
  Here's to the kid with the "perfect BOD,"

Chad

■ *THE BETTER LIFE INSTITUTE FAMILY HEALTH PLAN*

Leslie is fourteen and she is Tommy and Chad's sister:

Dearest Leslie,

    I like you. You are nice. You are a nice person and try hard to be nice to everyone. The Book says I must be positive. I will try very hard to be nice to Chad. He's terrible to me and tells me I'm fat and it's not true! He always teases me about my zits. But he has them and I don't tell him because it would hurt his feelings and I don't want to do that like he does to me.

    I will exercise with Mom to her new video tape and use the rebounder also. I will go to the after-school aerobics class when I don't have too much homework. I'm going to try to stop eating potato chips. Mom and I will plan the menu with Tommy and Chad and Daddy, and then I'll do the shopping as one of my major chores.

    I'll do the desserts because that's what I'm good at and I like desserts. I'll help Tommy with his homework and I'll exercise with Mom. I'll try to talk more with Daddy. He's so proper and I know he really hates my music, but, I'll try anyway.

    Everyone says these are my best years. If this is the best, the rest must be pretty awful so I'll make them better by thinking positive, like they say at church, not getting fat, and pray my zits go away.

Love,
Leslie

Tom, age unknown, is Tommy, Chad, and Leslie's father:

Dear Tom,

    I never thought I'd ever write a letter to myself, but here goes. I know I really need to get my act together. The last visit to the doctor was not so good. He read me the "riot act." I thought he was going to arrest me and throw me into jail! He's right, so is Phyllis and even sweet Leslie is getting on my back. Phyllis is doing wonderful things in the kitchen and it's really very easy to eat well. So no problem in that area.

    It's the exercise part that gets me. I am going to make a promise to myself that I promise to keep. I will ride my exercise bike at least three of five workdays and once on the weekend for at least thirty minutes. If it's nice outside, I'll take a walk—may pull one of the kids along. They can use the exercise too. Besides, I need to spend some more time with them. I think I'll get them to talk with me a little while I exercise.

    Chad has asked me to help him train for the 10K. I'll do my best. Maybe Leslie and I can learn to talk together like we used to when she was a little girl and not a teenager with problems. I'm really going to try.

I really am very tired after dinner, but I know how important it is for me to help Phyllis a little more. She's tired also. I will compliment her on her cooking more. I take that for granted and I won't take any "cheap shots" when she throws something together because she has no time to prepare a meal. I also promise to take the family out once a week on a weekday for a quick dinner. We now know how to eat well, and cheaply, in any kind of restaurant. I'll help plan the menus and I'll get the boys involved in what I always thought was women's work—it ain't so, McGee.

And last, but not least, I'm going to spend more time with each of the kids and Phyllis. I sort of lost perspective on that part of my life. I can kill two birds with one stone by taking one of them to the store each time I go there. I also promise to get everyone together to plan our family vacation. That conference idea is a good one.

See me in a few months (crazy!)—

Tom

Phyllis is Tom's wife and the mother of—well you know who they all are:

Dear Phyllis,

This is a wonderful idea—writing to myself. I can't wait to see what changes I'll have made when I open this up in a few months. Everyone is excited about the new health programs they are doing. I've been dreaming about losing those extra pounds and, by golly, I'm going to do it. I now know how, and it's easy. But, the best thing that is happening is my family is getting together and rallying around health and exercise.

Tom is actually paying attention to what he eats! I noticed Tommy brushed his teeth without being asked. And my two big ones are trying very hard to help everyone—hope it lasts, or at least they may stop fighting for a while.

As for little ole me, this girl will be in a size 10 once again and make sure my wonderful husband wines and dines me once a week— and not at some joint with cheeseburgers! I honestly do feel I can be a bit more imaginative about our meals and I promise to do this.

Leslie has been sniffing around the kitchen and I'll ask her to help out a bit—she loves to bake and has volunteered to shop and be in charge of desserts! Wonderful! I love the regular family meetings. It doesn't matter what we say, but we're saying it together and for each other! And I've learned that my children do truly care about each other even though they fight all the time. And they care so much about their grandparents.

THE BETTER LIFE INSTITUTE FAMILY HEALTH PLAN

Tom will always be Tom, but I think he could also be "Tom on the exercise bike." I think I'll spend more time with him when he's on the bike. We don't get enough little moments together. I'm going to try to get in a good thirty-minute walk at work as well as do the video with Leslie. She and I need one another. I truly do have the time, and it's better to spend it walking instead of eating . . . good idea, Phyllis!

So when we meet again, thanks to you my Guardian Angel, Phyllis will be a whole lot different—a little on the outside and a lot on the inside.

Love and thanks,
Phyllis

Index for Menus and Recipes

■ ■ ■ ■ ■ ■ ■ ■ ■ ■ ■ ■ ■ ■ ■ ■

About the Authors

■ ■

Steven M. Zifferblatt, Ph.D., is a recognized authority in the fields of physiology, fitness, and health. He formerly held research and faculty positions at the National Heart, Lung, and Blood institute and at Harvard and Stanford medical schools. He was associate director of the Pritikin Longevity Center where he created many of the behavioral and motivational concepts of The Pritikin Plan. In addition, he co-founded the LaCosta Lifestyle and Longevity Center, and is currently co-founder and director of the Better Life Institute.

Patricia M. Zifferblatt was also a co-founder of the LaCosta Lifestyle and Longevity Center and former program services director at the Pritikin Longevity Center. Currently co-founder and associate director of the Better Life Institute, she is a celebrated expert in the preparation of delicious and practical heart-healthy, low calorie foods for people of all ages. She has written several recipe books and has extensive experience as a public speaker and leader of workshops and seminars. She has nine children.

Norm Chandler Fox is an author, screenwriter, and journalist. A graduate of Harvard College and Columbia University, he has written books for Simon & Schuster and scripts for numerous network television shows, and is a contributing editor to *Los Angeles Magazine*. A freelance writer, his articles have been published in numerous national magazines. He also writes weekly columns for the Copley News Syndicate with an audience of six million readers.

About the Better Life Institute

■ ■ ■ ■ ■ ■ ■ ■ ■ ■ ■ ■ ■ ■ ■ ■ ■ ■

The Better Life Institute offers a variety of health habit change programs, a newsletter, and audio and video tapes designed to help families improve their diet and exercise habits. Current offerings include:

- *Five-day Residential Program*—a highly concentrated and intense program for people and families of all ages, sessions begin at 7:30 A.M. and end at 9:00 P.M. and include daily experience in exercise, cooking, shopping, and eating out as well as behavior change.
- *Corporate and Group Seminars*—designed by BLI to meet the needs of a particular company's employees and their families, topics include weight control, "family health power," surviving and thriving in restaurants and supermarkets, and the challenge of personal and health habit change.
- *BLI Medical Programs*—offered in several cities by physicians, group practices, and medical clinics, these programs are designed for specific patient groups.
- *Audio and Video Tapes*—available directly from the Better Life Institute for use in the home, these tapes teach the ABC's of health habit change and heart-healthy food preparation.
- *"The Better Life Longevity Digest"*—the monthly newsletter available from the Better Life Institute, provides practical tips on eating and exercise for the family.

For additional information and/or inquiries, contact the Better Life Institute, 220 Lyon Street, N.W., Suite 100, Grand Rapids, Michigan 49503; (616) 776-6490.